DATE DUE

~~DE 26 '00~~			
AG 2 9 '01			

DEMCO 38-296

OCCUPATIONAL LOW BACK PAIN
Assessment, Treatment and Prevention

Occupational Low Back Pain
Assessment, Treatment
and Prevention

MALCOLM H. POPE, DR. MED. SC., PH.D.
Director of Orthopaedic Research
Department of Orthopaedics and Rehabilitation
University of Vermont
Burlington, Vermont

GUNNAR B. J. ANDERSSON, M.D., PH.D.
Professor and Associate Chairman
Department of Orthopaedic Surgery
Rush Presbyterian-St. Luke's Medical Center
Chicago, Illinois

JOHN W. FRYMOYER, M.D.
Professor of Orthopaedics
Director, McClure
   Musculoskeletal Research Center
Department of Orthopaedics and Rehabilitation
University of Vermont
Burlington, Vermont

DON B. CHAFFIN, PH.D.
Center for Ergonomics
University of Michigan
Ann Arbor, Michigan

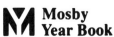 **Mosby**
Year Book

St. Louis   Baltimore   Boston   Chicago   London   Philadelphia   Sydney   Toronto

Dedicated to Publishing Excellence

Sponsoring Editor: James D. Ryan/Joyce-Rachel John
Assistant Director, Manuscript Services: Frances Perveiler
Production Project Coordinator: Karen Halm

5 6 7 8 9 0 V Y 95 94

Library of Congress Cataloging-in-Publication Data
Occupational low back pain: assessment, treatment and prevention/[edited by] Malcolm H. Pope . . . [et al.].

    p. cm.
    Includes bibliographical references.
    Includes index.
    ISBN 0-8016-6252-4
    1. Backache. 2. Occupational diseases. I. Pope, M. H. (Malcolm
Henry), 1941–
    [DNLM: 1. Backache. 2. Occupational Diseases. WE 755 O15]
RD771.B217O22 1991
362.1'97564—dc20
DNLM/DLC
for Library of Congress
    91-13224
    CIP

CONTRIBUTORS

Gunnar B. J. Andersson, M.D., Ph.D.
Professor and Associate Chairman
Department of Orthopaedic Surgery
Rush Presbyterian-St. Luke's Medical Center
Chicago, Illinois

Michele C. Battié, Ph.D.
Department of Orthopaedics
University of Washington
Bellevue, Washington

Don B. Chaffin, Ph.D.
Center for Ergonomics
University of Michigan
Ann Arbor, Michigan

John W. Frymoyer, M.D.
Professor of Orthopaedics
Director, McClure
   Musculoskeletal Research Center
Department of Orthopaedics and
   Rehabilitation
University of Vermont
Burlington, Vermont

Scott Haldeman, M.D., Ph.D.
Professional Corporation Consulting
   Neurology
Santa Ana, California

Rowland G. Hazard, M.D.
Medical Director
New England Back Center
Williston, Vermont

John D. Kemp, J.D.
Director of United Cerebral Palsy
Washington, D.C.

Thomas R. Lehmann, M.D.
Louisville Orthopaedic Clinic
Louisville, Kentucky

Leonard Matheson, Ph.D.
Director of Employment and Rehabilitation
   Institute of California
Santa Ana, California

Margareta Nordin, Ph.D.
Occupational and Industrial
   Orthopaedic Center
Hospital for Joint Diseases
New York, New York

Malcolm H. Pope, Dir. Med. Sc., Ph.D.
Director of Orthopaedic Research
Department of Orthopaedics and
   Rehabilitation
University of Vermont
Burlington, Vermont

Stover H. Snook, Ph.D.
Project Director of Ergonomics
Loss Prevention Department
Liberty Mutual Insurance Company
Hopkinton, Massachusetts

J.D.G. Troup, Ph.D.
Department of Orthopaedics
University of Liverpool
Liverpool, England

Gordon Waddell, M.D.
Consult Orthopaedic Surgeon
The Western Infirmary
Glasgow, Scotland

FOREWORD

It has been long recognized by occupational health and safety professionals that the incidence and severity of work-related low back pain result in excessive costs, both to the individual workers and to their employers. Controlling these costs, and the human suffering associated with low back pain requires a multidisciplinary team and a supportive, informed participative worker–management structure.

This text presents important concepts needed to identify and evaluate the variety of risk factors that are known to cause or exacerbate low back pain in different industries. This book reviews the relevant anatomy and pathophysiology needed to understand how various conditions cause both acute and chronic low back pain. What is special is that it extends beyond simply describing potential mechanisms of injury to emphasize how contemporary diagnostic tools and ergonomic-based intervention strategies can be used to return patients quickly to the workforce and prevent permanent low back pain. In this context, the book underscores the need to recognize that occupational low back pain and resulting disability can only be diagnosed and treated effectively when both patient and workplace attributes are considered, and that psychosocial factors often are as important as physical factors when determining the degree and type of resulting work limitation.

What is particularly desirable about this text in my opinion is its review of prevention strategies, including worker evaluation and selection methods, training and physical conditioning techniques, and designing jobs to be ergonomically less stressful to a worker's back. Given that most low back pain cannot be diagnosed and treated by traditional medical means, management and labor organizations must place much more emphasis on developing and evaluating types of prevention strategies described in this test. It is my firm belief that the greatest pay-off in reduced costs and human suffering will result from such actions.

John Triebwasser, M.D.
Director, Occupational Health and Safety
Ford Motor Company
Detroit, Michigan

FOREWORD

Low back disorders have long eluded a purely medical diagnosis. They are always job related, at least in the sense that the nature of the specific job influences the possibility and timing of a return to work. Thus an increase in disability pensions due to low back pain, now to be found in many Western societies, can probably not be explained in medical terms only. Conditions within a given society, such as availability of work and national insurance laws, are of obvious importance.

There are several good reasons for attending to people's need for health care closer to their place of work than has previously been the case. Demands made by the job—and the effects these have on the course of an illness and the chances of a return to work—are one such reason. There is often much to be gained by treating illnesses in the environment in which they have developed. The results of clinical investigations and treatment can then be used to make direct improvements in the work environment. As health costs escalate, Western societies increasingly pin their hopes on a broader approach to medical care and an emphasis on prevention of illnesses and disabilities.

Another reason why people's health needs should be met close to their place of work is that preventive measures call for considerable personal involvement. Individual habits must often be changed, and sometimes the entire lifestyle. This requires a learning process that must develop within the group with whom an individual shares customs and behavior patterns.

Health care at the place of work may fulfill an even more important function than that of dealing with job-related illness. In today's society, many people find the friendships they make at work to be among the most central and lasting friendships they have.

A recently concluded study on subchronic (8 weeks) low back pain patients at our Volvo Torslanda Plant clearly demonstrated the advantage of organizing activation programs in close vicinity to the work place, as well as of personal consideration being given by the physiotherapist to the type of work done by the patient. In this prospectively randomized study we found that manual workers who were trained for a specific type of job and who received no treatment other than a gradual and general increase in activation were able to return to work 7 weeks earlier on average than the control group patients, who received traditional low back treatment only. Furthermore, sick leave due to back pain was 4 months lower in the activated group over the subsequent 2 years, and permanent disability was down by 75%.

It is a great advantage to dispense health care within the environment where work is done and among those groups of people who do the work. Continuity is thus achieved, together with a greater understanding of the overall situation of the person seeking help. In addition, it is possible more directly to influence attitudes and habits.

It is my hope that this book will play a part in the creation of better working conditions and in the development of new methods for combatting occupational low back disorders.

Pehr G. Gyllenhammar
M.D. h c; D.Tech. hc
Chairman and Chief Executive Officer, AB Volvo
Gothenberg, Sweden

INTRODUCTION AND DEFINITIONS _____

Low back pain (LBP) has been called the nemesis of medicine and the albatross of industry. Although evidence of low back diseases can be identified in primitive man, most of the advances and understanding of the LBP problem have occurred in the past 50 years, and particularly in the past decade. As the social and economic costs of LBP have risen, interest has also increased, not only into the causation of LBP but also into methods of prevention. Despite this increased awareness, there has been widely dispersed literature for those interested in the specific problem of industrial LBP. Information has been disseminated in journals of orthopedics, biomechanics, engineering, industrial medicine and hygiene, physical and occupational therapy, and the law.

In 1981, we held a symposium on industrial low back pain which has now been repeated 10 times. Lessons were learned from these symposia. A diverse group is vitally interested in LBP. Physicians and surgeons, industrial nurses, physical and occupational therapists, engineers, representatives of the insurance industry, and labor and management all have been enthusiastic attendees. As anticipated, such a diverse group often had differences in perspective and also in the language by which they described their experiences with LBP. We have learned a great deal from all of these disciplines, most importantly that the ultimate solution to occupational LBP must involve all interested parties and is not solely a problem to be solved by doctors, labor, or management. We also have learned the importance of developing a communication system so that all participants have a commonality of understanding.

This book, then, represents an attempt to bring together in one place the scientific knowledge and its practical applications to the solution of industrial LBP. This information has been organized with the full recognition that it is to be used by a diverse readership. This book is organized into 5 parts. Part I presents the basic knowledge necessary to understand fully the problem of LBP. Chapters in this section describe the structure and function of the lumbar spine (the functional biomechanics), the occupational biomechanics of the lumbar spine (how overloading can occur), and clinical classification and descriptions of acute and chronic pain. The last chapter in this section concentrates on the definition of the problem in terms of its overall epidemiology or impact and cost. The occupational biomechanics chapter (Chapter 2) is, by necessity, quite technical; however, it forms the scientific basis for workplace design and evaluation. The concepts contained within this chapter will be useful to all readers. The last chapter in this section concentrates on the definition of the problem in terms of its overall epidemiology or impact and cost. Part II is an extension of this theme that breaks the problem down into considerations of the workplace and the worker. Part III deals with patient care and includes chapters on evaluation, treatment, and rehabilitation. These chapters are designed to be understandable to those without a medical background. Part IV focuses on selection and workplace evaluation with chapters on the overall concepts in prevention, considerations in worker selection, and a chapter on education and training. Further chapters in this section give practical advice about how to evaluate the workplace and how to design (or redesign) it. Part V deals with the important area of the legal aspects of LBP and contains useful information on impairment ratings, worker's compensation, and hiring practices. The Chapter 19 summary is designed to set the stage for future work and summarize our present knowledge.

Depending on the reader's experience and professional background, some sections of this book may represent new concepts or terminology. Although we have attempted to build a basis of understanding and definition within the text, a glossary of terms is provided as an additional aid to the reader. In every instance, we have tried to keep the illustrative material simple. Because there is a diversity of opinion contained within much of the scientific literature, we have incorporated these controversies, rather than attempted to preach a single-minded point of view. However, each chapter summary represents our carefully considered opinion as to the most useful theories and practices. For those who wish to explore further, fairly extensive bibliographies have been included.

Finally, it is clear that low back diseases are not a phenomenon of North America, but affect every country, particularly those that are highly industrialized. We have attempted to give an international perspective in all the material presented, with one exception. The law is so specific to each country that a review of compensation law, for example, in European countries alone would require a single volume. We therefore hope that our international readership will understand this obvious omission.

The participants in the symposia on LBP, and now the contributors to this book, have each been challenged by the problem of LBP, and bring to this effort a diversity of backgrounds and scientific experience. We hope you will enjoy their efforts, and we welcome your comments or criticisms.

Malcolm H. Pope, Dir. Med. Sc., Ph.D.
Gunnar B. J. Andersson, M.D., Ph.D.
John W. Frymoyer, M.D.
Don B. Chaffin, Ph.D.

CONTENTS _____

xiii

PART IV SELECTION AND WORKPLACE EVALUATION

PART V LEGAL ASPECTS

GLOSSARY OF TERMS _____

Accelerometer	Instrument that measures acceleration.
Analgesic	Pain-killing medication.
Anaphylactic	An allergic reaction.
Annular	Ring-shaped; related to annulus fibrosus of intervertebral disc.
Annulus fibrosus	Ring-shaped structure, outer part of intervertebral disc.
Anteroposterior	Pertaining to front and rear of body.
Anthropometric	Measurement of human body size and shape.
AP	Anteroposterior.
Apophyseal	Relating to projection from a bone; outgrowth without an independent center.
Arthropathy	Any disease affecting a joint.
Articular	Pertaining to a joint.
Autoimmune	Directed against the body's own tissues.
Axon	The axis of the nerve extending outward.
Biofeedback	The process of providing an individual with visual or auditory evidence of the status of an automatic body function.
Biomechanics	The application of principles of mechanics to better define human motions, forces, and moments and their limits.
CAT scan/CT scan	A view of a slice through the body using x-ray techniques.
Caudally	Inferiorly, toward the lower spine.
Chemonucleolysis	The administration of drugs to chemically remove portions of a disc.
Chronicity	State of being chronic (of long duration).
Claudication	Pain in the lower leg increased by walking.
Cohorts	Individuals who are members of the same group.
Chymopapain	Enzyme that dissolves soft tissue, especially intervertebral disc nucleus.
Compression fracture	A fracture (failure) of a vertebral bone caused by a force acting to squeeze the vertebra.
Diaphragm	A partition wall; the wall of muscle separating thorax and abdomen.
Diaphyseal	Relating to the shaft of a long bone.
Discitis	Inflammatory disease of the disc.
Discogenic	(Pain) caused by derangement of an intervertebral disc.

Discography	An x-ray photograph of an intervertebral disc containing an injected radiopaque contrast medium.
Dorsal	Related to back; posterior.
Electromyograph	Recording of the electrical output of the contraction of a muscle.
Endocrine	Denotes gland that internally secretes body chemicals.
Endogenous	Originating or produced within the organism.
End plate	The part of a vertebra that joins the intervertebral disc.
Epidemiology	Sum of what is known regarding epidemics (of disease or injury processes).
Erector spinae	Back muscles that extend the spine.
Ergonomics	Science that seeks the knowledge to adapt working conditions to suit the worker.
Etiology	Study of causes (of disease and injury).
Extensor	Any muscle that performs extension.
Facets	A pair of joints at each vertebral level; important for spine stabilization and bending capacity.
Fascia	Sheet of fibrous tissue that envelopes body beneath skin and encloses muscles.
Fibrosus	Formation of fibrous tissue.
Flexor	Any muscle that flexes a joint.
Ganglion	An aggregation of sensory nerve cells.
Herniated disc	Rupture of a disc, allowing the relatively fluid or gelatinous nucleus to push outward through the annulus.
HNP	Herniated nucleus pulposus, the gelatinous material in the center of the disc extends outwards.
Hypochondriasis	Morbid anxiety about health.
Idiopathic	Denoting a primary disease of unknown origin.
Innervation	Distribution of nerves, or degree of nerve stimulation.
Intervertebral	Situated between two adjacent vertebrae of the spine.
Ischemic	Relating to local diminished blood supply caused by mechanical obstruction.
Isometric	Of equal or constant magnitude.
Kinematics	Science of motion, including movements of body.
Lamina	A thin flat plate; part of the dorsal region of a vertebra.
Laminectomy	Excision of posterior arch (lamina) of a vertebra, commonly used approach to back surgery.
Latissimus dorsi	Superficially located broad flat muscles of the back.
LBP	Low back pain.
Lordosis	Curvature of spinal column as seen from the side (swayback).
Lumbar	Pertaining to the lower part of the spine; the last five vertebrae.
Lumbosacral	Pertaining to sacrum and lower back.

Magnetic resonance imaging (MRI)	An imaging technique using powerful magnets and radio waves to show proton densities of a slice through the body (sometimes called nuclear magnetic resonance).
Mechanoreceptor	A nerve receptor that is stimulated by mechanical pressure.
Morbidity	Proportion of disease to health in a community.
Necrosis	Death of one or more cells.
Neoplasms	New growth of cells or tissues, especially in cancerous conditions.
Nociceptor	A peripheral nerve organ or mechanism for the transmission of painful stimuli.
Nucleus pulposus	The central, more viscous portion of the intervertebral disc.
Orthosis	Orthopaedic device for assisting the function of part of the body without replacing it.
Osteoarthritis	A "wear-and-tear" arthritis affecting any joint.
Radiopaque	Impenetrable by x-rays.
Radiculopathy	Disease of the nerve root's ramus involving one of the primary blood or nerve vessels.
Retrospondylolisthesis	Misalignment of one vertebra relative to the adjacent vertebra characterized by backward displacement.
Sacral	Related to sacrum (tailbone).
Sacroiliac	Relating to the joint between the pelvis and the vertebral column.
Sagittal	Anatomic plane dividing body into left and right sides.
Scarification	Making a number of superficial incisions in the skin or other tissue.
Scoliosis	Abnormal curvature of vertebral column to one side, as seen from the frontal plane.
Segmental instability	An abnormal (excessive) motion or displacement between two adjacent vertebrae.
Somatization	Conversion of anxiety into physical symptoms.
Spasm	Involuntary muscular contraction.
Spinal stenosis	Reduction in the size of the spinal (neural) canal.
Spinous	Related to spine.
Spondylolisthesis	The condition of forward slippage of one vertebra on another.
Isthmic	The slippage is due to loss of the neural arch retention, secondary to a spondylolysis.
Degenerative/pseudo	Forward slippage, typically of L4 on L5 due to a degenerative process.
Congenital	A condition due to weakening of the bone, typically from a metabolic disease; rare.
Traumatic	In this text is defined as secondary to major trauma, as distinct from the isthmic type, which is due to subacute trauma.
Spondylolysis	A defect in the neural arch, typically at L5 and commonly believed to be due to repetitive low-grade trauma.

Spondylosis	Vertebral ankylosis; this term is also often applied nonspecifically to any spinal lesion of a degenerative nature.
Spondylotic	Usually refers to loss of disc height secondary to spinal degeneration.
Stenosis	Narrowing of any canal, especially the neural canal of the spine.
Stereophotograph	Two images viewed simultaneously to give the perception of depth or three-dimensional images.

PART I

Basis

1

Structure and Function of the Lumbar Spine

Malcolm H. Pope, Dr. Med. Sc., Ph.D.
John W. Frymoyer, M.D.
Thomas R. Lehmann, M.D.

OVERVIEW OF SPINE ANATOMY AND FUNCTION

The spine is a flexible multicurved column divided into five regions (Fig. 1.1): cervical (neck), thoracic (rib cage region, sometimes referred to as the dorsal region), lumbar (the low back, between the rib cage and the pelvis), sacral (five fused vertebrae that serve as an attachment to the pelvic girdle), and coccygeal (the tail, coccyx, which is not well developed in humans). Normally the cervical region has seven vertebrae, the thoracic twelve, and the lumbar five. The curves of the normal spine are illustrated in Figure 1.1. As seen in the side profile, the cervical and lumbar regions are in lordosis (lordotic curves); the thoracic, sacral, and coccygeal regions are in kyphosis (kyphotic curves). Hirsch and Nachemson[15] have suggested that the shape is important in absorbing energy and protecting the structures against impact.

In humans, the thoracic spine is partially splinted by the rib cage. The sacrum is rigid and the coccyx has no functional role. By contrast the cervical spine and lumbar spine not only support heavy loads but are flexible. It should not be surprising that these anatomic regions are the source of most spinal symptoms because of the greater functional demands.

The basic structure of the spine is similar in all of its subdivisions (Fig. 1.2). However, individual structures are more developed or less developed depending on the functional needs of that region. The descriptions to follow will be confined to the lumbar spine, where the components are generally larger and, therefore, consistent with the need to support more body weight and forces.

BASIC ANATOMY AND FUNCTION OF THE SPINE

The spine has four major interrelated functions: (1) support, (2) mobility, (3) housing and protection, and (4) control. As a support, the spine functions as a framework for the attachment of internal organs (facilitated by the rib cage). It also supports the upper and lower extremities, the trunk, the head, and external load moments. If the functional requirement were limited to support, the spine could be rigid, greatly simplifying its mechanical role. Because mobility is required for the many physical tasks of daily living and work, the spine structure is complicated. Thus, instead of a single rigid column, the spine is a flexible stack of rigid blocks with flexible soft tissue in between. The rigid blocks

3

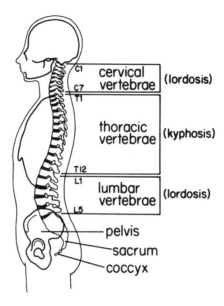

FIG 1.1.
The regions and curves of the normal spine.

are the vertebral bodies, and the flexible soft tissue structures in between each vertebra are the intervertebral discs. The basic functional unit of the spine is termed the motion segment (see Fig. 1.3). The motions of the individual spinal segments and the total motion of the spine and lumbar spine are shown in Figure 1.4. The largest motions of the lumbar spine are in forward bending (flexion), which occurs when touching the toes, and backward bending (extension), as when leaning back to view the sky. Other important motions are twisting, known as axial rotation, and lateral bending. More complex motions involve combinations of forward flexing, side bending, and twisting.

The housing function of the spine is to protect the spinal cord and nerves as they pass from the head to their point of departure to either the upper or lower extremities. The spinal

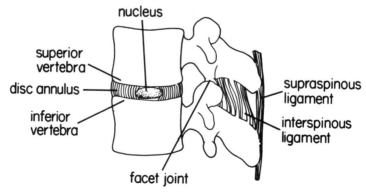

FIG 1.2.
The basic structural unit of the spine.

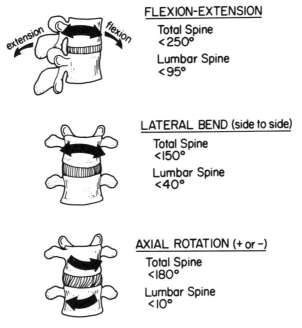

FLEXION-EXTENSION

Total Spine
<250°

Lumbar Spine
<95°

LATERAL BEND (side to side)

Total Spine
<150°

Lumbar Spine
<40°

AXIAL ROTATION (+ or −)

Total Spine
<180°

Lumbar Spine
<10°

FIG 1.3.
Motion segments of the lumbar spine.

cord terminates at the first or second lumbar vertebra, and the spinal canal beyond this point protects a fluid-filled sac containing nerve roots called the cauda equina. In cross section, the spinal canal or conduit is similar in construction to a house (see Fig. 1.5). The back of the vertebral body and disc serves as the foundation, the pedicles on either side serve as walls, and the laminae are the roof of this house.

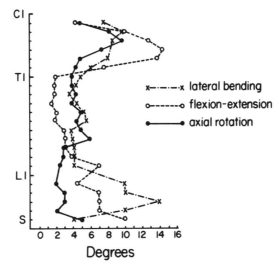

x———x lateral bending
o——————o flexion-extension
•————• axial rotation

Degrees

FIG 1.4.
Ranges of motion of the spine.

At a given level, the spine can be divided into anterior and posterior elements. The anterior segment includes the vertebral body, the disc, and the anterior and posterior longitudinal ligaments. The posterior elements are composed of the pedicles, the facet joints, and the posterior ligamentous and muscular attachments. Because of the need for mobility and flexibility, the roof of one vertebra joins to the adjacent vertebrae through a pair of interlocking joints (termed facet or zygoapophyseal joints), as illustrated in Figure 1.5. Although these joints are essential to normal motion, they also serve as a constraint. That is, depending on the planes of these joints, only certain motions may be allowed. The average motion by level is given in Figure 1.4.

The motion of each segment is controlled actively by muscles and passively by ligaments. These soft tissues attach directly to vertebral bodies, laminae, and specialized bony processes that act as lever arms. As depicted in Figure 1.5, each vertebra has a dorsally located spinous process and a pair of laterally placed transverse processes. The ligaments and muscles that connect these processes and the pelvis support the spine similar to the way guy wires support a radio tower.

SPINAL LOADING

The application of an external load results in deformations within the spinal structures and also produces movements between the structures. Quite strong forces are applied to spinal motion segments purely due to the mass of the trunk. For example (Fig. 1.6), if $L_2 = 0.05$ meter, $L_1 = 0.1$ meter, and $W = 40$ kg, then the muscle force (M) is 800 N (newtons) and the disc force (D) is 1200 N. Each spinal motion segment is normally subjected to a variety of loads and resultant forces, as illustrated in Figure 1.7.

Since the pattern of injury observed in the spine is a function of the type and magnitude of forces present, it is important to understand these forces and the types of deformations and tissue failures they eventually produce.

A downward force (stress) perpendicular to the surface of the upper vertebra compresses the disc and causes it to bulge. As the compressive load increases, pressure within the disc also increases. If the compressive force were increased, failure should occur at some point. In the laboratory, application of compressive load results in failure of the vertebral end plate, usually toward its center. This mechanism of injury most commonly results from a fall that lands a person in the seated posture and produces a compression fracture. This type

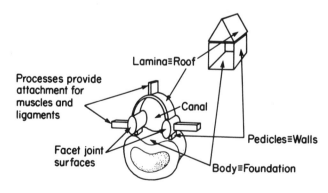

FIG 1.5.
The housing function of the spine.

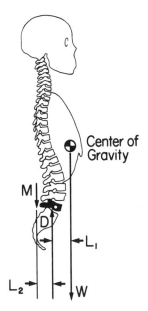

M = Dorsal muscle force
D = Disc reaction force
W = Weight of trunk
D = W + M
$L_2 M = L_1 W$

FIG 1.6.
Simple model of the spine.

of failure may be modified by the spine being loaded in flexion or extension. Flexion tends to cause anterior collapse of the end plate, a point where the bone structure is weaker. Forces sufficient to cause end-plate failure may also result from the act of lifting grossly excessive loads. This concept and the prevention of end-plate failure is explored further in Chapter 14.

A second type of loading is tension. Tensions tend to pull apart the structure being loaded, and the cross-sectional area of the structure decreases. Depending on the material that makes up the structure, tension loading may produce an elastic recoil. These principles are most evident in the highly elastic structure of the rubber band. In the spine, the ligaments are loaded in tension. In spinal extension, the anterior ligaments are stretched; while in flexion, the posterior ligaments are stretched. Overstretching any ligament may cause rupture of either individual ligament fibers or the entire ligament. Collectively, these failures are called sprains. When there is major spinal trauma, as might occur in a severe fall or vehicular injury, ligaments do rupture completely, usually accompanied by frank dislocation of the vertebra. However, the role of ligament strains in most occupational low back injuries is controversial (see Chapter 2). Ligaments contain pain fibers, and healing spinal ligaments are noted at autopsy, which adds credence to their role in low back pain.

Twisting motions of the spine produce strains in the tissues. In the normal lumbar spine, the facets tend to restrict torsion. In the laboratory, application of the torsional stresses produce fragmentation and disruption of the disc. Twisting also leads to large disc loads and

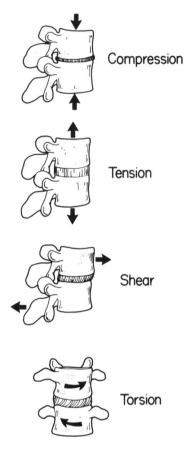

FIG 1.7.
Loads and resultant forces on spinal motion segments.

muscle forces.[25] Torsional injuries may be one of the earliest causes of acute low back pain episodes.[9]

Shear loading is produced by attempted translation of structures. For example, as the spine flexes, there is a tendency for a vertebra to slide forward relative to its next lowest neighbor. Shear stresses occur in the lumbar spine because of the lordotic curvature of this region, particularly at the lumbosacral junction (see Fig. 1.1), and is thought to be an important mechanism for lumbar disc herniation.[15]

In real life, we load our spines in many directions. Consider a worker transferring an object from a low pallet on the right to a higher table on the left. During the course of moving the object, the spine may be subjected to compressive loads (associated with the initial lift), lateral bending forces, torsional loads, and shear. Each force occurs in different phases of the lifting cycle and in different combinations. These complex forces are difficult to analyze in the workplace and difficult to replicate in the laboratory. By separating specific activities into their component parts, one can obtain a fairly accurate assessment of the types of loads involved and the resultant loads to which the vertebral structures have been subjected. This type of analysis, presented in the next chapter, involves the application of basic engineering principles coupled with an understanding of spinal stresses and strains. It is the cornerstone of the concepts presented in subsequent chapters regarding education, prevention, and workplace design.

INDIVIDUAL SPINAL STRUCTURES: THE SUPPORT SYSTEM

Let us now consider the individual spinal structures and how they respond to motion and load.

The Vertebral Bodies

The vertebral bodies are short cylindrical bones with a kidney-shaped cross section, as shown in Figure 1.8. They are the key element in the load-bearing system of the spine. The core of the vertebral body is made primarily of cancellous bone that has a honeycomblike construction. Since a functional characteristic of bone is to grow in a direction to withstand forces, the directions of trabeculae reveal the normal forces acting on the vertebra (see Fig. 1.8).

The vertically directed trabeculae support the compressive loads in the main vertebral body (see Fig. 1.8). At the upper and lower surfaces of the body oblique trabeculae sweep up or down to aid in this compressive load-bearing function. These trabeculae come together at the pedicles to resist the tensile forces there. The trabeculae sweep up and down to the superior and inferior facets to support the compressive and shear forces in the facets, and outward to the spinous process to withstand the tensile and bending forces applied to the spinous process.

As already noted, the type of failure resulting from an injury may relate to whether the spine was loaded in flexion or extension, with flexion tending to cause anterior collapse where the trabeculae are weaker (Fig. 1.9).

Krenz and Troup[19] found that the pressure was higher in the center of the end plate than in the periphery during compressive loading. Failure results from the nucleus (central part of the disc) rupturing the end plate. This is of particular significance for older workers who have diminished bone strength, usually the result of osteoporosis. In osteoporosis there is a reduction of bone volume. This reduction of bone volume is inversely related to the load necessary to produce a vertebral fracture.[13] In life the vertebrae are filled with blood, and thus it is possible that they behave like hydraulically strengthened shock absorbers,[18] which may result in greater strength in life than in laboratory observations.

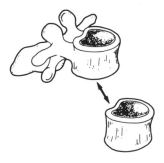

FIG 1.8.
The vertebral body and cross section.

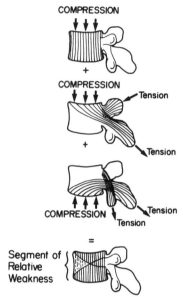

FIG 1.9.
Trabecular directions in the vertebrae.

The Posterior Elements and the Facet Joints (Apophyseal Joints)

Posteriorly the vertebral arch attaches to the vertebral body. The vertebral arch is made of the pedicles, lamina, facet joints, and spinous and transverse processes (Fig. 1.5). At the site where the lamina takes origin from the pedicles, the lamina is narrowed. This area is referred to as the pars interarticularis or isthmus. Whereas pedicles require major forces to fracture, the pars is a frequent site of a fatigue (stress) fracture, termed spondylolysis.[16] Such fractures may heal by fibrous union, which weakens the motion segment and sets the stage for a condition termed spondylolisthesis, discussed in Chapter 3.

The articulations between one vertebral roof and its neighbor are termed facet joints. The upward (cephalad or toward the head) extension of the roof is the superior articular process, the downward extension of the roof the inferior articular process. The facet joints are the right and left articulations of the superior and inferior articular processes, which are lined with hyaline cartilage. The facets are particularly important in resisting torsion and shear, but they also play a role in compression. Normally, the facets and discs together contribute about 80 percent of the torsional load resistance, with the facets contributing one-half of that amount.[9] Hutton, Stott, and Cyron[16] found similar load share between facet and disc under shear loads.

Lorenz, Patwardhan, and Vanderby[20] found that approximately 25 percent of the axial compressive load is transmitted through the facets. This load bearing was reduced markedly by excision of a single facet.

The amount of load bearing by the facet joints is related to whether the motion segment is loaded in flexion or extension. Thus, the difference in intradiscal pressures between erect sitting and erect standing (discussed in Chapter 14) can be explained in part by load bearing of the facet joints while in extension or lordosis. Theoretically, then, the disc would be protected from both torsional and compressive loads when the motion segment is in extension (or lordosis). Excessive loading of the spine in extension, however, may cause failure of this secondary load-bearing mechanism; that is, loads transmitted through the facet joints may produce high strains in the pars interarticularis leading to spondylolysis.

The Intervertebral Disc

The disc forms the primary articulation between the vertebral bodies. Its major role in weight bearing is shown by the fact that the area increases as a direct function of body mass in all mammals.[33] As already noted, the function of load bearing in shear, compression, and torsion is shared among the discs and the facet joints that collectively form the three-joint complex.

The disc, which is avascular, is composed of two morphologically separate parts. The outer part (Fig. 1.10), called the annulus fibrosus, is made up of about 90 sheets bonded to each other. Each sheet is made of collagen fibers that are oriented vertically at the peripheral layer but become progressively more oblique with each underlying sheet. The fibers in adjacent sheets run somewhat at 30-degree angles to each other. The lamination of the annular layers strengthens the annulus much like the plies strengthen an automobile tire. The central part of the disc is called the nucleus pulposus. In the younger individual, it is nearly 90 percent water, with the remaining structure being comprised of the fibrous materials collagen and proteoglycans, which are specialized materials that bind water. In the young healthy disc, a positive pressure is present within the nucleus pulposus at rest and increases as loads are applied to the spine. This pressure approximates to 1.5 times the mean applied pressure over the entire area of the end plate.[24] Disc pressures have been extensively studied in various postures and seating configurations (discussed fully in Chapter 14).

In axial compression, the increased intradiscal pressure is counteracted by annular fiber tension and disc bulge, rather analogous to the bulging in the sides of a tire (Fig. 1.11). Some disc space narrowing also occurs.[17] In flexion, extension, and lateral bending the same process occurs, although it usually focuses on a specific segment of the circumference of the disc. This process is associated with a small displacement of the nucleus posteriorly to the end-plate motion. The disc is an avascular structure and relies on passive diffusion driven by osmotic pressure for nutrition.[30] This nutrition can be affected by changes in end-plate permeability. Thus, ongoing smoking and vibration decrease permeability (nutrition), and exercise enhances it.

In axial rotation (i.e., torsion of the disc), the annular fibers in one direction are stretched significantly, whereas those on the opposite side are shortened or crimped. Mathematical

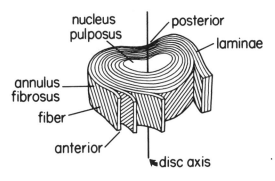

FIG 1.10.
The intervertebral disc.

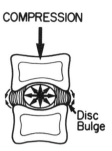

FIG 1.11.
Tire analogy.

models based on the geometry of the lumbar disc demonstrate that torsion produces stress concentration at the region of the posterior lateral annulus, which is a common site of disc herniation.[4,18,29] Torsional loading of spinal segments in the laboratory produces fissures in the annulus in the same posterolateral location. This fissuring may be accompanied by tracking of the nuclear material into the defects. This mechanical load does not produce a frank rupture, however. These events are suspected of being one of the common early causes of acute low back pain, but acute ruptures of lumbar intervertebral discs can only be produced in the laboratory by combining flexion and lateral bending motions.

Farfan[9] believes that compression failures promote disc degeneration. Normally the adult disc is avascular, but end-plate microfractures can result in vascular ingrowth, the formation of granulation tissue, and alterations in the chemistry and mechanical behavior of the disc. This concept is central to a controversial diagnosis termed disc disruption syndrome, discussed in Chapter 15.

The Effects of Surgery and Other Treatments on the Mechanics of the Disc

Although the clinical role of spine surgery is discussed in Chapter 7, it is important to recognize some effects of common treatments and operations on the mechanics of the disc and spine. For example, removal of the nucleus involves making a defect in the annulus. Such a defect has been shown by Seroussi et al.[28] to lead to abnormal bulging of the annulus. The presence of such defects would produce abnormal stress concentrations and theoretically could predispose the disc to further herniation.

Analysis of patients following disc excision or chymopapain injection almost always reveals narrowing at the operated or injected interspace, often accompanied by peripheral osteophyte formation. These observations imply altered compressive load-bearing capability of the motion segment. It is possible that over a lifetime the altered mechanics resulting from disc space narrowing may contribute to narrowing of the spinal canal and to spinal stenosis.

The House

The housing function of the spine is to serve as a conduit to protect the nervous system (see Fig. 1.5). The main conduit is the spinal canal, which traverses the spine from the head to the tailbone. In cross section the spinal canal is divided into areas or zones. Of particular importance is the area directly under the facet joint called the lateral recess (or subarticular recess). The height of the roof in the lateral recess is less than that in the central canal. The spinal nerve passes through the lateral recess (under the medial or inner aspect of the facet joint) as it starts to exit the spinal cord. Therefore, enlargement or hypertrophy of the facet joint can compress the spinal nerve in its lateral recess (lateral recess stenosis). That area of the main conduit other than the right and left lateral recesses is the central spinal canal. The central canal has a large variation in size in the general population and may vary by sex and race.[8] Workers with smaller central canals may be more subject to clinical symptoms in the presence of a herniated nucleus pulposus.[26] In the absence of a herniated nucleus pulposus, narrowing of the central canal from congenital or developmental origins or enlargement of the posterior elements (facet joints and ligamentum flavum) can lead to compression of the cauda equina (central spinal stenosis). The cauda equina are the nerves traveling inside the spinal sac (dura and arachnoid) through the spinal canal from the termination of the spinal cord (at about L1) to the sacrum. Schonstrom has demonstrated that the canal has to be constricted well below 100 mm^2 in a cross-sectional area before cauda equina constriction becomes significant.[27]

Additional conduits are present at each segmental level for the exit of the spinal nerve from the main conduit. This exiting conduit is called the intervertebral foramen. The roof of the foramen is the facet joint; the floor is the intervertebral disc and adjacent vertebral bodies. The upper and lower borders of the foramen are the pedicles of the adjacent vertebra. The intervertebral foramen houses the posterior root ganglion, which is an enlargement of the spinal nerve. This ganglion is enlarged because it contains the nucleus of the sensory nerve cell and thus is extremely pain sensitive[14] and the center of neurochemical activity related to pain.[31] The foramen may also become constricted secondary to lateral disc herniations, hypertrophic changes within the motion segment, and unstable shifts of the vertebrae (foramenal stenosis).

INDIVIDUAL SPINAL STRUCTURES: THE CONTROL SYSTEM

We have discussed the spinal structures that provide the basic functions of load bearing, mobility, and housing. These structures, unlike most other joints, depend on other tissues for their stability. This is most dramatically illustrated in the paralyzed individual when buckling of the spinal column occurs, producing severe scoliosis. The muscles are the inherent stabilizers, whereas the ligaments are the passive element of support, much like cables supporting a radio tower.

Ligaments

Various investigators have shown that ligaments are vital for the structural stability of the spinal system. The ligaments are also the primary tensile load-bearing elements. In general they act as passive, elastic check reins preventing excessive motion. Because ligaments (unlike muscles) are passive structures, their tension depends on their length. Ligaments also have a property known as viscoelasticity, which means their deformation and type of failure depends on the rate at which loads are applied. Their strength also depends upon the number of deformations applied. Repetitive loading cycles may cause fatigue and failure.[32]

The posterior and anterior longitudinal ligaments both traverse the length of the spine, adding to the support of the vertebral body and disc (Fig. 1.12). They are interlinked at each level by the disc. These ligaments together with the outer fibers of the annulus are richly supplied by nerve fibers, which are typical of pain-sensitive nerve endings.

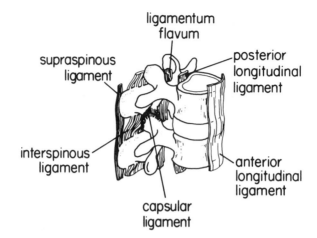

FIG 1.12.
The ligaments of the spine.

The remaining ligaments support and link the posterior elements. Of great functional importance is the ligamentum flavum, which joins the lamina of adjacent vertebrae. The ligamentum flavum is highly elastic and strong compared to other ligaments, and its high content of elastic fibers gives it a yellow appearance (hence it is sometimes called the yellow ligament). Its elastic properties allow it to lengthen with spine flexion and shorten with extension. In patients with severe spine degeneration, it becomes thickened and less elastic. These changes produce narrowing of the spinal canal in extension, because the ligament buckles into the spinal canal.

The tip and edges of the spinous process are joined by the interspinous and supraspinous ligaments. Because they are far from the disc and therefore act on long moment arms, these ligaments have an important functional role in resisting spine flexion. Similarly, intertransverse ligaments join the transverse processes of the vertebra.

The capsular structures around the apophyseal or facet joints are of functional importance in low back pain (LBP). These capsules include separate thickenings at the front and back, which have different functions. These capsular ligaments appear to limit the excursion of the facet joints, although their stabilizing functions have not yet been validated. Like all other joints, they are richly supplied with pain-sensitive nerve endings, but the facets have no nerves. Therefore, pain from degenerated joints would have to be initiated by a mechanical strain or chemical irritation of these capsular structures. Facet joint pain has been thought to be a common cause for chronic LBP but newer studies have questioned the importance of the facets in low back pain, as discussed in Chapter 7.

The Musculature

Without muscular support, the spine is unstable. The spinal musculature consists of flexors and extensors. The flexor muscles are made up of the psoas, which attaches directly to the vertebral bodies anterolaterally, and the abdominal muscles, which flex the spine through their attachments to the rib cage and pelvis.

The abdominal muscles are made up of the midline and anterior rectus abdominus muscles and the anterior and laterally placed layers of the internal and external oblique and transverse abdominal muscles. The extensor muscles (erector spinae, multifidi, and intertransversarii) attach to the outriggers (spinous processes and transverse processes) and other parts of the posterior elements. Their fibers may attach intrasegmentally (between adjacent vertebrae only) or intersegmentally (bridging multiple motion segments). The lumbar erector spinae consist of the iliocostalis lumborum and longissimus thoracis. The lumbar fibers arise from the accessory processes and the L1–L4 transverse processes and insert in the ileum.[21] When both sides contract symmetrically, they produce extension of the spine. When right and left sides contract and relax asymmetrically, lateral bending is produced. Both flexor and extensor muscles work together symmetrically.

In the upright posture, the dorsal muscles are electrically fairly inactive. With increased flexion, they become more active due to the increased load moment, but at large flexion angles they become silent (Fig. 1.13). From the standpoint of prevention and therapy, strengthening these muscles and training them to hold the spine in comfortable postures may allow function even in the presence of disease. Muscles can be strengthened and trained under the voluntary control of the patient.

From a standpoint of prevention and therapy, the muscles are vital structures of the spine. Most important, they are the motors that power the spine and are under voluntary control. They position the spine and stabilize it during awkward work postures, and they provide the power necessary for lifting and carrying. Gregersen and Lucas[11] showed how an excised spine with ligaments intact, but without muscles, buckles under very small compressive forces. Various animal models of the spine, when the mechanical function of

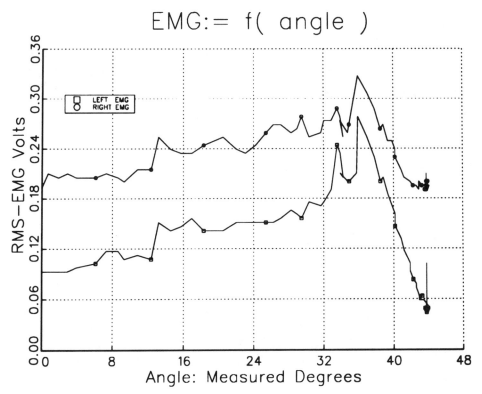

FIG 1.13.
Flexion/relaxation phenomenon.

the muscles has been disrupted, have shown how spinal stability is delicately controlled by the musculature. Changes in muscular strength or changes of muscle balance may lead to an increased risk of LBP.

Chaffin[5] has demonstrated that workers with inadequate lifting strength working in relatively stressful lifting tasks have higher low back injury rates than workers with less stressful lifting tasks. Apparently, when lifting near the strength limit of these muscles, excessive strain may be transmitted to other soft tissues (e.g., the ligaments and discs). Not all studies have confirmed these relationships; for example, Battié[3] found no relationship between isometric strength and later disabling low back pain episodes in aircraft assembly workers. It is possible that with muscle fatigue the probability of injury is increased. The ability to respond quickly to sudden loading may help prevent spine injury. When one of two workers carrying a load drops his share, a sudden load is transferred to the other worker. When muscles are fatigued, the possibility of injury increases because of an alteration in the ability to respond to these conditions.

Other Support Structures

Both the abdominal and thoracic cavities have been shown to become pressurized during strenuous activity (Fig. 1.14). The abdominal cavity can be pressurized by mechanical contraction of the muscles of the abdominal wall together with the diaphragm. Concomitant closing of the glottis (Valsalva maneuver) results in further pressurization.[6] This increased pressure tends to force the pelvic wall (floor of abdominal cavity) and the lung's diaphragm (roof of abdominal cavity) apart. Bartelink[2] and Morris, Lucas, and Bresler[23] suggest

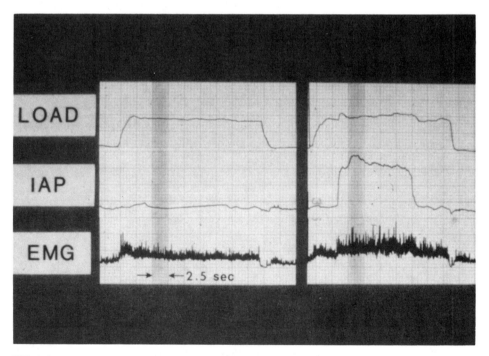

FIG 1.14.
Chart paper tracing showing that abdominal pressurization during lifting does not necessarily reduce dorsal muscle tension.

that this mechanism tends to extend the spine and thus reduce the contraction force required in the extensor muscles. In turn, this force rebalancing is said to reduce the compressive load bearing of the disc.[12] This assertion is controversial, since the abdominal muscles must contract, producing a flexion moment, in order to produce the intraabdominal pressure.

Another mechanism of action might be through the lumbodorsal fascia. Farfan[9] has suggested that the lumbodorsal fascia can change the length of the dorsal ligament by means of a laterally directed force from the oblique musculature. This is said to shorten this ligament. Farfan postulated that this is the mechanism by which intraabdominal pressure creates extension moments about the spine and thus assists in compressive load bearing. Thus, the muscles control compressive load bearing by acting through the ligaments. The importance of the lumbodorsal fascia has recently been questioned by McGill and Norman.[22] The general concept of spinal support from the abdomen has led to a rationale for flexion exercises, the wearing of corsets, and the protection of the spine by a belt for weight lifters. Davis[7] has used this concept in the determination of safe loads to be used in industry. In lifting, there is a linear relationship between the amount of weight lifted and the intraabdominal pressure that can be measured in the stomach or rectum.[1,7,13] Such relationships do not take into account the altered mechanics when the spine is located in a flexed or axially rotated position. Other measurements in those positions[10] have shown that an increase in intraabdominal pressure may not decrease the activity of the dorsal musculature. Thus, one would presume that the net axial loading of the disc is not reduced (Fig. 1.13). Therefore abdominal pressurization per se does not appear to have direct beneficial effects.

SUMMARY

The spine is a flexible multicurved column that has four primary functions: load bearing, mobility, control, and protective housing of the spinal cord. The dual roles of motion and support complicate the structure. The vertebral body and the disc have the primary role in compressive load bearing. The disc is composed of a fibrous laminated construction filled with a gel. Compressive forces increase the disc pressure and cause the disc to bulge. The vertebral bodies are made of trabecular bone that is oriented so as to provide support against the normal forces on the vertebrae. The vertebrae are filled with blood and may act as hydraulic shock absorbers. The ligaments have a primary role in tensile load support, and in the industrial environment such tensile load support can occur in many of the ligaments' movements. Mechanical overload may result in ligament sprain. The facet joints combined have a load-bearing function in compression and shear. The muscles have a role in control of posture and position and act as the motors to lift and move weights. They also provide the major stabilizing effect of the spine structures.

REFERENCES

1. Andersson GBJ, Ortengren R, Nachemson A: Intradiskal pressure, intra-abdominal pressure and myoelectric back muscle activity related to posture and loading. *Clin Ortho Rel Res* 1977; 129:156.
2. Bartelink DL: The role of abdominal pressure in relieving the pressure on the lumbar intervertebral discs. *J Bone Joint Surg* 1957; 39:718.
3. Battié M: *The Reliability of Physical Factors as Predictors of the Occurrence of Back Pain Reports. A Prospective Study within Industry* (thesis). University of Goteburg, 1989.

4. Broberg KB, von Essen HO: Modeling of intervertebral discs. *Spine* 1980; 5:155.
5. Chaffin DB: Human strength capability and low-back pain. *J Occupational Med* 1974; 16:248.
6. Davis PR: The causation of herniae by weight-lifting. *Lancet* 1959; 2:155.
7. Davis PR: The use of intra-abdominal pressure in evaluating stress on the lumbar spine. *Spine* 1981; 6:90.
8. Eisenstein S: Lumbar vertebral canal morphometry for computerised tomography in spinal stenosis. 1983; 8:187.
9. Farfan HF: *Mechanical disorders of the low back*. Philadelphia, Lea & Febiger, 1973.
10. Gilbertson LG, Krag MH, Pope MH: Investigation of the effect of intra-abdominal pressure on the load bearing of the spine. *Trans Ortho Res Soc* 1983; 8:177.
11. Gregersen GG, Lucas DB: An in vivo study of the axial rotation of the human thoracolumbar spine. *J Bone Joint Surg* 1967; 49A:247.
12. Grew ND: Intraabdominal pressure response to loads applied to the torso in normal subjects. *Spine* 1980; 5:149.
13. Hansson T: *The Bone Mineral Content and Biomechanical Properties of Lumbar Vertebrae* (thesis). University of Goteborg, 1977.
14. Howe JF, Loeser JD, Calvin WH: Mechanosensitivity of dorsal root ganglia and chronically injured axons: A physiological basis for the radicular pain of nerve root compression. *Pain* 1977; 3:25.
15. Hirsch C, Nachemson A: A new observation on the mechanical behavior of lumbar discs. *Acta Orthop Scand* 1954; 23:254.
16. Hutton WC, Stott JRR, Cyron BM: Is spondylolysis a fatigue fracture? *Spine* 1977; 2:202.
17. Kazarian L: Dynamic response characteristics of the human vertebral column: An experimental study of human autopsy specimens. *Acta Orthop Scand [Suppl]* 1972;146:1.
18. Kraus H: Stress analysis, in HF Farfan (ed): *Mechanical Disorders of the Low Back*. Philadelphia, Lea & Febiger, 1973, p 112.
19. Krenz J, Troup JDG: The structure of the pars inter-articularis of the lower lumbar vertebrae and its relation to the etiology of spondylolysis with a report of a healing fracture in the neural arch of a fourth lumbar vertebra. *J Bone Joint Surg* 1973; 55:735.
20. Lorenz M, Patwardhan A, Vanderby R: Load-bearing characteristics of lumbar facets in normal and surgically altered spinal segments. *Spine* 1983; 8:122.
21. Macintosh JE: *The Biomechanics of the Lumbar Musculature* (thesis). Department of Anatomy, University of Queensland, St Lucia, Australia, 1988.
22. McGill SM, Norman RW: Partitioning of the L4–L5 dynamic moment into disc, ligamentous and muscular components during lifting. *Spine* 1986; 11:666.
23. Morris JM, Lucas DB, Bresler B: Role of the trunk in stability of the spine. *J Bone Joint Surg* 1961; 43:327.
24. Nachemson A, Morris JM: In vivo measurements of intradiscal pressure. Discometry, a method for the determination of pressure in the lower lumbar discs. *J Bone Joint Surg* 1964; 46:1077.
25. Pope MH, Andersson GBJ, Broman H, et al: Electromyographic studies of the lumbar spine musculature during the development of axial torque. *J Orthop Res* 1986; 4:288.
26. Porter RW, Hibbert C, Wellman P: Backache and the lumbar spinal canal. *Spine* 1980; 5:99.
27. Schonstrom N, Bolender NF, Spengler DM, et al: Pressure changes within the cauda equina following constriction of the dural sac—an in vitro experimental study. *Spine* 1986; 9:604.
28. Seroussi RE, Krag MH, Muller DL, et al: Internal deformations of intact and denucleated human lumbar discs subjected to compression, flexion, and extension loads. *J Ortho Res* 1988; 7:122.
29. Spilker RL: Mechanical behavior of a simple model of an intervertebral disk under compressive loading, *J Biomech* 1980; 13:895.

30. Urban J, Holm S, Marondas A, et al: Nutrition of the intervertebral disc: An in vivo study of the soluto transport, *Clin Orthop* 1977; 129:101.
31. Weinstein JN: Mechanisms of spinal pain: The dorsal root ganglion and its role as a mediator of low back pain. *Spine* 1986; 11:999.
32. Weisman G, Pope MH, Johnson RJ: Cyclic loading in knee ligament injuries. *Am J Sports Med* 1980; 8:24.
33. Wilder DG, Krag MH, Pope MH: *Atlas of Mammalian Lumbar Vertebrae—Pictorial and Dimensional Information*. Springfield, Charles C. Thomas, 1991.

2

Occupational Biomechanics of the Lumbar Spine

Gunnar B.J. Andersson, M.D., Ph.D.
Don B. Chaffin, Ph.D.
Malcolm H. Pope, Dir. Med. Sc., Ph.D.

The preceding chapter has dealt with the biomechanics of the spine and its motion segments in broad context. Additional data are important to understand the biomechanics of the spine as it relates to work and work environment. Occupational biomechanics of the spine, as presented here, form the basis for subsequent discussion on workplace evaluation (Chapter 12) and workplace design (Chapter 14). As noted in the introduction, this chapter is necessarily technical and dependent on engineering concepts. The basic message, however, should be of interest to all readers.

The forces and moments acting on the lumbar spine come from body segment weights, movements of the trunk and extremities, and any external loads being handled or applied. These forces and moments must be equilibrated by internal forces, mainly contractions of the trunk muscles and resistances of the soft tissues. Pressures within the trunk cavities may also aid in this respect, as discussed in Chapter 1.

In the following pages we discuss the forces and moments on the spine as they relate to body posture and to the handling of materials and tools. We also discuss how externally applied forces, such as vibration, can influence the spine and its substructures. As such the chapter is introductory to the subject. The interested reader is referred to Chaffin and Andersson[30] for more detailed aspects of occupational biomechanics.

BIOMECHANICS OF POSTURE

In any discussion of the influence of postural factors on the load on the spine there are three issues to consider: (1) basic posture, (2) postural symmetry, and (3) postural constraint.

At the workplace, standing and sitting are the two basic forms of posture. The main advantages of standing are mobility, reach, and exertion of force, while sitting is less stressful for the legs, less energy consuming, less demanding on the blood circulation to the legs, and more stable for precision work. There are also disadvantages to sitting work postures, especially with respect to the back and neck. Ergonomic problems cannot be solved by simply providing a chair, only by a well thought-out and all-inclusive workplace design.

Even the most comfortable posture should not be maintained for long periods: static loading of muscles and joint tissues will occur which can often lead to discomfort.

Standing Postures

Muscular activity is required to maintain an upright posture, but as long as the body segments are well aligned with respect to the center of gravity, the activity is small.[4,6,7–11,14,27,41,66]

Any shift in the center of gravity of the trunk requires active counterbalancing by muscle force to maintain equilibrium.[14,58] Muscle forces are also required to counterbalance the moment caused by an outstretched arm, an external weight, or any other force applied to the trunk, head, and upper extremities.[13,84] The combined effect of all these forces upon the lumbar spine produces a moment that must be counterbalanced by the spinal muscles to maintain equilibrium. In this book this moment is referred to as the load moment. While the load moment is illustrated in Figure 2.1 for sagittally symmetric situations, a much more complex situation occurs when asymmetry prevails. In such postures—lateral flexion, rotation, and combinations thereof—other appropriate muscles contract. The asymmetry in muscle force is illustrated in Figure 2.2, from a study by Andersson et al.[14] In rotation and lateral bending, high levels of activity occur contralateral to the direction of postural asymmetries, while the activities on the ipsilateral side are much smaller. This asymmetry in muscle activity can lead to unequal stress concentrations on the different component structures of the spine. To maintain low muscle forces and consequently low stresses on the spine structures when standing, an upright symmetric posture should always be advocated, and all loads should be handled as close to the body as possible. Disc pressure measurements obtained in vivo when standing indicate that the load on the L3 disc in a person weighing 150 lb (70 kg) is about 107 lb (500 N).[7–11,68]

When a person leans forward, an increase in pressure occurs parallel to the increase in load moment.[14,84] The electromyographic activity of the dorsal muscles increases with increasing forward flexion up to full flexion, where the activity diminishes and then is absent. This is referred to as the flexion relaxation phenomenon. In the fully flexed posture, the individual is literally hanging on the posterior spinal ligaments.

Sitting Postures

Sitting is a position in which the weight of the body is transferred to the supporting area mainly by the ischial tuberosities of the pelvis and their surrounding soft tissues. Depending on the chair and posture, some proportion of the total body weight is also transferred through the legs to the floor as well as to the backrest and armrests.

Three different types of sitting may be distinguished: anterior, middle, and posterior sitting postures. In the middle posture, the trunk's center of mass is directly above the ischial tuberosities. This posture is quite unstable due to the ischial tuberosities acting as a pivot. In a relaxed middle posture, the lumbar spine is either straight or in slight kyphosis. The anterior (forward-leaning) posture is adopted most often when desk work is performed. In the anterior posture, the center of mass is in front of the ischial tuberosities, whereas in the posterior (backward-leaning) posture, the center of mass is behind the ischial tuberosities. That posture is obtained by a backward rotation of the pelvis resulting in kyphosis of the lumbar spine. It is a posture typically assumed in rest chairs and in chairs with reclining backrests, such as lounge chairs.

In general the posture of a seated person depends not only on the design of the chair but on sitting habits and the task to be performed. The height and inclination of the seat of the chair; the position, shape, and inclination of the backrest; and the presence of other types of support all influence the resulting posture. The chair should also permit regular and easy

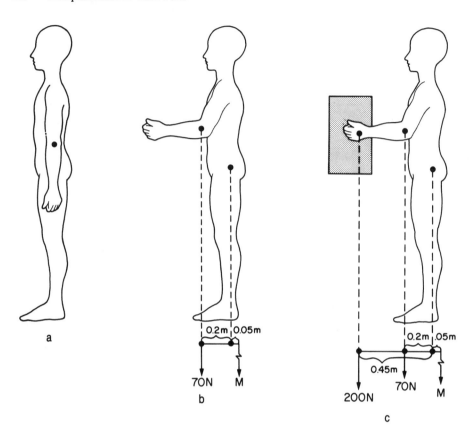

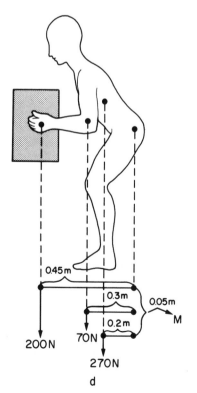

FIG 2.1.
(a) In upright standing the body segments are well aligned with respect to the center of gravity, and little muscular effort is required to maintain equilibrium. **(b)** An elevated arm causes a load moment of about 70 N × 0.2 m (14 Nm), which must be equilibrated by the back muscles acting with an average moment arm of 0.05 m (muscle tension = 280 N). An additional object with a weight of 200 N held at 0.45 M **(c)** causes an additional moment of 90 Nm (total muscle tension = 2080 N). When leaning forward holding no weight **(d)** the trunk moment (270 × 0.2 = 54 Nm), arm moment (70 × 0.3 = 21 Nm), and with weight of hand at 37 Nm, the hand moment (37 × 0.45 = 17 Nm) act together, causing a total load moment of 92 Nm (muscle tension = 1840 N). An additional weight **(e)** causes an additional moment of 200 × 0.45 = 90 Nm, (plus 92 Nm body load moment) altogether 182 Nm (muscle tension = 3640 N).

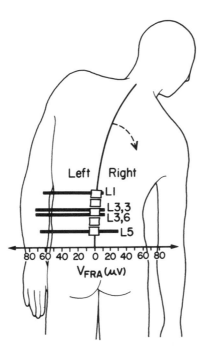

FIG 2.2.
Myoelectric activity (EMG) recorded in lateral bending. A weight was held in the right arm. Note high activity levels on the convex side (contralateral to the load) and low levels on ipsilateral side. (Adapted from Andersson GBJ, Ortengren R, Herberts P: Quantitative electromyographic studies. *Orthop Clin N Am* 1977; 8:85.)

alterations in posture, since continuous sitting in one position is a risk factor for LBP. Grieco,[50] in an address to the Ergonomics Society, focused his attention on the problem of *postural fixity*, that is, of remaining in the same posture for long periods of time. This problem (also discussed in Chapter 6) is often exaggerated in offices and electronic and small parts assembly workplaces, where movements are limited or stereotyped.

To facilitate transitions between certain tasks, an intermediate posture, *semisitting*, is often desirable. In semisitting, a higher than normal chair is used, usually with a forward-sloping seat that requires a person to lean on it, dividing the weight between the buttocks and feet[61] (Fig. 2.3). These seats result in a tendency for the person to slide forward, resulting in an increase of muscle activity.

Information on the biomechanics of sitting comes from radiographic studies, studies of the myoelectric activity of muscles (electromyography, or EMG), disc pressure measurements, and studies of seat pan pressure.

Radiographic studies show that the pelvis often rotates backward and the lumbar spine flattens during sitting without back support.[3,16,25,29,57,83,93] Andersson et al. studied the influence of different types of backrests on pelvic rotation and on the lumbar lordosis angle. In this study changes in pelvic rotation influenced the shape of the lumbar spine because the sacral-horizontal angle changed, that is, the foundation of the lumbar spine changed (Fig. 2.4). There must be compensation for this change in angle to keep the trunk upright.

To influence pelvic rotation a forward-tilted seat was proposed by Burandt,[25] Carlsoo,[28] and Mandal.[64] These measures minimize hip flexion and lumbar kyphosis. The lordosis of

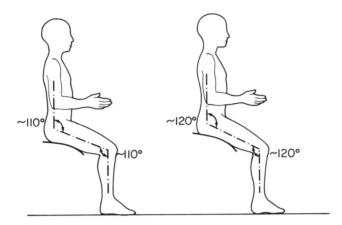

FIG 2.3.
A semisitting posture allows for rapid changes from sitting to standing. (Adapted from Engdahl, S. "Specification for Office Furniture" in B. Jonsson, (ed) *Sitting Work Postures,* (in Swedish) National Board of Occupational Safety and Health, 1978;12:97–135.)

the lumbar spine can also be maintained by a well designed low-back support according to Akerblom,[3] Keegan,[57] and Schoberth.[83] Bendix[21,22] used a statometric approach to determine the effect of the angle of the seat on the lumbar curvature. He found that the lumbar curve did change toward lordosis (less kyphosis) when a forward-sloping seat was used. A similar effect was also obtained by raising the seat.[22]

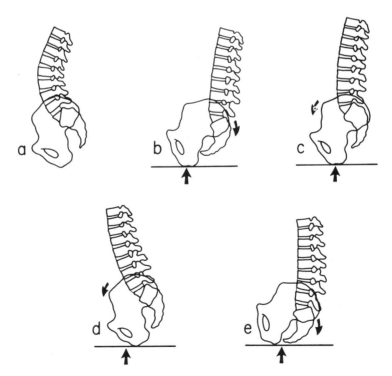

FIG 2.4.
Changes in pelvic rotation influence the shape of the lumbar spine.

In vivo pressures measured within a lumbar disc in a sitting posture without a lumbar support have been found to be about 35 percent higher than those in a standing posture.[68,70] To study the influence of supports, disc pressure has also been measured in subjects sitting in different chairs with different back supports.[4,8–11] These studies confirmed that disc pressure is considerably lower in standing than in unsupported sitting (Fig. 2.5). Among different unsupported sitting postures, the lowest pressure was found in sitting with the back straight. The reasons for this increased pressure in sitting postures are (1) an increase in the trunk load moment when the pelvis is rotated backward and the lumbar spine and torso are rotated forward and (2) the deformation of the disc itself, caused by the lumbar spine flattening.

When supports were added to the chair, disc pressure was found to be influenced by several factors (Fig. 2.6). Inclination of the backrest backward from vertical resulted in a decrease in disc pressure. An increase in lumbar support resulted also in a decrease in disc pressure. The decrease was generally larger when the backrest-seat angle was small. Studies performed by placing the back support in an office chair at different lumbar levels showed a slightly lower pressure when the support was at the level of the fourth and fifth lumbar vertebrae than when it was positioned at the first and second vertebrae. The use of armrests always resulted in a decrease in disc pressure, but this was less pronounced when the backrest-seat angle was large. The disc pressure measurements may be interpreted as follows: (1) when backrests are used, part of the body weight is transferred to them when a

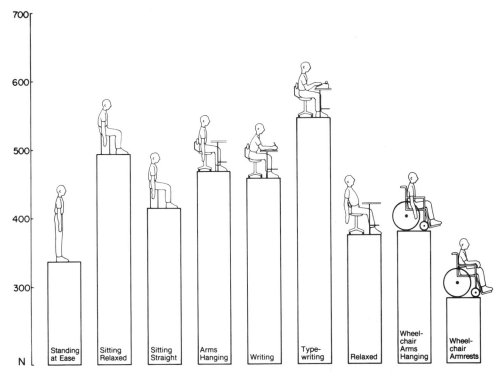

FIG 2.5.
Disc pressure measurements in standing, unsupported sitting, office work activities, and with and without armrests. (Adapted from Andersson GBJ, Ortengren R, Nachemson A, et al: Lumbar disc pressure and myoelectric back muscle activity during sitting. IV: Studies on a car driver's seat. *Scand J Rehab Med* 1974; 6:128.)

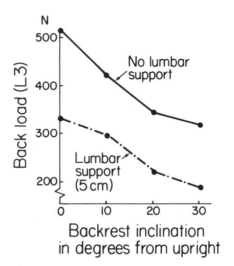

FIG 2.6.
The disc pressure decreases when the backrest inclination is increased and when a lumbar support is used. (Adapted from Andersson et al, 1974. See Fig. 2.5 for full reference.)

person leans back, reducing the load on the lumbar spine caused by the upper body weight; (2) an increase in backrest inclination (leaning the backrest more backward) means an increase in load transfer to the backrest and results in a reduced disc pressure; (3) the use of armrests supports the weight of the arms, reducing the disc pressure; and (4) the use of a lumbar support changes the posture of the lumbar spine toward lordosis and hence reduces the deformation of the lumbar spine and corresponding disc pressure (Fig. 2.7).

Typical seated office work has also been studied. In writing at a desk, a decrease in disc pressure was noted (Fig. 2.5) compared to the performance of other tasks. This was

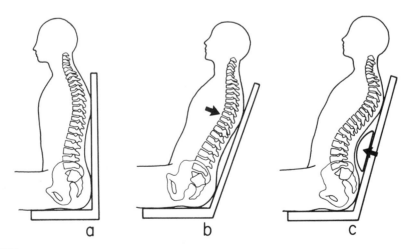

FIG 2.7.
When backrests are used an increasing part of the body weight is transferred to the backrest (*b*). The use of a lumbar support changes the posture of the lumbar spine toward lordosis (*c*).

expected, since the arms can be well supported by the desk. Other office activities, such as typing and lifting a phone at arm's length, increased the pressure because of larger external load moments imparted to the spine during such tasks.

Electromyography has been used to study the activity of back muscles in sitting. The EMG activity levels are important because high activities indicate muscle contractions. Generally, similar activity levels have been recorded in standing and sitting postures without a back support.[7,9,28,46,81] There is general agreement that, in sitting, myoelectric activity (EMG) decreases when: (1) the back is slumped forward in full flexion,[3,46,55,62,63,83] (2) the arms are supported,[7,8,28,47,81] or (3) a backrest is used.[3,7,8,28,47,59,81]

Of these three support parameters, backrest inclination has been found to be very important, with EMG levels and disc pressure both decreasing as the backrest-seat angle is increased[59,81] (as illustrated in Fig. 2.8[7]). Andersson et al.[7-11] also found that myoelectric activity not only decreased in the lumbar region but also in the thoracic and cervical areas of the spine when backrest inclination was increased. When the angle was greater than 110 degrees there was little further effect on the EMG levels. The influence of a lumbar support on muscle activity was small, whereas it was considerable on disc pressure. Hosea et al.[53] extended the studies by Andersson et al. by recording the myoelectric activities of several back muscles while subjects were driving over a 3.5-hour period. The myoelectric activity decreased when the backrest inclination increased in all areas of the spine. Lumbar supports of 3 and 5 cm did not significantly influence activity levels, but at 7 cm an increase in myoelectric activity of the lumbar erector spinae muscles occurred. The lowest myoelectric activities were recorded at 120 degrees of backrest inclination and 5 cm of lumbar support.

Yamaguchi, Umezawa, and Ishinada[99] also found that muscle activity decreased when the seat inclination was increased backward. Bendix et al.[23] also studied the effect of seat angle and tiltability on erector spinae myoelectric activity. No differences were found between a forward-sloping seat, a backward-sloping seat, and a tiltable seat. Further, no difference was found between high and low fixed-seat chairs.[21] Studies of the so-called Balans Chair, which induces sitting in a semikneeling posture, show that this posture actually results in increased muscle activity of lumbar and cervical muscles and increased blood flow to the feet compared to a standard chair.[60] The effect of different locations of the

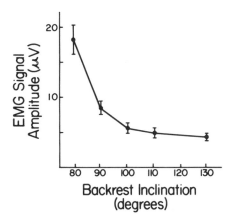

FIG 2.8.
The myoelectric (EMG) activity decreases when the backrest inclination is increased. (Adapted from Andersson GBJ, Ortengren R: Lumbar disc pressure and myoelectric back muscle activity during sitting. III: Studies on a wheelchair. *Scand J Rehab Med* 1974; 6:122.)

backrest was studied by Lundervold[62,63] and Floyd and Roberts.[45] They found that the myoelectric activity was lower when the back support was located in the lumbar region than when placed in the thoracic, thus confirming Akerblom's[3] observation that a support in the lumbar region reduced the load moments on the spine.

The relationship between seat height and table height has also been investigated. Too high or too low a seat has been found to increase muscle activity.[61,62,63] Bendix[20] studied the acceptability of seats of variable heights. Subjects disfavored low seats, and posture also became more constrained with less spontaneous body movements. In another study a tiltable seat was compared to a forward-sloping (10-degree) and a backward-sloping (5-degree).[88] The tiltable seat was preferred to the others.

Leg support is critical to better distribution and reduction of the load on the buttocks and the back of the thighs. To accomplish adequate leg support the feet should rest firmly on the floor or foot support so that the weight of the lower legs is not supported by the front part of the thighs resting on the seat. When a chair is so high that the feet do not reach the floor, there may be uncomfortable pressures on the back of the thighs.[3,26,83] These pressures can also be minimized by providing a "waterfall" profile at the front of the seat. All of these concepts provide the basis for optimal seat design, discussed in Chapter 14.

RECUMBENT POSTURE

A significant portion of each day is spent in the recumbent position. There is much opinion but only scant scientific data supporting optimal sleeping postures and bedding. The usual teaching has stressed the importance of lying supine on a relatively firm bedding surface, thus giving overall support to the spine while avoiding areas of excessive focal pressure on bony prominences. Flexion at the knees and hips is thought to decrease further stresses on the spine and supportive musculature. The only real direct evidence favoring this position comes from measurements of interdiscal pressure (usually at the L3–L4 level) that show the lowest measurements in the supine, hip-knee flexed posture. In this position, the iliopsoas muscles are also relaxed. Patients with acute and chronic low back conditions often observe that this is the position of maximal comfort. In particular, individuals with advanced spinal stenosis and spinal claudication often can find comfort only in this position, presumably because in it the canal dimensions are greatest. The position also reduces lumbar lordosis and theoretically decreases stresses on the facet joints and their capsules. However, not all individuals or patients with low back complaints find this posture comfortable. Indeed, some patients are more comfortable in the prone position, an observation emphasized by the proponents of extension exercise programs for the relief of certain low back conditions. The theoretical reason that the extended posture is comfortable for some patients is based on the assumption that a posteriorly bulging annulus becomes less bulged in extension as the nucleus pulposus moves into a more forward position, and also that the spinal cord and nerve roots are relaxed.

In the side-lying position, particularly when bedding is soft, increases are observed in intradiscal pressure. Typically, the side-lying posture is associated with some element of twisting, thus placing abnormal stresses on the facet capsules and producing torsional stresses on the annulus fibrosus. Despite these theoretical mechanical consequences many people, with or without low back pain, adopt this sleeping posture. Possibly one reason for comfort of this position is the associated hip and knee flexion. There may be insufficient evidence, however, to justify insistence on a single recumbent body posture because no basis exists to indicate which posture might or might not reduce the risk of low back episodes, and it is not practical to alter many individuals' normal sleeping habits. It does seem reasonable for individuals whose complaint is sharp spinal stiffness or pain on arising from bed to try a variety of resting postures to determine the most comfortable one. Based on the limited scientific evidence, the knee-hip flexed supine posture seems to be the most useful starting point.

The question of optimal bedding design is equally elusive. Clearly there is a great deal of commercial interest in promoting one or another alternative in bed design, both for the prevention and for the relief of low back diseases. Among the most popular current fads is the waterbed. Again, the evidence is scant and largely based on uncontrolled consumer reports. It seems logical that supportive mattresses and springs would have adequate structural integrity to give uniform body support and would not force the individual into an abnormal posture. For example, a stomach sleeper lying on inadequate bed support is forced into a position of hyperextension. Similarly, side-lying sleeping postures under these circumstances would tend to accentuate the lateral bend and axial rotation. Perhaps the simplest and most efficient sleeping surface is that advocated by some Scandinavians: thick plywood support with a foam rubber surface of six to eight inches.

BIOMECHANICS OF MANUAL MATERIALS HANDLING

Contrary to popular opinion, manual material handling has not been replaced by automation in modern industries. People are still lifting heavy loads in both employment and leisure activities. One of the parts of the body that is often the most highly stressed during lifting is the low back, specifically the lower lumbar segments of the spinal column and their associated muscles and ligaments. These stresses can be estimated by biomechanical models.

What follows is an introduction to modeling the L5/S1 motion segment during load lifting in industry. Through the use of such models one can begin to understand the complex interrelated mechanical factors that cause low back injuries. More detailed discussions of the mechanics of the spine are presented in Schultz et al.[84,85] and Chaffin and Andersson.[30]

Biomechanical Modeling of Load-Lifting Activities

It is evident from papers by, among others, Andersson et al.[5,13] and Chaffin[32] that the estimation of stresses on various parts of the musculoskeletal system during lifting activities requires a complex model that accounts for such factors as (1) instantaneous positions and accelerations of the extremities, head, and trunk; (2) changes in spinal geometry; and (3) strength variations within different muscle groups and people.

Recent efforts have been made to extend an early biomechanical model of the human body created by Plagenhoef[75] for sports activities to include (1) an estimate of the stresses in the lumbosacral disc; (2) the addition of external loads on the hands (e.g., in a materials-handling task); and (3) an evaluation of the effects of various muscle-group strengths on the performance of the person being studied. In accomplishing this, several computerized biomechanical models have evolved. A description of one of these models follows, along with some results obtained by using the model to study various whole-body lifting activities.

The model to be described has been referred to as the 2D Static Strength Prediction Program™. It was developed by the Center of Ergonomics at the University of Michigan, which has used and refined it over the last 20 years. As the name implies, this particular model was developed to evaluate various static situations, such as holding a weight or pushing or pulling on an unmoving object with both hands. In addition to these applications the model can be used to analyze the more normal slow motions used in heavy materials handling by formulating the input data to describe a sequence of static positions with very small changes in each successive position during a movement. This type of "pseudodynamic" analysis assumes that the effects of acceleration and momentum are negligible.

The 2DSSPP model is also restricted to symmetric sagittal plane activities; thus, a rotation or lateral deviation of the body cannot be analyzed. A 3D Static Strength Prediction Program is available for such analysis.[65,82,84,85]

The 2DSSPP model develops estimates of the forces and load moments at each of the major articulations of the extremities and back by treating the body as a series of seven solid links that articulate at the ankles, knees, hips, L5/S1 disc, shoulders, elbows, and wrists, as shown in Figure 2.9. Each of the links in the model is considered to have a mass estimated from body weight proportionality constants presented by Dempster and Gaughran[38] and Clauser, McConville, and Young.[33] The distribution of the mass within each link is based on the data of Dempster.[37] The length of each link is established from over-the-body measurements, with reference landmarks described by Dempster.[37] Specifically, the body measurements needed as input data are body stature, body weight, center of gravity of the hand-to-wrist distance, lower arm length, lower leg length, foot length, and elbow height when standing erect. From this data the link lengths (i.e., the straight-line distances between the articulation points of rotation) are estimated based on the empirical relationships developed by Dempster and co-workers.[38,39]

A task being analyzed with the 2DSSPP model is described by two types of data. First, any external force that may be exerted against the hands is measured and considered in the model as a vector acting at the center of gravity of the hands. For example, if a person is

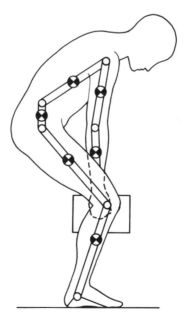

FiG 2.9.
The static sagittal plane (SSP) model. Wrist joint not shown.

holding a 21-lb (10-kg) box, it is entered into the program as a 21-lb force acting downward (i.e., a force acting in respect to some defined reference axis). The second type of information required by the model is a description of the posture of interest. These data are obtained by measuring the joint angles from either a lateral photograph (or similar) of a person in the position of interest or from an articulated drawing-board body template placed in the "task" position.

These data are sufficient for the model to compute the load moments and forces at each of the six major articulations of the body. The remainder of the discussion focuses on the development and use of a model that transforms the externally produced forces and load moments acting on the L5/S1 disc into predictions of compression and shear forces acting on the disc. Specifically, the compression force on the disc is estimated as a function of (1) posterior muscle actions, (2) body weight and load effects, and (3) abdominal pressure against the diaphragm.

Compressive forces on the lumbar spine caused by the abdominal muscles per se are assumed to be negligible since Bartelink[18] found that the rectus abdominis, which could mechanically cause a spinal compressive force, was relatively inactive during lifting activities. The abdominal pressure was therefore attributed to the oblique and transverse muscles, which are not well positioned to assist or hinder directly in sagittal plane flexion or extension of the trunk. Rather, they act to create pressure against the diaphragm, which causes erection of the torso.

The line of action of the muscles of the lower lumbar spine are assumed in the example to act parallel to the force of compression on the intervertebral discs with a moment arm of (5.0 cm), 2.0 in. as illustrated in Figure 2.10. The estimate of the magnitude of the muscle force required to maintain a particular trunk position is accomplished by dividing the estimated L5/S1 load moment caused by the body weight above the L5/S1 disc plus the weight of the load in the hands (after the abdominal pressure effect has been subtracted) by the 5.0 cm moment arm assumed for the back muscles. This logic assumes that the bending strength of the column is caused only by the spinal muscles and that the facet joints do not resist compression in the lumbar column during a lifting act when in the posture shown in Figure 2.11.

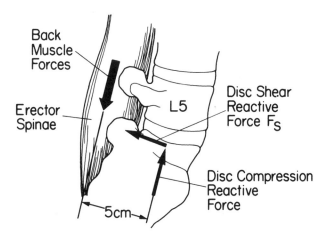

FIG 2.10.
Forces acting around disc.

Some Numerical Examples

To assist in understanding the biomechanics of the spine, the 2DSSPP model has been used to study various lifting situations. The results of these simulations are now described.

Case 1. Lifting a 500 N load close to the body. For this case we assume a common lifting posture, illustrated in Figure 2.11. Here the trunk is in forward flexion (30 degrees from vertical). In an average-sized male, the resulting load moment at the hips is 200 Nm because of the weight (BW) of the trunk, neck, head, and arms and the 500-N load (FH) held in the hands. The abdominal pressure F_{abdom} is predicted to be about 160 N based on the hip load moment and the angle between the trunk and thighs.

The static moment equilibrium equation results in the following estimate of the erector spinae forces.

$$F_{musc} = \frac{(BW \times B) + (FH \times H) - (F_{abdom} \times A)}{M} = 3.5 \text{ KN}$$

The compressive force (F_{comp}) on the superior surface of the sacrum is estimated for a pelvic angle α of 66 degrees by solving the static force equilibrium equation, which gives

$$F_{comp} = (\sin 66° \times BW) + (\sin 66° \times FH) - F_{abdom} + F_{musc} = 4.1 \text{ KN}$$

It should be noted that the erector spinae muscle force F_{musc} is the primary source of compression force on the disc during a volitional lifting activity. By stooping over further, the effect of the body weight and the load held in the hands is shifted still further from a

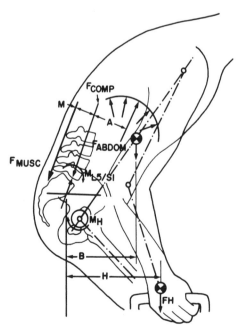

FIG 2.11.
Case 1. Lifting close to body.

compression force to a shearing force that is in part resisted by the lumbar facet joints and their associated ligaments. Such shear force could cause or aggravate problems in these structures. This will be further illustrated with other numerical examples later in the chapter.

The major point is that the erector spinae muscles are essential to the stability of the column, but their actions create high compression forces within the spine. Studies of cadaver spinal column strengths[44,74,88] indicate that such forces could cause microfractures of the cartilage end plates and/or annulus fibrosus that might then initiate or aggravate disc degeneration.

The role of abdominal pressure in relieving the compression load on the spinal column during lifting has been proposed[67] to be a major source of column support. Data obtained by Asmussen and Poulsen[17] however, appear to limit the general effectiveness of this reflex mechanism. A maximum limit of 150 mm Hg appears possible with highly trained individuals, although 90 mm Hg is probably a more reasonable limit for the normal population. It should be noted, though, that this spinal relief may not be possible when a person is carrying a load for a sustained period. If assumed to be a well developed reflex in an individual, abdominal pressurization probably can relieve approximately 15 to 20 percent of the lumbar spinal column compression during lifting.

Case 2. Lifting variable loads close to body. As a more general case, let us use the body position shown earlier in Figure 2.11 but vary the load from zero to 600 N. The predicted L5/S1 compression forces for each load resulting from this procedure are shown in Figure 2.12. Even with moderate loads held reasonably close to the body, high compression forces occur at the lumbosacral level. Perhaps this explains why one epidemiological study[31] has shown that some people had an increased incidence of low back pain when lifting weights not exceeding 200 N (44 lbs) in their jobs.

Case 3. Lifting loads with two different postures. It is often stated that lifting with the legs straight and the back stooped over is much more stressful on the lower back than lifting with a near vertical back, using the legs for the major lifting action. Unfortunately this rule, though widely quoted and sometimes valid, is not generally applicable. One reason for suspecting that the rule may be wrong is that observations of people lifting loads[72,73] have

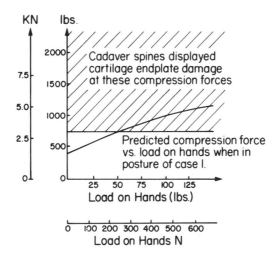

FIG 2.12.
Predicted forces compared to end-plate damage.

shown that people who have been repeatedly instructed to lift in this manner do not follow these instructions; rather, they more often stoop over and lift with their backs, using only a small degree of knee flexion.

The numerical example that follows illustrates two alternative postures to be used when lifting a bulky object that cannot pass easily between the knees. The load is located 37 cm in front of the ankles and 37 cm above the floor. The static load on the hands is 130 N (30 lbs) with a dynamic component added to represent the initial load accelerations (at about 100 ms into the lifting action). In dynamic load lifting, when the load is horizontally forward of the feet, a person normally lifts the load in a direction toward the torso rather than only vertically, as was assumed in Cases 1 and 2. The two postures assumed in the example are shown in Figure 2.13, with the predicted L5/S1 compression forces shown under each figure.

The back-stooped posture used in lifting a bulky load actually reduces the compressive loading on the L5/S1 disc below that predicted for lifting with a more vertical back. The reasons for the larger compression forces in lifting with the back near vertical in this example are (1) the load moment arm is increased and (2) the vertical component of both the body weight and hand forces add more directly to the compressive forces on the more vertical spine. Of course the shearing forces are greater in lifting with the back flexed. Also, depending on the precise curvature of the lumbar spine during the lift, the articular facet capsules and the posterior ligaments may be overstrained, especially with the more flexed torso posture required when performing a stoop type of lift.

In short, it appears that people often lift loads with their backs rather than their legs. In so doing, they minimize the energy necessary to move the body-load mass combination, as described by both Brown[24] and Park.[73] Although it is commonly believed that "back lifting" is more stressful than "leg lifting," this does not appear to be so in regard to compression loading of the column, especially in lifting loads that are larger than can be brought between the knees or loads that are located horizontally away from the feet. Disc pressure measurements[15] have shown the pressure to be similar in comparisons of "back-lift" and "leg-lift" methods, provided the moment arm to the load was kept constant.

If a person can maintain the torso in a completely erect position while lifting, then the compressive force is minimized on the L5/S1 disc. Because of limited shoulder strength and arm reach, this normally requires a small object held close to the body. The most important principle in load lifting is to minimize the horizontal distance of the load from the L5/S1 disc, especially if the load is heavy. The effect of varied H distances is illustrated in Figure

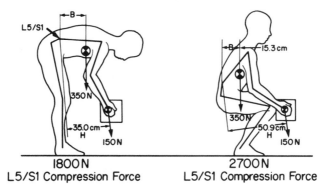

FIG 2.13.
Comparison of straight- and bent-leg lifting.

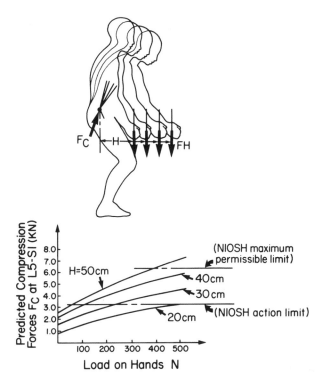

FIG 2.14.
Effect of moment arm on disc load.

2.14. Also shown are the NIOSH (National Institute for Occupational Safety and Health) limits to compression forces.[69] Clearly a heavy load held close to the body is much less hazardous to the back than one lifted further away from the body.

Cyclic Loading

Cyclic loading, or vibration, has been shown to have many and varied effects on the human. Dupuis and Zerlett[42] give an extensive description. The fatigue life of the tissues is of importance for the spine. Fatigue, which is defined as a loss of strength resulting from intermittent stresses over time, may lead to material failure. This may occur with relatively small stresses compared to those required for a static stress failure. A material's fatigue life (the number of loading cycles it can withstand) depends on the range of stress imposed. For most materials, there is a stress below which the material's fatigue life may be considered infinite. Even a small increase in stress over that limit may cause a significant decrease in the material's fatigue life. For instance, in one polymer of polytetrafluoroethylene, a 10 percent increase in stress range causes a 73.2 percent decrease in its fatigue life.[80] Under cyclic loading, microdamage is initiated and gradually increased until mechanical failure occurs. In living tissues, repair processes compensate for microdamage. Failure only occurs when the repair process cannot compensate for the damage process.

A mechanical softening caused by cyclic loading similar to that in polymers has also been demonstrated in ligaments by Weisman, Pope, and Johnson.[95] A ligament, although a biological connective tissue, consists of collagen, a polymer composed of polypeptide chains.[48] After cyclic loading of a ligament in one of a pair of knees, the ultimate strength of the ligament was significantly less than its contralateral, unstressed fellow. The amount of softening in the ligament was related to the cyclic stress. Hutton et al.[54] found that a cyclic shear force may cause a fatigue failure of the neural arch of the vertebra.

Cyclic loading of the spine induces "vibrocreep," which has been defined as the acceleration of creep under vibration.[56] Vibrocreep was demonstrated in cadaveric specimens, and it may be assumed to occur in living subjects. Adams and Hutton[2] cyclically loaded mature spinal motion segments in combined axial loading and bending. End-plate fractures were common, and some discs prolapsed.

Mechanical studies have also been performed to evaluate the effect of vibrating the whole human in various postures, in single or multiple directions. With mounting epidemiologic evidence associating low back pain with vibration environments (Chapter 6), there has been an increasing focus on the mechanical effect of occupational vibrations on the lower back. Most of this work has been related to seating and motor vehicles.

Simons[87] and Dupuis and Zerlett[42] looked at the seated environment as a design problem. They suggested it was necessary to record the three-dimensional motions, analyze the data with human tolerances in mind, and design a seat to protect the operator. If possible, measures should be taken to reduce vibration transmission. Unfortunately, good vibration tolerance data have yet to be determined for all people. The most serious consequence of providing a seat in a vehicle is that the most effective isolation mechanism humans have—their legs—is lost, yet the alternative (to drive the vehicle while standing) is clearly unacceptable.

Basic studies of vibration of the human have focused on the following mechanical parameters: resonant frequency, transmissibility, impedance, spinal muscle activity, and effects on the materials comprising the spine.

The natural frequency is the frequency at which an object freely vibrates after it has been struck mechanically, a bell being a good example. The frequency at which a simple spring-mass system freely vibrates is proportional to the square root of the stiffness divided by the mass in a single degree of freedom system.[86] For a given mass, natural frequency depends on stiffness. When a structure having a particular natural frequency is moved by some periodic oscillating force at the structure's natural frequency, a condition called resonance occurs, which has major mechanical consequences. In this situation, it takes very little additional energy to keep the structure vibrating at its natural frequency, and the associated stress can lead to the structure's mechanical failure (e.g., the Tacoma Narrows bridge collapse or an opera singer's voice shattering a glass). Failure occurs because the structure oscillates at its maximum possible excursion, thus creating the greatest possible strains on its components. As a result, the structure is at its greatest susceptibility for fatigue failure.

In a vehicle, the primary source of vibration is the interaction of the vehicle and the ground surface, but any component of the vehicle—engine, wheels, or drive shaft—for example, may be a source. In some cars driving at 50 to 60 mph over California expressways, the joints in the concrete slabs that are placed at 15-ft intervals can lead to a 6-Hz continuous vibration. In helicopters, the rotor and wind buffeting also have vibration effects, and in semitrailers, interaction between the trailer and the tractor may be an important source. Under some conditions, the natural frequency of the vehicle's suspension is approached, resulting in a violent response from the vehicle. Over very smooth ground the vehicle component (tires, for example) may excite the chassis and again the vibration may be excessive.

The natural frequency of a single-degree-of-freedom structure can be determined by two means: acceleration transmissibility and driving point impedance. Using the acceleration transmissibility method (transmissibility $= Acc_{out}/Acc_{in}$) to determine the output acceleration in the simple structure caused by a given input or driving acceleration. At resonance, the ratio of Acc_{out} exceeds Acc_{in}. In mechanical driving point impedance studies, the driving force is divided by the structure's resultant velocity. Resonance occurs when both the driving force and resultant velocity are in phase and the impedance/frequency curve reaches a maximum.[51] Figure 2.15 illustrates the mechanical impedance of the body as a function of frequency and body posture.[79]

Vibrational transmission may also be characterized by transfer functions, describing the relationship of input acceleration and measured output acceleration at a point in the body. In frequency ranges were attenuation is low, resonances occur, causing increases in the transfer function magnitude. Figure 2.16 shows some data obtained when standing and sitting subjects are exposed to vertical vibrations. In a standing subject the first resonance occurs at the hip, shoulders, and head at about 5 Hz. In sitting subjects resonance occurs at the shoulders at 5 Hz and to some degree also at the head. Further, a significant resonance from shoulders to head occurs at about 30 Hz.

Mechanical studies to determine the resonant frequency of the seated human operator subjected to vertical vibration have been summarized by Dupuis and Zerlett.[42] They generally found that resonant frequencies occur between 4 and 6 Hz when the upper torso is vibrating vertically with respect to the pelvis, and between 10 and 14 Hz in the case of bending vibrations of the upper torso with respect to the lumbar spine, producing a back slap against a seat back. Some of these studies also reported resonant frequencies of standing and supine subjects and resonant frequencies of seated subjects as affected by side-to-side or fore-aft vibrations.[52]

The degree to which the operator moves in a vibration environment is demonstrated by the magnitude of the acceleration transmissibility at the frequency of interest. At the resonant frequency the acceleration transmissibility is the greatest. Work reported by Dupuis and Zerlett[42] showed transmissibilities greater than 1.0 for the first resonant frequency of the seated operator. This indicates that the resultant motion exceeds the input

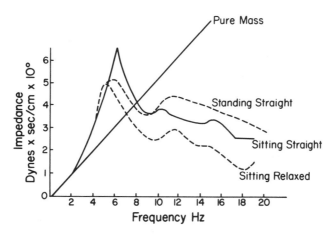

FIG 2.15.
Mechanical impedance of the body as a function of frequency and body posture (From Rao BKN, Ashley C: Subjective effects of vibration, in Tempest W (ed): *Infrasound and Low Frequency Vibration*. London, Academic Press, 1976.)

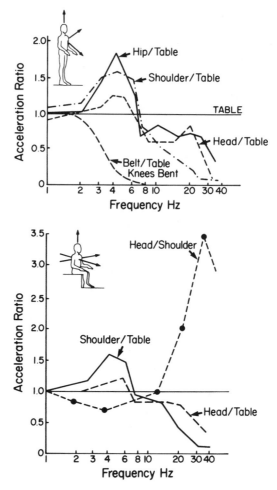

FIG 2.16.
Top figure: Transmissibility of vertical vibration from table to various parts of the body of a standing human subject as a function of frequency. **Bottom figure:** Transmissibility of vertical vibration from table to various parts of a seated human subject as a function of frequency. (Adapted from G. Rasmussen, Human body vibration exposure and its measurement, *Bruel & Kjaer Technical Review,* No 1-1982.)

motion and that the biological structures are being stretched maximally. Using accelerometers implanted in the lumbar region, Panjabi et al.[71] and Pope et al.[77] showed that the resonant frequency in the lumbar region of the vertically vibrated, seated operator was 4.5 Hz, indicating that maximum strain was occurring in the seated operator's lumbar region at resonances of 4.5 Hz. These studies demonstrated that much of the dynamic response is due to the combined rotation and vertical compression of the pelvis-buttocks system.

Driving point mechanical impedance evaluation gives information on aspects other than frequencies of resonance and phase shift between driving force and resulting velocity. It can also show the mass, stiffness, and damping characteristics of the system being tested. Studies of impedance, primarily of the seated human subjected to longitudinal vibration and secondarily of the human in other positions with other applied forces, were reported by Bastek et al.[19]; Coermann[34]; Coermann et al.[35]; Dieckmann[40]; Edwards and Lange[43];

Goldman and von Gierke[49]; Pope et al[76]; Radke[78]; Seidel et al.[86]; Vogt, Coermann, and Fust[94]; and Wilder et al.[96,97,98] Changes in impedance of the subject may indicate a softening of the system and an increased susceptibility to damage as a result of material and muscular fatigue.

The muscular effort of driving is considerable. This is a result of the forces necessary to maintain posture, control the vehicle, and resist its movements.[91] The components of vibration and shock may not be enough to cause acute injury, but lateral thrusts may add to the spinal stress. Thus, there may be a symbiotic effect of vibration and posture.

SUMMARY

It appears from radiographic, disc pressure, and myoelectric data that the load on the spine increases when sitting without a lumbar support compared to when standing. Reduced low back stress levels may be expected, however, from the use of proper back supports. The most important factor in reducing low back stress is the backrest, and the most important parameter in backrest design is its inclination angle. By addition of a separate lumbar support, the load moments on the back may be reduced further, particularly in an upright sitting posture. Such support should be placed in the lumbar region to achieve a more normal lordotic curvature when sitting. To provide as much comfort as possible, the support should be adjustable in height and size. The evidence presented also shows that supporting the arms and ensuring that the seat is adjustable to the proper height can reduce low back stress further.

Moderate loads may produce high compression forces in the lumbar spinal discs. Both epidemiological and cadaver data indicate that compression forces in the ranges observed in industry may produce structural failures in the weight-bearing cartilage end plates. Some researchers believe that the resulting microfractures and scarring are a major factor in accelerating the natural aging and degeneration of the spinal discs.

Lifting recommendations are based on a concern for minimizing compression forces incurred by the spinal column when lifting loads in the sagittal plane. Much more research is needed to understand the pathobiomechanics of load lifting, especially with regard to asymmetric and highly dynamic motions. Simple biomechanical models of the type described in this chapter are able, however, to assist in determining how the many anatomical, postural, and load-related variables combine to affect injury-producing stresses in common load-lifting situations. These models, though admittedly crude at this time, have provided much of the knowledge now used to develop the job design guidelines discussed later in this book.

Vibration affects the spine by causing vibrocreep of the disc and mechanical fatigue of spinal tissues. The postures in driving can cause muscular fatigue, probably shifting loads to the soft tissue, and this is exacerbated by the vibrational environment. Many vehicles excite the natural frequencies of the human spinal system.

REFERENCES

1. Adams MA: Anatomische und Physiologische Grundlagen zur Gestaltung von Sitzen, in E Grandjean (ed): *Sitting Posture*. London, Taylor, 1969, pp 6–17.
2. Adams MA, Hutton WC: Gradual disc prolapse. *Spine* 1985; 6:241.
3. Akerblom B: Standing and sitting posture. With special reference to the construction of chairs. Nordiska Bokhandelin, Stockholm, doctoral dissertation, 1948.

4. Andersson GBJ: *On Myoelectric Back Muscle Activity and Lumbar Disc Pressure in Sitting Postures* (thesis). Gothenburg, Sweden, University of Gothenburg, 1974.
5. Andersson GBJ, Chaffin DB, Herrin GD, et al: A biomechanical model of the lumbosacral joint during lifting activities. *J Biomech* 1985; 18:571.
6. Andersson GBJ, Ortengren R: Myoelectric back muscle activity during sitting. *Scand J Rehab Med [Suppl]* 1974; 3:73.
7. Andersson GBJ, Jonsson B, Ortengren R: Myoelectric activity in individual lumbar erector spinae muscles in sitting. A study with surface and wire electrodes. *Scand J Rehab Med [Suppl]* 1974; 3:91.
8. Andersson GBJ, Ortengren R, Nachemson A, et al: Lumbar disc pressure and myoelectric back muscle activity during sitting. I: Studies on an experimental chair. *Scand J Rehab Med* 1974; 6:104.
9. Andersson GBJ, Ortengren R: Lumbar disc pressure and myoelectric back muscle activity during sitting. II: Studies on an office chair. *Scand J Rehab Med* 1974; 6:115.
10. Andersson GBJ, Ortengren R: Lumbar disc pressure and myoelectric back muscle activity during sitting. III: Studies on a wheelchair. *Scand J Rehab Med* 1974; 6:122.
11. Andersson GBJ, Ortengren R, Nachemson A, et al: Lumbar disc pressure and myoelectric back muscle activity during sitting. IV: Studies on a car driver's seat. *Scand J Rehab Med* 1974; 6:128.
12. Andersson GBJ, et al: The sitting posture: An electromyographic and discometric study. *Orth Clin N Am* 1975; 6:105.
13. Andersson GBJ, Ortengren R, Schultz A: Analysis and measurement of the loads on the lumbar spine during work at a table. *J Biomech* 1980; 13:513.
14. Andersson GBJ, Ortengren R, Herberts P: Quantitative electromyographic studies of back muscle activity related to posture and loading. *Orthop Clin N Am* 1977; 8:85.
15. Andersson GBJ, Ortengren R, Nachemson A: Quantitative studies of back loads in lifting. *Spine* 1976; 1:178.
16. Andersson GBJ, Murphy RW, Ortengren R, et al: The influence of backrest inclination and lumbar support on the lumbar lordosis in sitting. *Spine* 1979; 4:52.
17. Asmussen E, Poulsen E: On the role of the intra-abdominal pressure in relieving the back muscles while holding weights in a forward inclined position. *Commun Dan Natl Assoc Infant Paral* 1968; 28:3.
18. Bartelink DL: The role of abdominal pressure in relieving the pressure on the lumbar intervertebral discs. *J Bone Joint Surg* 1957; 39:718.
19. Bastek R, et al: Comparison of the effects of sinusoidal and stochastic octave-band-wide vibrations—A multi-disciplinary study. I: Experimental arrangement and physical aspects, II: Physiological aspects, III: Psychological investigations. *Intl Arch Occup & Envir Health* 1977; 39:143.
20. Bendix T: Adjustment of the Seated Workplace—with Special Reference to Heights and Inclinations of Seat and Table. Copenhagen, Laegeforeningens Forlag, 1987.
21. Bendix T: Seated trunk posture at various seat inclinations, seat heights and table heights. *Human Factors* 1986, 26:695–703.
22. Bendix T, Biering-Sorensen F: Posture of the trunk when sitting on forward inclining seats. *Scand J Rehab Med* 1983; 15:197–203.
23. Bendix T, Winkel J, Jessen F: Comparison of office chairs with fixed forwards and backwards inclining, or tiltable seats. *Eur J Appl Physiol* 1985; 54:378–385.
24. Brown JR: Lifting as an Industrial Hazard. Toronto, Ontario Department of Labour, Labour Safety Council of Ontario, 1972.
25. Burandt U: Röntgenuntersuchung über die Stellung von Becken und Wirbelsäule beim Sitzen auf vorgeneigten Flächen. *Ergonomics* 1969; 12:356.
26. Bush CA: Study of pressures on skin under ischial tuberosities and thighs during sitting. *Arch Phys Med* 1969; 50:207.

27. Carlsoo S: The static muscle load in different work positions: An electromyographic study. *Ergonomics* 1961; 4:193.
28. Carlsoo S: Writing desk, chair and posture of work (in Swedish). Dept of Anatomy, University of Stockholm 1963.
29. Carlsoo, S: *How Man Moves.* London, Heinemann, 1972.
30. Chaffin DB, Andersson GBJ: *Occupational Biomechanics.* New York, J Wiley & Sons, 1990.
31. Chaffin DB, Park KS: A longitudinal study of low-back pain as associated with occupational weight lifting factors. *Am Ind Hyg Ass J* 1973; 34:513.
32. Chaffin DB: Computerized models for occupational biomechanics, in *Biomechanics X-A,* Internat Series on Biomech, 6A:3, Champaign, Illinois, Human Kinetic Publishers, 1987.
33. Clauser CE, McConville JT, Young JW: *Weight, Volume, and Center of Mass of Segments of the Human Body.* Wright Patterson Air Force Base, Ohio, Aerospace Medical Research Laboratory, AMRL Tech Report No 69–70, 1970.
34. Coermann RR: The mechanical impedance of the human body in sitting and standing position at low frequencies. Aerospace Medical Research Labs, Wright Patterson Air Force Base, Ohio, Acoustic Systems Div Tech Report No 61–492, 1961.
35. Coermann RR, Ziegenrucker GH, Wittwer AL, von Gierke HE: The passive dynamic mechanical properties of the human thorax-abdomen system and of the whole body system. *Aerospace Med* 1960; 31:443.
36. Davis PR, Troup JDG, Burnard JH: Movements of the thoracic and lumbar spine when lifting: A chrono-cyclophotographic study. *Anat* (London) 1965; 99:13.
37. Dempster WT: Space requirements of the seated operator. Wright Air Development Center, WADC Tech Report No 55–159, 1955.
38. Dempster WT, Gaughran GRL: Properties of body segments based on size and weight. *Am J Anat* 1967; 120:33.
39. Dempster WT, Sherr LA, Priest JG: Conversion scales estimating humeral and femoral lengths and lengths of functional segments in the limbs of American Caucasoid males. *Hum Biol* 1964; 36:246.
40. Dieckmann D: A study of the influence of vibration on man. *Ergonomics* 1958; 1:347.
41. Donish ER, Basmajian JV: Electromyography of deep back muscles in man. *Am J Anat* 1972; 133:25.
42. Dupuis H, Zerlett G: *The Effects of Whole-Body Vibration.* Heidelberg, Germany Springer-Verlag, 1986.
43. Edwards RG, Lange KO: A mechanical impedance investigation of human response to vibration. AD-609-006, Wright Patterson Air Force Base, Aerospace Medical Research Laboratory, Dayton, Ohio, AMRL-TR-64-91, 1964.
44. Evans FG, Lissner HR: Strength of intervertebral disc. *J Bone Joint Surg* 1954; 36:185.
45. Floyd WF, Roberts DF: Anatomical and physiological principles in chair and table design. *Ergonomics* 1958; 2:1.
46. Floyd WF, Silver PHS: The function of the erectores spinae muscles in certain movements and postures in man. *J Phys* (London) 1955; 129:184.
47. Floyd WF, Ward JS: Anthropometric and physiological considerations in school, office and factory seating, in Grandjean E (ed): *Sitting Posture.* London, Taylor and Francis, 1969, pp 18–25.
48. Fung YC. *Biomechanics: Mechanical Properties of Living Tissues.* New York, Springer-Verlag, 1981.
49. Goldman DE, von Gierke HE: The effects of shock and vibration on man. Bethesda, Md, Naval Medical Research Inst, Lecture and Review Series, American National Standards Institute No S3-W-39.
50. Grieco A: Sitting posture: An old problem and a new one. *Ergonomics* 1986; 29:345–362.
51. Hixson EL: Mechanical impedance and mobility, in Harris CM, Crede CE (eds): *Shock and Vibration Handbook.* New York, McGraw-Hill, 1976.

52. Hornick RJ, Boettcher CA, Simons AK: The effect of low frequency high amplitude, whole body, longitudinal and transverse vibration upon human performance. Milwaukee, Wisc, Bostrom Research Labs, contract No DA-11-022-509-ORD-3300, 1961.
53. Hosea TM, Simon SR, Delatizky J, et al: Myoelectric analysis of the paraspinal musculature in relation to automobile driving. *Spine* 1986, 11:928–936.
54. Hutton WC, Stott JR, Cynn BM: Is spondylolysis a fatigue fracture? *Spine* 1977; 2:202.
55. Jonsson B: The functions of individual muscles in the lumbar part of the spinae muscle. *Electromyography* 1970; 10:5.
56. Kazarian LE: Dynamic response characteristics of the human vertebral column. *Acta Orthop Scand [Suppl]* 1972; 146.
57. Keegan JJ: Alterations of the lumbar curve related to posture and seating. *J Bone Joint Surg* 1953; 35:589.
58. Klausen K: The form and function of the loaded human spine. *Acta Phys Scand* 1965; 65:176.
59. Knutsson B, Lindh K, Telhag H: Sitting—an electromyographic and mechanical study. *Acta Orthop Scand* 1966; 37:415.
60. Lander C, Korbon GA, DeGood DE, Rowlinson JC: The Balans Chair and its semi-kneeling position: An ergonomic comparison with conventional sitting position. *Spine* 1987; 12:269–272.
61. Laurig W: Der Stehsitz als Physiologisch günstige Alternative zum Reinen Steharbeitsplatz. *Arbeitsmed Sozialmed Arbeitshyg* 1969; 4:219.
62. Lundervold AJS: Electromyographic investigations of position and manner of working in typewriting. *Acta Physiol Scand [Suppl]* 1951; 84:1.
63. Lundervold AJS: Electromyographic investigations during sedentary work, especially typewriting. *Brit J Phys Med* 1951; 14:32.
64. Mandal AC: Work-chair with tilting seat. *Lancet* 1975; 1:642.
65. McGill SM, Norman RW. Partitioning of the L4–L5 dynamic moment into disc, ligamentous and muscular components during lifting. *Spine* 1986; 11:666.
66. Morris JM, Benner G, Lucas DB: An electromyographic study of the intrinsic muscles of the back in man. *J Anat* 1962; 95:509.
67. Morris JM, Lucas DB, Bresler B: Role of the trunk in stability of the spine. *J Bone Joint Surg* 1961; 43:327.
68. Nachemson AL, Elfstrom G: Intravital dynamic pressure measurements in lumbar discs. A study of common movements, maneuvers and exercises. *Scand J Rehab Med [Suppl 1]* 1970; 2:1.
69. National Institute for Occupational Safety and Health: A work practices guide for manual lifting, Cincinnati, Oh, US Dept of Health and Human Services, Tech Report No 81-122, 1981.
70. Okushima H: Study on hydrodynamic pressure of lumbar intervertebral disc. (in Japanese) *Arch Jap Chir* 1970; 39:45.
71. Panjabi MM, Andersson GBJ, Jorneus L, et al: In vivo measurement of spinal column vibrations. Presented at Proceedings of Am Soc Biomech, Rochester, MN, Sept, 1983.
72. Park K, Chaffin DB: A biomechanical evaluation of two methods of manual load lifting. *AIIE Trans* 1974; 6:105.
73. Park KYS: *A Computerized Simulation Model of Postures During Manual Materials Handling* (thesis). Ann Arbor, Univ of Michigan, 1973.
74. Perey O: Fracture of the vertebral endplate in the lumbar spine: An experimental biomechanical investigation. *Acta Orthop Scand [Suppl]* 1957,25:1–72.
75. Plagenhoef SC: Methods for obtaining kinetic data to analyze human motions. *Res Quart Amer Assoc Health Phys Educ* 1966; 37:103.
76. Pope MH, Wilder DG, Frymoyer JW: Vibration as an aetiologic factor in low back pain. Proc Inst Mech Engs Conf on Low Back Pain, Inst Mech Engs Paper No C121/80, 1980.

77. Pope MH, Wilder DG, Jorneus L, et al: The response of the seated human to sinusoidal vibration and impact. *J Biomech Eng* 1987; 109:279.
78. Radke AO: International view of tractor seating. New York, Soc Automotive Engineers, No 730794, 1973.
79. Rao BKN, Ashley C: Subjective effects of vibration, in Tempest W (ed): *Infrasound and Low Frequency Vibration*. London, Academic Press, 1976.
80. Riddell MN, Koo GP, O'Toole JL: Fatigue mechanisms of thermoplastics. Soc Polymer Engineers, 22nd Annual Tech Conf, *Polymer Eng Sci* 1966; 6:363.
81. Rosemeyer B: Electromygraphiche Untersuchungen der Rücken- und Schultermuskulatur im Stehen und Sitzen unter Berücksichtigung der Haltung des Autofahrers. *Arch Orthop Unfallchir* 1971; 71:59.
82. Schanne FJ Jr: *A Three-Dimensional Hand Force Capability Model for a Seated Person*, (thesis) vols I, II. Univ of Michigan, Ann Arbor, 1972.
83. Schoberth H: *Sitzhaltung, Sitzschaden, Sitzmöbel*. Heidelberg, Germany, Springer Verlag, 1962.
84. Schultz AB, Andersson GBJ, Ortengren R, et al: Analysis and quantitative myoelectric measurements of loads on the lumbar spine when holding weights in standing postures. *Spine* 1982; 7:390.
85. Schultz AB, Andersson GBJ, Ortengren R, et al: Loads on the lumbar spine: Validation of biomechanical analysis by measurements of intradiscal and myoelectric signals. *J Bone Joint Surg* 1982; 64:713.
86. Seidel H, et al: On human response to prolonged repeated whole-body vibration. *Ergonomics* 1980; 23:191.
87. Simons AK: Tractor ride research. *SAE Quart Trans* 1952; 6:357.
88. Sonoda T: Studies on the compression, tension, and torsion strength of the human vertebral column. *J Kyota Prefect Med Univ* 1962; 71:659.
89. Stayner RM: *Vibration and the Tractor Driver*. CIGR-COISTA Congress, Flerohof, Netherlands, (from Tractor Dept, Natl Inst Agric Eng, Silsoe, Bedford, England), 1974.
90. Stayner RM, Hilton DJ, Moran P: *Protecting the Tractor Driver from Low Frequency Ride Vibration*. Inst Mech Eng No 200/75, 1975, pp 39.
91. Steidel RF: *An Introduction to Mechanical Vibrations*, ed 2, rev. New York, John Wiley & Sons, 1979.
92. Troup JDG: Driver's back pain and its prevention. A review of the postural, vibratory, and muscular factors, together with the problem of transmitted road-shock. *Appl Ergonomics* 1978; 9:207.
93. Umezawa F: The study of comfortable sitting postures, (in Japanese). *J Jap Orthop Assoc* 1971; 45:1015.
94. Vogt HL, Coermann RR, Fust HO: Mechanical impedance of the sitting human under sustained acceleration. *Aerospace Med* 1968; 39:675.
95. Weisman G, Pope MH, Johnson RJ: Cyclic loading in knee ligament injuries. 1980; *Am J Sports Med* 8:24.
96. Wilder DG, Frymoyer JW, Pope MH: The effect of vibration on the spine of the seated individual. *Automedica* (in press).
97. Wilder DG, Pope MH, Frymoyer JW: Cyclic loading of the intervertebral motion segment, in Hansen EW (ed): *Proc Northeast Bioeng Conf*, Dartmouth, Hanover, NH, 1982.
98. Wilder DG, Woodworth BB, Frymoyer JW, Pope MH: Energy absorption in the human spine, in Igor Paul (ed): *Proceedings Eighth Northeast Bioengineering Conference*, MIT, Cambridge, Mass, March, 1980, pp 442–445.
99. Yamaguchi Y, Umezawa F, Ishinada Y: Sitting posture: An electromyographic study on healthy and notalgic people. *J Jap Orthop Assoc* 1972; 46:277.

3

Clinical Classification

John W. Frymoyer, M.D.
Gunnar B.J. Andersson, M.D., Ph.D.

INTRODUCTION

Numerous classification systems have been developed to categorize low back complaints. The historic absence of uniform systems has been a major barrier to research, treatment, and the development of rational schemes for impairment rating. Two main approaches are currently used, the first based on symptoms, the second based on pathoanatomic causation.

SYMPTOM DIAGNOSIS

The most comprehensive system based on symptoms is that developed by the Quebec Task Force.[73] This task force represented all of the various medical disciplines involved in occupational health as well as lawyers and other nonmedical professionals. Table 3.1 outlines their system, which is applicable to all anatomic regions of the human spine.

Category 1 represents the majority of patients with a low back disorder. Typically, it is aggravated by mechanical factors such as activity, worsens over the day, and is relieved by rest.[7,15,75] Such back pain often develops in the industrial setting, following acute or chronic repetitive loading events. Acute low back pain may also develop from minor postural changes, such as bending or twisting from simple coughing or, as in the majority of cases, from an unknown event. Examination typically reveals loss of lumbar lordosis, varying degrees of back muscle tightness and spasm, and restriction of spinal motion. Neurologic signs and symptoms are absent. Nonspecific and commonly used diagnoses for this patient group include low back strain or sprain, implying a muscular or ligamentous injury. This etiology may or may not be correct and is almost never verifiable.

Category 2 is consistent with pain distributions induced by mechanical stimuli or injection of noxious substances such as hypertonic saline into muscle, facet joints, ligaments, and bone. The classic experiments of Lewis and Kellgren,[54] Kellgren,[42] and others[35,55] mapped these pain distributions, which are frequently referred to as sclerotome pain. All of the structures that produce this type of pain derive their neurologic innervation from the posterior primary rami.

Category 3, which radiates distally into the leg(s), may arise from three sources: structures innervated by the posterior primary rami[59]; increased tension, compression, or inflammation of an anterior primary rami, termed monoradiculopathy; or as the result of more diffuse changes in the space available for the cauda equina and/or nerve roots, resulting in the symptom of neurologic claudication or a mono- or polyradiculopathy. The

TABLE 3.1
Two Important Means for the Classification of Low Back Disorders: Duration of Symptoms and Working Status*

Classification	Symptoms	Duration of symptoms from onset	Working status at time of evaluation
1	Pain without radiation		
2	Pain + radiation to extremity, proximally	a (<7 days)	W (working)
3	Pain + radiation to extremity, distally†	b (7 days–7 weeks)	I (idle)
4	Pain + radiation to upper/lower limb neurologic signs	c (>7 weeks)	
5	Presumptive compression of a spinal nerve root on a simple roentgenogram (ie, spinal instability or fracture)		
6	Compression of a spinal nerve root confirmed by Specific imaging techniques (ie, computerized axial tomography, myelography, or magnetic resonance imaging) Other diagnostic techniques (eg, electromyography, venography)		
7	Spinal stenosis		
8	Postsurgical status, 1–6 months after intervention		
9	Postsurgical status, >6 months after intervention 9.1 Asymptomatic 9.2 Symptomatic		
10	Chronic pain syndrome		W (working)
11	Other diagnoses		I (idle)

*From Spitzer WO, LeBlanc FE, Dupuis M, et al: Scientific approach to the assessment and management of activity-related spinal disorders: A monograph for clinicians. Report of the Quebec Task Force on Spinal Disorders *Spine* 1987;12 (suppl. 7) S1–S59. Used by permission.

monoradiculopathies are typically called sciatica when the nerves involved are the L5 or S1 roots or, less commonly, femoral radiculopathy when the involved nerve roots are L2, L3, or L4. Neurologic claudication has the same distribution of pain within the limb but has the specific attribute of being increased by walking and relieved by cessation of walking. The patient with neurologic claudication typically must sit down for pain relief, whereas the patient with vascular claudication can obtain relief in the standing position. Category 3 does not present with specific neurologic signs.

Category 4 increases the specificity of the diagnosis for a mono- or polyradioculopathy by incorporating neurologic signs, such as a positive nerve root tension sign or loss (or reduction) of reflex, sensation, or motor power. In the instance of a monoradiculopathy, the presence of these signs accurately identifies a lumbar disc herniation in 70% of patients.[34] When nerve root tension signs, such as a contralaterally positive straight leg raising test, are present the probability of lumbar disc herniation approaches 98%.[67]

Category 5 accounts for other causes of nerve root and cauda equina compression that can be observed on routine, plane radiographic evaluation. Included in this category are obvious spinal fractures that compromise the bony spinal canal, as well as the more subtle problem of segmental instability, which is discussed later in this chapter.

Category 6 introduces the utilization of imaging techniques which are both sensitive and specific to the causation of mono- and polyradiculopathies. These techniques include myelography, computerized tomography (CT) scans, and magnetic resonance imaging (MRI) as well as nonimaging techniques such as electromyography.

Category 7 specifically refers to the most common cause of polyradiculopathy and claudication: spinal stenosis, which is revealed by these same imaging techniques.

Categories 8 and 9 refer to the small subset of patients who have undergone one or another surgical intervention for spinal disorders, most commonly a disc operation. The separation of the postoperative period into 1 to 6 months and greater than 6 months is important because most patients with simple disc operations should have recovered and returned to work within 6 months of the intervention. Similarly, the separation of Category 9 into asymptomatic and symptomatic has highly significant implications for causation and prognosis for long-term recovery, a topic that is covered in Chapter 10.

Category 10, chronic pain syndrome, has been recognized as a major problem not only in low back disorders but in a variety of other chronic pain syndromes such as neck pain, chronic headache, and causalgia. For the majority (80%) of patients with chronic low back pain, an anatomic cause is not identified.[28,79] For some patients, however, there is an anatomic causation, such as arachnoiditis (diffuse scarring of the cauda equina) or focal nerve root fibrosis. One school believes that patients with no demonstrable anatomic causation have a behavioral problem, possibly a variant of depression, and these patients therefore are often labeled as suffering from "psychologic" low back pain or "compensation neurosis" if the onset of symptoms is associated with a potentially compensable "injury" in the workplace.[20,71,83] The psychologic test most commonly used to reveal underlying psychopathology is the Minnesota Multiphasic Personality Inventory (MMPI), a 389-item questionnaire. Patients with chronic disabling low back pain (LBP) often show abnormal findings in one or more scales of the MMPI, typically hysteria hypochondriasis, somatization, and depression. A typical example of these findings is shown in Figure 3.1. These individuals may also be preoccupied with health and may be angry at the health professionals who care for them.[28,75] It is unclear whether the psychologic abnormalities are the cause or the result of continued low back symptoms. Prospective studies of low back pain in industry[9] as well as prospective clinical studies attempting to identify patients who will become disabled by low back pain[30] suggest that many of the psychologic attributes associated with the disability actually precede the condition. This topic and alternative tests used to identify such individuals are presented in Chapter 10.

Another school of thought, one with a neurophysiologic emphasis, suggests chronic pain may have a neuroanatomic causation.[82] This issue is discussed in Chapter 4.

Category 11 contains all other known causes of low back pain. Although it is a very extensive list, it accounts for only a minority of patients with low back disorders, and these conditions are rarely seen in an occupational setting.

Reference to Table 3.1 also demonstrates two other important means for the classification of low back disorders: duration of symptoms and working status.

Based on duration, symptoms are usually divided into acute, subacute, and chronic. The Quebec Task Force suggests acute symptoms last 7 days or less; subacute, 7 days to 7 weeks; and chronic, more than 7 weeks. Others[26,61] use somewhat different time sequences: acute, less than 1 month; subacute, 1 to 3 months; and chronic, greater than 3

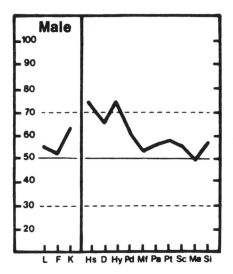

FIG 3.1.
A typical Minnesota Multiphasic Personality Inventory profile is shown for a patient who has anxiety, hypochondriasis, and depression. These scales are listed as the Hy, Hs, and D scales, respectively, and they create the inverted V, which is said to be characteristic of the population at risk for poor outcomes from surgical and nonsurgical treatments.

months. Figure 3.2 demonstrates the normal recovery curve after an acute episode of low back pain and makes the important point that all but 5 to 10% of patients recover within 3 months. Failure to recover over that period has significant implications for the increased probability of a chronic pain syndrome: less than 20% of patients who fall into the chronic pain syndrome group are given a definitive diagnosis,[65] particularly when the complaint is low back pain only. We believe, however, that before a patient is labeled as suffering from chronic pain syndrome, one well-planned and comprehensive diagnostic evaluation should be performed. This is necessary because a few specific etiological entities hide behind the label "chronic low back pain." For example, Wiesel[88] studied 109 patients derived from an initial population of 5,362 individuals who developed chronic symptoms. Fourteen of the patients were found to have a significant pathoanatomic cause for their continued complaints, including spinal tumors and treatable spondyloarthropathies.

Another subset of patients are those who have recurrent pain complaints. It is estimated that 60% of patients who have an acute low back episode and recover will have a recurrence, usually within the first 2 years.[7,76,77] Patients with sciatica have an increased risk of recurrence. If the recurrent complaints are nondisabling or minimally disabling, the prognosis is generally favorable. When their symptoms are recurrent and significantly disabling, however, the patients are likely to have many of the attributes of chronic pain syndrome.[26]

Similarly, the second subclassification by work status has major implications for prognosis. Beals and Hickman[4,5] studied the natural history of individuals disabled by low back pain. Figure 3.3, derived from their published data, shows the rapidly diminishing likelihood that the individual will ever return to work. Thus, at 1 year of continued disability only 20% of the individuals ever return to work, whereas at 2 years the probability is

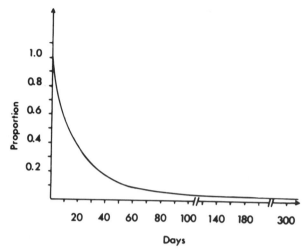

FIG 3.2.
The normal recovery curve following an acute low back episode is displayed. Notice the very rapid improvement that occurs in the majority but the continuing symptoms, which are classified as chronic. (From Andersson GBJ, Svensson H-O: The intensity of work recovery in low back pain. *Spine* 1983;8:880. Used by permission.)

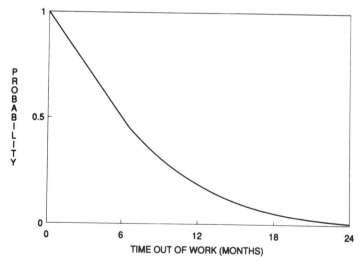

FIG 3.3.
The natural history of disabling low back pain is demonstrated as measured by the capacity for returning to work in the future. Notice the very rapid decline in that potential, so that by two years there is virtually no chance that the person will ever return to work without a specific therapeutic intervention.

virtually zero. As shown in Chapter 10, newer, aggressive rehabilitation programs may significantly alter this ominous prognosis, but duration is still a major prognostic factor.

To understand the value and application of the Quebec classification let us consider two patient examples. The first is a 35-year-old man with low back and left leg pain radiating down the lateral aspect of the leg and foot, accompanied by numbness and the physical finding of a positive straight leg raising test, reproductive of his pain complaint at 30 degrees. He is not working. At this point his classification is 4,b,I (Table 3.1). On this information alone, it is possible to predict with 75% accuracy that he has a lumbar disk herniation, most likely at L5–S1. A lumbar CT scan is performed because he has failed to respond to bedrest and medication. This confirms the clinical impression of L5–S1 disc herniation, and the patient is now reclassified as 5,b,I. Assuming no major psychologic dysfunction, there is an 85 to 90% rate of recovery following a simple disc operation. Three months after the surgery he has returned to work and is reclassified as category 8,W. This case illustrates how the Quebec classification may be used dynamically and accurately to represent the altering condition of the patient.

For comparison, let us consider a 48-year-old man who has the following history: low back pain occurred at work after he picked up a 25-pound carton. Despite bedrest, medication, and physical therapy, he continues to complain of disabling low back pain 3 months later and is unable to work. Physical examination reveals only restricted spinal motion; lumbar MRI is normal. At this point he is categorized as 1,c,I, and it can be predicted he will soon become category 10 unless vigorous rehabilitation is undertaken. Further medical, laboratory, and imaging analyses are unlikely to reveal a pathoanatomic causation for his symptoms.

LOW BACK PAIN OF KNOWN ETIOLOGY

The other main classification method is by etiology, including degenerative, congenital, inflammatory, neoplastic, and metabolic causations. As already noted, this system is presently applicable only to some 20% of patients with low back pain, but it has major significance for treatment and prognosis of those patients. This system also complements a symptom diagnosis system such as the Quebec classification. The majority of patients with certain pathoanatomic causes for pain fall into Quebec categories 4, 5, 6, and 7. A small but important minority are found in category 11.

DEGENERATIVE SPINAL DISORDERS

Degenerative spinal disorders are the most common pathoanatomic causes of low back pain, mono- and polyradiculopathies, and claudication. While this is true, it is important not to assume that degeneration is synonomous with back pain and is, indeed, the cause in an individual patient. Degeneration is often present in people without low back pain. Spinal degeneration encompasses clinically insignificant age-related radiographic changes observed in the spine, well-delineated diagnostic categories such as herniated intervertebral disc, some types of spinal stenosis, as well as less certain diagnoses such as the facet and disc disruption syndromes and segmental instability.

Age-Related Spinal Degeneration

It is critical to place normal, age-related spinal degeneration in perspective as a background against which to consider clinically significant degenerative syndromes. The following information is important.

1. All human spines degenerate with time.[18,22,43,57,70,81] Most autopsy specimens show the onset of gross and microscopic evidence of intervertebral disc degeneration by the third decade of life. These pathologic changes accompany alterations in the disc's chemical composition, such as decreased water content, increased collagen, and decreased mucopolysaccharides.[18] A recent study has suggested that the onset of changes occurs earlier in the male and affects the L3–L4 and L4–L5 disc equally.[57] Other studies suggest the changes occur more commonly in L4–L5 and L5–S1.

2. Radiographic changes, such as disc space narrowing and spinal osteophytes, lag behind the histologic and chemical events. These degenerative changes (Fig. 3.4) are equally prevalent in patients with and without low back pain.[28,43] It is also important to recognize that the presence of a narrowed intervertebral disc does not correlate with the risk for or presence of a disc herniation. In fact, disc space narrowing, in one study, was a negative predictor for lumbar disk herniation at that level.[34]

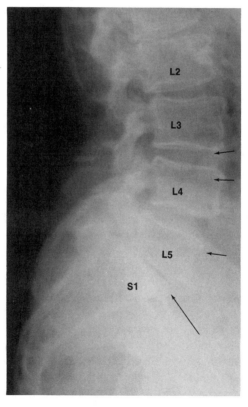

FIG 3.4.
A lateral spinal radiograph is demonstrated. Note the presence of narrowing of the L5–S1 (*large arrow*) disc space and the presence of bony spurs projecting from the anterior aspects of the vertebral bodies (*small arrows*). This x-ray was taken for another reason in an individual who has no history of back pain.

The issue of disc herniation is of even greater importance in the interpretation of sensitive imaging studies such as CT and magnetic resonance imaging. The presence of "diffuse" disc bulging is equally common in those with and without a history of back pain.[86,87] Of greater interest is that 20 to 30% of asymptomatic patients have evidence of disc herniation on structural (imaging) exams. In clinical practice, therefore, the patient's symptoms and signs must be carefully correlated with an imaging study. A positive image without fitting clinical symptoms and signs is not enough to make a clinical diagnosis. It is also important not to confuse normal, age-related radiographic changes with the diagnosis of spinal degeneration, which is often viewed by the lay public as a progressive and unrelenting problem. The overuse of degeneration as a diagnosis may also lead to self-imposed and unnecessary restrictions in physical activity.

Herniated Nucleus Pulposus

The classic description of herniated nucleus pulposus (HNP) (Fig. 3.5), commonly and erroneously called a slipped disc, was first published by Mixter and Barr.[58] The syndrome is characterized by sciatica, usually accompanied or preceded by LBP. Physical examination reveals the presence of one or more objective neurologic changes such as reflex asymmetry, sensory change in the distribution of a nerve root, or muscle weakness. The clinical diagnosis requires the presence of a positive nerve root tension test, of which the straight leg raising test is most commonly used (see Chapter 8 for a complete description of these tests). A positive straight leg raising test should reproduce the sciatic pain below the knee. The degree of elevation necessary to produce sciatic symptoms approximates the degree of nerve root tension. Between 0.3 and 1% of patients who have lumbar disc herniations also have a massive extrusion of nuclear material sufficient to interfere with nerve control of bladder and bowel function (Fig. 3.6).[51,72] Although uncommon, the cauda equina syndrome is a true surgical emergency since failure to decompress the lesion may result in permanent loss of bladder and bowel control.

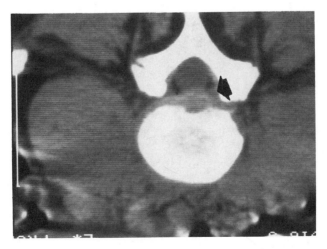

FIG 3.5.
This figure demonstrates a typical herniated nucleus pulposus as seen on a lumbar CT scan (computerized tomogram). The arrow points to the disc bulge (1), which is encroaching on the nerve root on the left side. This patient presented with typical symptoms of an L5–S1 disc with S1 radioculopathy and, following conservative management, was successfully treated by surgical removal of the disc.

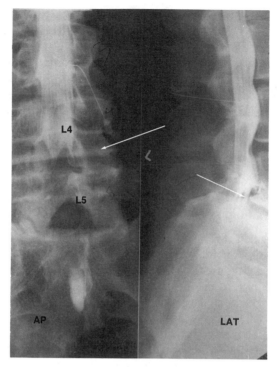

FIG 3.6.
A myelogram showing complete blockage of the dye (*arrow*) at the level of L4–L5 on the anteroposterior and lateral radiographs. This patient presented with acute symptoms of low back pain accompanied by bilateral lower extremity paralysis, numbness, and loss of sacral sensation, with incontinence of bladder (not of bowel). He was surgically decompressed as an emergency and has regained all function.

It is important to realize that the majority of patients who meet the clinical criteria of HNP recover from acute symptoms and have minimal residual functional or work capacity impairment. Patients who have had a known disc herniation, however, are more likely to have a recurrent herniation.

Spinal Stenosis

Spinal stenosis is defined as a narrowing of the spinal canal and/or nerve root foraminae. Narrowing of the cross-sectional dimensions of the lumbar spinal canal may occur at one or many levels of the lumbar spine (Fig. 3.7).[2,63,80] When multiple levels are involved, typical symptoms include recurrent or continued LBP aggravated by specific body postures and/or physical exertion. As stenosis increases, extension of the spine may become more painful and relief may be sought in flexion. Neurogenic claudication is a common symptom, but reflex, motor, and sensory changes are often confusing because of the involvement of multiple nerve roots, and such changes may be completely absent. Unlike lumbar disc herniations, positive nerve root tension signs, such as the straight leg raising test, are often absent. Diffuse narrowing of the spinal canal may have many causes,[2] but most commonly the stenosis results from degeneration with posterior osteophytes projecting into the spinal canal, hypertrophy of the articular facets, and buckling of the ligamentum flavum (Fig. 3.8).

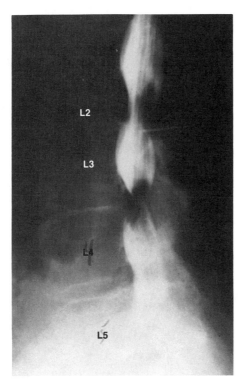

FIG 3.7.
A lateral radiograph of a myelogram taken in a patient who has claudication on walking and a long history of low back pain. Note that the dye column is extremely narrowed at L2–L3, L3–L4.

A second group of stenotic lesions are associated with more focal degenerative disease. Degenerative spondylolisthesis (Fig. 3.9) is the most common of these and typically affects females during the fifth and sixth decades of life. It occurs most commonly at the L4–L5 level and may be associated with diabetes.[66] Radiographic surveys have shown that as many as 9.1% of females and 5.8% of males have this deformity, although many have no symptoms.[78] Some authorities believe the cause of degenerative spondylolisthesis is a rotational deformity[19,48] rather than a straightforward displacement.

In other patients disc space collapse leads to backward displacement (retrospondylolisthesis) (Fig. 3.10), which may lead to compromise of the nerve root canals or central spinal stenosis. Another group has severe disc space collapse but neither forward nor backward displacement. The accompanying degenerative changes may produce focal stenosis. The condition is characterized as isolated disc resorption and is most commonly observed at the L5–S1 level.[13]

A third group of patients are characterized as having predominantly lateral recess (nerve root canal) stenosis. In this situation, the combination of facet hypertrophy and varying degrees of disc bulge reduce the space available at the affected disc level(s) and compromise the nerve root. This may present as a mono- or polyradiculopathy, and the symptom of neurologic claudication is less likely to be present.[46,53] Ken[44] and others[47,53] have emphasized the interrelationships between spinal stenosis and disc herniations. When the spinal canal and lateral nerve root canal are narrowed, a relatively small disc herniation can

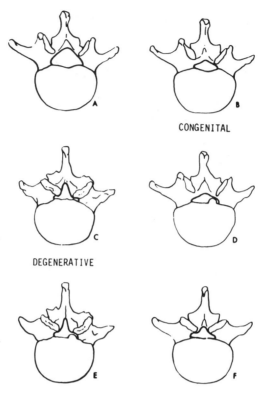

CONGENITAL

DEGENERATIVE

FIG 3.8.
Spinal stenosis is a result of many pathologic processes, which are shown here. (From Arnoldi CC, Brodsky AE, Cauchoix J, et al: Lumbar spinal stenosis and nerve root entrapment syndromes: Definition and classification. *Clin Orthop* 1976;115:4. Used by permission.)

produce clinically significant symptoms, such as sciatica, which would not have occurred if the canal had been of adequate dimensions (Fig. 3.11).

These various local and more generalized stenotic deformities may occur together and in combination.

Two other conditions of minimal importance in the industrial setting are idiopathic vertebrogenic sclerosis and diffuse idiopathic spinal hyperostosis (DISH). The former is characterized by severe low back pain, severe disc space narrowing, and diffuse sclerosis of the vertebral body adjacent to the disc. It usually affects the L4 vertebral body, and women are affected four to five times more often than men.[85] In contrast, DISH affects multiple vertebrae, is most common in men, and is characterized radiographically by diffuse flowing osteophytes, which bridge over a minimum of three vertebral levels. Patients commonly have general metabolic conditions such as diabetes or gout.

Degenerative Conditions of Less Certain Significance

Three diagnoses are commonly considered causes of low back pain, with or without radiculopathies: segmental instability, facet syndrome, and disc disruption syndrome.

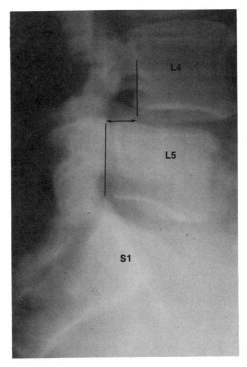

FIG 3.9.
This 60-year-old female has a long history of low back pain and now presents with increased low back pain as well as claudication on walking. The radiographs show the fourth lumbar vertebra anteriorly displaced relative to the fifth lumbar vertebra, the classic location for a degenerative spondylolisthesis.

Segmental Instability

Many patients with low back pain have recurring episodes of increasing severity, sometimes transiently associated with nerve root irritation and usually triggered by increasing but minor mechanical overloads.[26,48] Morgan and King[60] concluded that as many as 25% of all patients with low back pain have this condition, but others have found it to be far less prevalent, affecting fewer than 1% of patients.[74] Radiographic criteria associated with this diagnosis have included the presence of disc space narrowing, spinal osteophytes projecting away from the disc space, and the so-called traction spur.[56] The most important criterion has been abnormal shifts in the alignment of vertebrae observed on lateral spinal radiographs taken in flexion and extension (Fig. 3.12).[17,50] Others[23] have observed similar shifts when the spine is sequentially overloaded by a backpack and then placed in traction. Attempts to classify segmental instability associated with spinal degeneration have not been uniformly adopted.[29] Despite the absence of certain clinical and radiographic criteria, segmental instability remains one of the most common indications of lumbar spinal fusion.

Facet Syndrome

Sixty years ago it was proposed that many causes of low back pain originated from the facet joints. The discovery of the clinical syndrome of lumbar disc herniation focused attention on the disc as the dominant cause of most back symptoms. Mooney and Robertson[59] repopularized this diagnosis. They described a patient group characterized by

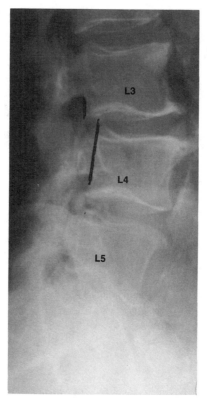

FIG 3.10.
This patient had pain on extension with intermittent nerve root symptoms affecting the L3–L4 level. The radiographs show that the vertebral body of L3 is shifted posteriorly on that of L4, creating a so-called retrospondylolisthesis, which is part of a degenerative process. Note the different direction of slippage in this radiograph compared to that shown in Figure 3.9.

pain in spinal extension or rotation, with referral of pain to the upper buttocks or sometimes even into the legs. Spinal radiographs were normal. Injection of hypertonic saline into the facet joints reproduced the symptoms and was sometimes associated with transient loss of a reflex. Relief of pain followed injection of the facet with local anesthetic. In other patients, radiographic evidence of degeneration of the facets was present; this group was given the diagnosis of facet arthritis. Treatment with anti-inflammatory medication and, in some instances, local cortisone injection into the affected joint, was associated with symptom relief. Since this original description, there have been a number of attempts to characterize the clinical syndrome precisely and evolve rational therapy. A comprehensive analysis of over 400 patients led to the conclusion that facet syndrome cannot be classified with any certainty.[41] There is little doubt, however, that frank degeneration of the facets may be associated with three clinically important conditions: (1) Degeneration of the facets is part of the overall process of spinal degeneration and significantly contributes to pain in patients with multilevel spinal osteoarthritis; (2) Degeneration of the facets with associated development of osteophytes projecting into the lateral recess and central spinal canal is a significant part of degenerative spinal stenosis; (3) Degeneration of the facets is sometimes associated with a ventrally projecting synovial cyst, which impinges on the nerve root and, thus, is part of the differential diagnosis of sciatica.[52,62]

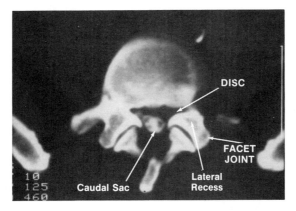

FIG 3.11.
When narrowing of the spinal canal and the lateral recesses is present, a smaller disc herniation often produces symptoms of great severity. This particular patient had left S1 nerve root pain. Notice the relatively small disc and the facet overgrowth that has occurred at the L5–S1 level (arrows).

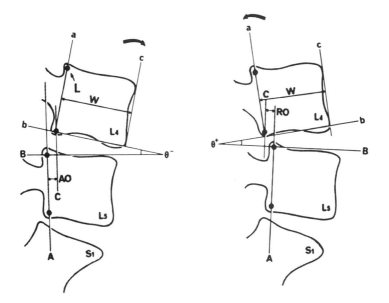

FIG 3.12.
To determine the amount of horizontal displacement on the flexion-extension views, first find and mark on each vertebra of the motion segment the remnants of Luschka's joints (*L*). Join the landmarks of the upper vertebra by a line (line *a*), and repeat the procedure for the lower vertebra (line *A*). From the lower landmark of the upper vertebra a line drawn parallel to lines A and C (*AO* for anterior olisthesis and *RO* for retrolisthesis) is the amount of horizontal displacement of the vertebra above, not taking magnification into account. To obviate inaccuracies due to the x-ray magnification factor, the horizontal displacement is measured in percentage of displacement. Draw a line (line *c*) from the anterior border of the upper end plate on the proximal vertebra. Measure the horizontal midbody width (*W*) of the upper body between lines *a* and *c*. The percentage of horizontal displacement is *HD%* = (*AO* or *RO/W*) × 100. To measure angular displacement, draw line *b* perpendicular to line *a* from the inferior landmark of the vertebra below. The angle between the two lines is the angular displacement in degrees. (From Dupuis PR, Yong-Hing K, Cassidy JD, et al: Radiologic diagnosis of degenerative lumbar spinal instability. *Spine* 1985;10:262. Used by permission.)

Disc Disruption Syndrome

Crock[14] described the disc disruption syndrome as characterized by severe, unrelenting, mechanical low back pain following a compression injury (typically the patient has fallen in a sitting position). In his patient group he also noticed systemic symptoms such as weight loss. Spinal radiographs were usually normal, and the diagnosis depended on discography (for issues relating to discography and its clinical significance, see Chapter 8). Injection of radiopaque contrast media into the disc most faithfully reproduced the patient's pain and also demonstrated disruption of the normal disc architecture (Fig. 3.13**a** and **b**). Treatment of this condition is by anterior interbody lumbar fusion. Disc disruption syndrome is currently a source of controversy and uncertainty, but clearly it does not have a major role in occupational low back disorders.

Congenital Abnormalities

In the normal embryologic development of the spine, defects in the formation of spinal structures may occur. The majority of these abnormalities have minimal significance but are often erroneously believed to cause low back pain. Most of the common congenital abnormalities occur equally in the LBP- and non-LBP-affected population (Table 3.2).

Spina Bifida Occulta.—As the neural arch forms, incomplete closure may occur, accompanied by partial or complete absence of the spinous process. In a small subgroup (1 in 100,000) the bony defect is accompanied by a herniation of the neural elements through the defect. This condition is termed meningomyelocele and is associated with a variety of neurologic defects usually apparent at birth.

Segmentation Abnormalities.—Wide variations exist in the number and shape of lumbar vertebrae. In lumbarization, the first sacral segment has the appearance of a lumbar vertebra, and so there are six rather than five lumbar segments. In sacralization, the fifth lumbar vertebra may be incorporated into the sacrum, resulting in only four mobile lumbar vertebrae. Sometimes the incorporation occurs only on one side (hemisacralization), and in a small patient group this may be associated with the development of a false joint between the ilium and the elongated transverse process of the fifth lumbar vertebra (Fig. 3.14). In general, segmentation abnormalities are not associated with an increased risk of back pain, although some patients with hemisacralization may have pain arising from the false joint. In patients with sciatica and segmentation abnormalities, precise localization of the affected level may be more difficult.

Conjoined Nerve Roots.—Anatomic variants may also occur in neural structures. For example, nerve roots may be conjoined. This condition has minimal significance, except as a possible cause of sciatica, and may pose additional technical problems in surgical interventions. It may also confuse readers of structural examinations, particularly myelograms.

Spondylolysis and Spondylolisthesis

We include spondylolysis and spondylolisthesis under congenital abnormalities, although many of these deformities do not have a congenital basis. Spondylolisthesis may be broadly defined as forward displacement of one vertebra relative to the next lower lumbar segment. This condition can arise from numerous causes (Table 3.3).[91] The most common form is isthmic spondylolisthesis, which involves an acquired or congenital defect in the

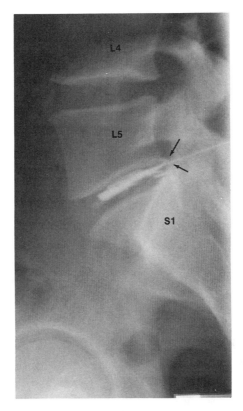

FIG 3.13a.
Discography remains a controversial study. In this patient with chronic low back pain, injection of the disc totally reproduced not only his back pain but his leg symptoms, which up to that point had not been defined by either CT scan or MRI. This figure shows the lateral discogram, which has complete disruption of the architecture of the disc with some extravasation of dye (*arrows*) posteriorly.

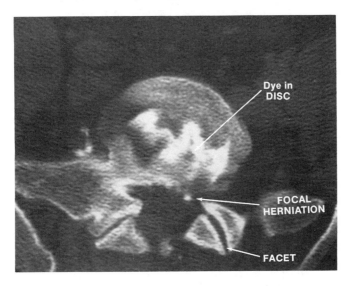

FIG 3.13b.
Demonstrates the disruption of the architecture. Note the dye between the various lamellae of the annulus, as well as the filling of a focal protrusion on the left side.

TABLE 3.2

Prevalence of Congenital Abnormalities in Five Case Studies*

Anomaly	Case 1	Case 2	Case 3	Case 4	Case 5
No anomaly	55.7%	88.0%	72.9%	—	—
Transitional vertebrae	23.4%	6.68%	9.7%	14.3%	15.7%
Narrowed L-S disc	7.6%	—	57.2%	12.8%	71.25%
Lamina defects	6.3%	4.14%	8.1%	—	3.25%
Spina bifida	8.8%	1.20%	10.8%	—	—
Facet asymmetry	13.9%	—	21.9%	—	2.0%

*From Willis, TA: Anatomical variations and roentgenographic appearance of low back pain in relation to sciatic pain. *J Bone Joint Surg* 1941;23:410–416. Used by permission.

neural arch at the pars interarticularis. This is called spondylolysis and may be unilateral or bilateral (Fig. 3.15). The presence of the defect varies widely in the population, ranging from 1 to 10%.[45] The most common site is forward slippage of L5 on S1, and the lesion, unlike degenerative spondylolisthesis, is far more common in males than in females. Significantly, continuation of forward slippage ceases with adulthood and, thus, patients

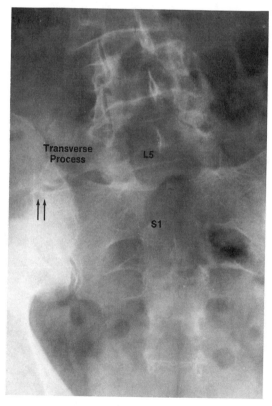

FIG 3.14.

This patient has a known scoliosis and presents with very focal pain, referable, it was thought, to a hemisacralization, secondary to an elongated transverse process articulating with the ilium (*arrow*). Injection of this false joint totally relieved the patient's symptoms. Usually this is a coincidental finding of no significance.

TABLE 3.3
Causes of Spondylolisthesis

Type I:	Dysplastic spondylolisthesis
Type II:	Isthmic spondylolisthesis
Type III:	Degenerative spondylolisthesis
Type IV:	Traumatic spondylolisthesis
Type V:	Pathologic spondylolisthesis

with the common L5–S1 lesion do not have an unstable spine.[21] A far more uncommon site is at L4–L5. This patient subgroup does appear to have continued slippage after adulthood and often may require spinal fusion.[32]

Rather than a frank congenital abnormality, the development of spondylolysis and subsequent isthmic spondylolisthesis is thought to be caused by a fatigue failure of the neural arch. In some patients, particularly athletic teenagers, onset of low back pain is associated with increased radioisotope uptake within the neural arch, and a bony defect is not observed on routine spinal radiographs. In these patients, bracing may resolve the symptoms, and the actual defect may never develop, that is, the fracture heals. Because spondylolysis is more common in athletes such as football linemen and female gymnasts, repetitive flexion-extension forces have been thought to be the fatiguing load. This theory is furthered by the laboratory observation that bony defects may be produced by repetitive cyclic loading of vertebral specimens.[39,91] There is no evidence, however, of an occupational causation of spondylolysis or spondylolisthesis, except in the rare instance of a major traumatic event that produces the actual acute fracture.

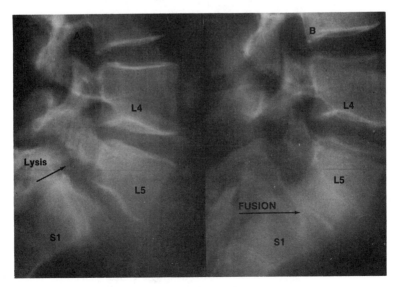

FIG 3.15.
A typical isthmic spondylolisthesis, in which the fifth lumbar vertebra has slipped forward on the first sacral vertebra. Dislocation is far more common than isthmic spondylolisthesis, whereas degenerative spondylolisthesis usually affects the L4 or L5 lumbar level. Moreover, the former condition is more common in males than in females. This patient required an interbody fusion.

The importance of these conditions for industry are minimal. Spondylolysis is equally common in populations with and without back pain. Workers with spondylolisthesis, however, are somewhat more susceptible to low back pain. Whether or not this susceptibility makes it worthwhile to perform preemployment screening is debatable (see Chapter 13).

Spine Trauma

Acute fractures and fracture dislocations indicate the application of an external load that exceeds the strength of the tissues. The resulting injury is a function of the magnitude and velocity of the applied load and the direction(s) of that load application.[37,84] A variety of classifications that are beyond the scope of this chapter have been devised,[16] but the more frequently seen types are presented here.

The most common fracture—a compression fracture—is the result of a fall in the seated position (Fig. 3.16). Such fractures are usually quantified by the degree of vertebral body collapse that occurs. Because of structural characteristics, the anterior part of the body is usually more compressed than the posterior. If the force magnitude is great, actual bursting of the vertebral body may occur, with bony fragments impinging on the spinal cord or cauda equina and producing varying degrees of neurologic involvement, ranging from partial to complete paralysis. When a twisting force is also applied, disruption of spinal ligaments and

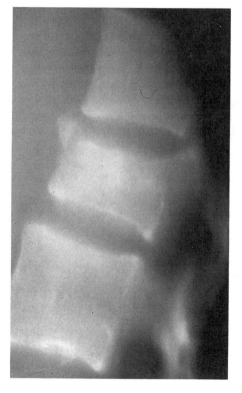

FIG 3.16.
This patient fell, landing in a seated position. A typical compression fracture is demonstrated with loss of anterior vertebral height. He recovered with any exercise and a brace.

facet joints may occur, and partial or complete dislocation results. Such injuries significantly destabilize the spine, frequently require operative stabilization by spinal fusion, and
are commonly associated with neurologic injury (Fig. 3.17). A third general group involves
shearing forces most often seen in vehicular trauma, in which an across-the-lap seat belt
fixes the lower spine.

Another mechanism of spinal injury is a direct blow to the spinous process or transverse
processes that produces fractures of these structures. This mechanism of injury is common
in mining and quarrying operations and, when the forces are great, may be associated with
injuries to kidneys and other abdominal structures. A less common mechanism of injury is
a violent, self-imposed twisting, where the force of the muscle contraction actually pulls
apart the transverse process.

With the exception of very severe (greater than 50% of vertebral body height)
compression fractures, burst fractures, and fracture-dislocations, most of these injuries do
not require operative treatment, heal uneventfully, and are compatible with the resumption
of the worker's normal occupation. Obviously, the neurologic dysfunction associated with
more severe injuries has major implications for the worker's capacity and is incompatible
with any form of heavy manual or standing occupation.

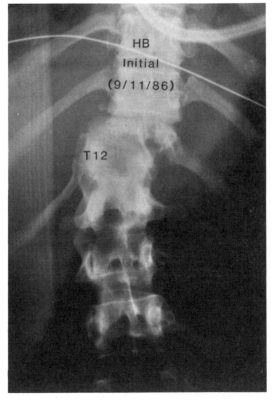

FIG 3.17.
This patient fell from scaffolding at an estimated height of 10 feet, twisting the back. The AP radiograph
demonstrates a complete dislocation of the 11th and 12th thoracic vertebrae. The patient was paraplegic
initially and has never recovered. This is the appearance of a severe fracture dislocation of the spine.

Inflammatory Lesions

Inflammatory lesions include those of infectious and noninfectious etiology.

Spinal Infections

Acute or chronic bacterial infections of the spine are relatively uncommon but may occur spontaneously or after spinal surgery. Acute infections are the result of blood-borne bacteria reaching the vertebrae or, less commonly, the epidural space. Such blood-borne infections are rare in an otherwise healthy individual. Predispositions include diabetes, the use of corticosteroids or other immunosuppressive drugs, and recent genitourinary surgery. Intravenous drug abusers and patients with AIDS are also at risk. Staphylococci are the most commonly cultured bacteria, but a variety of other organisms are becoming more common.

Another group of infections are caused by tuberculosis, which is common in underdeveloped countries but still exists in this country in miners and quarry workers.[36] Postoperative infections occur after disc surgery in 1 in 200 patients and more commonly involve the disc space.[25,64,72]

The history of these patients varies considerably from very acute, severe systemic illness with pain and fever to an insidious onset with minimal, if any, systemic symptoms. An acute onset is most common with blood-borne bacterial infections, whereas insidious onset is typical of tuberculosis. A distinctive characteristic is the complaint of pain at night. Physical examination varies widely, ranging from restricted spinal motion and muscle spasm to excruciating pain. In the small subset of patients with epidural abscesses, neurologic dysfunction may be rapidly progressive and constitute a surgical emergency.[3] In other patients with vertebral osteomyelitis, neurologic dysfunction may be either insidious or acute, but in either case it usually constitutes an indication for surgical intervention.

Early in the course of these infections the spinal radiographs may be normal, and diagnosis depends on radioisotope scans or magnetic resonance imaging. Later, destruction of the vertebral bodies may occur, with collapse and obliteration of the disc space. (Associated laboratory findings are discussed in Chapter 8.) The future of these patients and their ability to return to their occupations depend on the underlying disease that may have predisposed to the condition and the successful eradication of the infection by appropriate antibiotics, with or without associated surgical intervention. Many patients, particularly those with postoperative disc space infections, ultimately resume fairly normal activities.[64]

Inflammatory Causes of Noninfectious Etiology

Common inflammatory lesions affecting the lumbar spine are the spondyloarthropathies, of which ankylosing spondylitis is most prevalent. Ankylosing spondylitis affects 2% of the population.[10,11,38] The patient is typically a male less than 40 years of age. The onset of back pain is insidious, accompanied by early awakening and spinal stiffness, particularly in the morning. These symptoms often improve as the day progresses. Physical examination reveals decreased chest expansion and reduced spinal mobility. Radiographic studies are often normal for years but eventually demonstrate erosive changes at the sacroiliac joints, and in severe cases complete ankylosis (fusion) of the spine may occur (Fig. 3.18). Laboratory studies may be normal, but more commonly there are mild elevations of the erythrocyte sedimentation rate, and in 95% a specific serum antigen, the HLA-27B antigen, is present. A positive serologic test alone is not diagnostic, however, because 5 to 12% of the male population have this finding, most of whom do not have the disease.

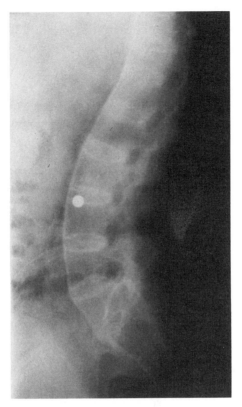

FIG 3.18.
Ankylosing spondylitis initially may show only erosive changes at the sacroiliac joints. When it is advanced, as shown here, complete bony fusion of the entire spine may occur, producing the appearance of the "bamboo spine." Although the patient's entire thoracic and lumbar spine is completely fused, he nevertheless has been able to function quite normally in work and can almost touch his toes because of normal hip mobility.

Other types of spondyloarthropathy include Reiter's syndrome (a disease characterized by genitourinary inflammation [urethritis], eye inflammation [uveitis], and sacroiliitis)[12] and spondylitis associated with inflammatory bowel diseases such as ulcerative colitis[31] or psoriasis (a scaling skin condition).[92]

The majority of these patients are able to carry on normal occupational activities. In the more severely affected individuals, limitation of spinal mobility or involvement of other joints, such as the hips, may preclude all but sedentary occupations.

Another group of patients are presumed to have inflammatory disorders, called fibromyalgia or myofascial pain syndrome. This controversial diagnosis is characterized by its proponents as often associated with minor trauma or sprains. The general presentation is nonspecific, chronic low back pain, sometimes radiating into the lower legs in a sclerotome distribution. The important diagnostic finding is the presence of trigger points, which are localized areas of tissue density within muscle and fascia that are tender.[6,8,68,69] Relief of symptoms by localized anesthesic injections into the trigger point is thought to be diagnostic. Sleep disturbances are common. Almost half of the patients report that they are awakened during the night, and fatigue is often a significant functional problem. Others believe fibromyalgia and myofascial pain are simply variants of idiopathic chronic low back pain and doubt the existence of a specific diagnostic category.[33] In general the treatment of this condition, if it exists, is similar to the overall management of chronic, nonspecific low back pain.

Metabolic Disorders

The vertebrae are affected by numerous metabolic disorders, but the most important is osteoporosis, a condition characterized by loss of total bone mass.[24] The condition most commonly affects women over 50 and is more likely to occur if the individual is of northern European descent, is of small stature, has had an early menopause, and is a smoker. Other causes include malfunction of the thyroid and adrenal glands, long-term use of corticosteroids, and disuse as the result of extended bedrest treatment.[49] Males are far less commonly affected than females. The major consequence of osteoporosis is weakening of the bone, which makes the individual more susceptible to compression fractures. Awareness of this problem in older working women or in males, particularly those treated with long-term corticosteroids, is important, and it may be necessary to reduce the affected individual's lifting and bending requirements.

Neoplasms

Tumors may involve osseous or neural structures that produce pain or neurologic dysfunction. They present a minor problem to the working population and are rare before age 50. The most common tumors are the result of metastatic spread from some other primary site, usually breast cancer in the female; prostatic cancer in the male; or lung, kidney, or thyroid cancer in both sexes. Multiple myeloma is the most common primary malignant bone tumor, but a variety of other, rarer primary bone or neural tumors may cause low back pain or sciatica. Bony malignant tumors often present with the insidious onset of pain, although acute pain may occur if structural weakening causes a compression fracture. The characteristic pain complaint is night pain that awakens the patient. The spinal radiograph is often diagnostic, but early in the development of a tumor bone scan, CT scan, or MRI may be required for diagnosis. The effect of a spinal tumor on the patient's occupation is highly variable and largely a function not only of the local tumor involvement but also of the overall course of the disease in patients with metastatic malignancies. Some tumors are responsive to hormonal manipulation (breast, prostate), radiation therapy, or surgical excision and spinal stabilization and may be compatible with long-term employability. The majority of patients with tumors, however, need minimal requirements for manual labor.

PAIN AS A KEY TO DIAGNOSIS

In this chapter we have stressed a variety of pain presentations. The majority of patients have mechanical low back pain characterized by accentuation by activity and relief by rest. There are, however, two distinctive patterns of pain that should alert the examiner to the possibility of a more serious spinal disorder. Night pain, particularly when it is unrelenting, is suggestive of an expanding lesion affecting bone, and spinal tumors or infections should be suspected. Morning pain, particularly that which awakens the patient, accompanied by stiffness that improves, highly suggests spondyloarthropathy. Clearly, the pattern of pain referral to the extremities as well as the character of the pain helps identify the more common degenerative conditions.

SUMMARY

The lumbar spine is susceptible to a broad variety of pathologic conditions, but the majority of patients do not have a definable pathoanatomic causation for their pain, if strict diagnostic criteria are employed. The Quebec classification overcomes the reliance on classic pathoanatomic classification systems and has the important attribute that not only is the pain pattern characterized, but the duration and effect on work status are incorporated. In the majority of patients, duration of symptoms and work status are more important in defining treatment and employability than is the actual diagnosis. The examiner must keep in mind, however, that there is a small subgroup of patients who have a clear diagnosis for their symptoms, which is more likely when sciatica or claudication accompany the complaint. The patient's pain complaint must be carefully evaluated and may give important clues to the causation. Because radiographic abnormalities are so common in asymptomatic individuals, the most important lesson in clinical diagnosis is to correlate the radiographic studies with the patient's clinical complaint rather than give a radiographic diagnosis of spinal degeneration or disk degeneration, which may result in needless disability.

BIBLIOGRAPHY

1. Andersson GBJ, Svensson H-O: The intensity of work recovery in low back pain. *Spine* 1983; 8:880.
2. Arnoldi CC, Brodsky AE, Cauchoix J, et al: Lumbar spinal stenosis and nerve root entrapment syndromes: Definition and classification. *Clin Orthop* 1976; 115:4.
3. Baker AS, Ojemann RG, Swartz MN, et al: Spinal epidural abscess. *N Engl J Med* 1975; 293:463.
4. Beals RK: Compensation and recovery from injury. *West J Med* 1984; 140:233.
5. Beals RK, Hickman NW: Industrial injuries of the back and extremities. Comprehensive evaluation—an aid in prognosis and management: A study of one hundred and eighty patients. *J Bone Joint Surg* 1972; 54:1593.
6. Bennett RM: Fibrositis: Evolution of an enigma. *J Rheumatol* 1986; 13:676.
7. Bergquist-Ullman M, Larsson U: Acute low back pain in industry. *Acta Orthop Scand [Suppl]* 1977; 170:1.
8. Bernard TN Jr, Kirkaldy-Willis WH: Recognizing specific characteristics of nonspecific low back pain. *Clin Orthop* 1987; 217:266.
9. Bigos SJ, Battié MC: Surveillance of back problems in industry, in Hadler NM (ed): *Clinical Concepts in Regional Musculoskeletal Illness*. Orlando, Fla., Grune & Stratton, 1987, p. 299.
10. Calin A, Porta J, Fries JF, et al: Clinical history as a screening test for ankylosing spondylitis. *JAMA* 1977; 237:2613.
11. Calin AC: Ankylosing spondylitis, in Kelley WN, Harris ED Jr, Ruddy S, et al (eds): *Textbook of Rheumatology*. Philadelphia, Saunders, 1981a.
12. Calin AC: Reiter's syndrome, in Kelley WN, Harris ED, Ruddy S, et al: (eds): *Textbook of Rheumatology*. Philadelphia, Saunders, 1981b.
13. Crock HV: Isolated lumbar disk resorption as a cause of nerve root canal stenosis. *Clin Orthop* 1976; 115:109.
14. Crock HV: Internal disc disruption: A challenge to disc prolapse fifty years on. *Spine* 1986; 11:650.
15. Damkot DK, Lord J, Pope MH, et al: Relationship between work history, work environment, and low back pain in males. *Spine* 1984; 9:395.
16. Denis F: The three-column spine and its significance in the classification of acute thoraco-lumbar spinal injuries. *Spine* 1983; 8:817.

17. Dupuis PR, Yong-Hing K, Cassidy JD, et al: Radiologic diagnosis of degenerative lumbar spinal instability. *Spine* 1985; 10:262.

18. Eyre D, Benya P, Buckwalter J, et al: Intervertebral disc: Basic science perspectives, in Frymoyer JW, Gordon SL (eds): *New Perspectives on Low Back Pain*. Chicago, American Academy of Orthopaedic Surgeons, 1989.

19. Farfan HF: Effects of torsion on the intervertebral joints. *Can J Surg* 1969; 12:336.

20. Fordyce WE: *Behavioral Methods for Chronic Pain and Illness*. St. Louis, CV Mosby, 1976.

21. Fredrickson BE, Baker D, McHolick WJ, et al: The natural history of spondylolysis and spondylolisthesis. *J Bone Joint Surg* 1984; 66:699.

22. Friberg S, Hirsch C: Anatomical and clinical studies on lumbar disc degeneration. *Acta Orthop Scand* 1949; 19:222.

23. Friberg O: Lumbar instability: A dynamic approach by traction-compression radiography. *Spine* 1987; 12:119.

24. Frost HM: The evolution of pathophysiologic knowledge of osteoporoses. *Orthop Clin N Am* 1981; 12:475.

25. Frymoyer JW: The role of spine fusion. Question 3. *Spine* 1981; 6:284.

26. Frymoyer JW: Back pain and sciatica. *N Engl J Med* 1988; 318:291.

27. Frymoyer JW: Epidemiologic aspects of back pain. In Turczyn KM, Drury TS, Ganz A (eds): *Pain Data Available from the National Center for Health Statistics: An Evaluation of Adequacy, Epidemiologic Uses and National Data Needs*, in *Vital and Health Statistics*, series 4. Public Health Service, National Center for Health Statistics, in press.

28. Frymoyer JW, Pope MH, Clements JH, et al: Risk factors in low-back pain. An epidemiological survey. *J Bone Joint Surg* 1983; 65A:213.

29. Frymoyer JW, Selby DK: Segmental instability: Rationale for treatment. *Spine* 1985; 10:280.

30. Frymoyer JW, Cats-Baril W: Predictors of low back pain disability. *Clin Orthop* 1987; 221:89.

31. Good AE: Enteropathic arthritis. In Kelley WN, Harris ED, Ruddy S, et al (eds): *Textbook of Rheumatology*. Philadelphia, Saunders, 1981.

32. Grobler LJ, Wiltse LL, Frymoyer JW: Personal communication, 1989.

33. Hadler NM: A critical reappraisal of the fibrositis concept. *Am J Med* 1986; 81:26.

34. Hakelius A, Hindmarsh J: The significance of neurological signs and myelographic findings in the diagnosis of lumbar root compression. *Acta Orthop Scand* 1972; 43:239.

35. Hirsch C, Ingelmark B-E, Miller M: The anatomical basis for low back pain: Studies on the presence of sensory nerve endings in ligamentous, capsular and intervertebral disc structures in the human lumbar spine. *Acta Orthop Scand* 1963; 33:1.

36. Hoffman GS: Mycobacterial and fungal infections of bones and joints. In Kelley WN, Harris ED, Ruddy S, et al (eds): *Textbook of Rheumatology*. Philadelphia, Saunders, 1981.

37. Holdsworth F: Fractures, dislocations, and fracture-dislocations of the spine. *J Bone Joint Surg* 1970; 52:1534.

38. Hollander JL: Arthritis and allied conditions, in Hollander JL (ed): *A Textbook of Rheumatology*, ed 7. Philadelphia, Lea & Febiger, 1966.

39. Hutton WC, Stott JRR, Cyron BM: Is spondylolysis a fatigue fracture? *Spine* 1977; 2:202.

40. Inglemark BE, Lindstrom J: Asymmetries of the lower extremities and pelvis and their relations to lumbar scoliosis. *Acta Morph Scand* 1963; 5:221.

41. Jackson RP, Jacobs RR, Montesano PX: Facet joint injection in low back pain: A prospective statistical study. *Spine* 1988; 13:966.

42. Kellgren JH: The anatomical source of back pain. *Rheu Rehab* 1977; 16:3.

43. Kellgren JH, Lawrence JS: Osteo-arthritis and disk degeneration in an urban population. *Ann Rheu Diseases* 1958; 17:388.

44. Ken YH, Kirkaldy-Willis WH: The pathophysiology of degenerative disease of the lumbar spine. *Orthop Clin N Am* 1983; 14:491.

45. Kettelkamp DB, Wright DB: Spondylolysis in the Alaskan Eskimo. *J Bone Joint Surg* 1971; 53:563.
46. Kirkaldy-Willis WH: The relationship of structural pathology to the nerve root. *Spine* 1984; 9:49.
47. Kirkaldy-Willis WH, Wedge JH, Yong-Hing K, et al: Pathology and pathogenesis of lumbar spondylosis and stenosis. *Spine* 1978; 3:419.
48. Kirkaldy-Willis WH, Farfan HF: Instability of the lumbar spine. *Clin Orthop* 1982; 165:110.
49. Kleerekoper M, Tolia K, Parfitt AM: Nutritional, endocrine, and demographic aspects of osteoporosis. *Orthop Clin N Am* 1981; 12:547.
50. Knutsson F: The instability associated with disk degeneration in the lumbar spine. *Acta Radiol* 1944; 25:593.
51. Kostuik JP, Harrington I, Alexander D, et al: Cauda equina syndrome and lumbar disc herniation. *J Bone Joint Surg* 1986; 68:386.
52. Kurz LT, Garfin SR, Bjorkengren AG, et al: Intraspinal synovial cysts: Radiologic documentation of their facet communication. *Orthop Trans* 1986; 10:510.
53. Lee CK, Rauschning W: Lateral lumbar spinal canal stenosis: Classification, pathologic anatomy and surgical decompression. *Spine* 1988; 13:313.
54. Lewis T, Kellgren JH: Observations relating to referred pain, visceromotor reflexes and other associated phenomena. *Clin Sci* 1939; 4:47.
55. McCall IW, Park WM, O'Brien JP: Induced pain referral from posterior lumbar elements in normal subjects. *Spine* 1979; 4:441.
56. Macnab I: The traction spur: An indicator of segmental instability. *J Bone Joint Surg* 1971; 53:663.
57. Miller JAA, Schmatz C, Schultz AB: Lumbar disc degeneration: Correlation with age, sex, and spine level in 600 autopsy specimens. *Spine* 1988; 13:173.
58. Mixter WJ, Barr JS: Rupture of the intervertebral disc with involvement of the spinal canal. *N Engl J Med* 1934; 211:210.
59. Mooney V, Robertson J: The facet syndrome. *Clin Orthop* 1976; 115:149.
60. Morgan FP, King T: Primary instability of lumbar vertebrae as a common cause of low back pain. *Brit J Bone Joint Surg* 1957; 39:6.
61. Nachemson AL, Andersson GBJ: Classification of low back pain. *Scand J Work Envir Health* 1982; 8:134.
62. Onofrio BM, Mih AD: Synovial cysts of the spine. *Neurosurg* 1988; 22:642.
63. Paine KWE: Clinical features of lumbar spinal stenosis. *Clin Orthop* 1976; 115:77.
64. Pilgaard S: Discitis (closed space infection) following removal of lumbar intervertebral disc. *J Bone Joint Surg* 1969; 51:713.
65. Pope MH, Wilder DG, Stokes IAF, et al: Biomechanical testing as an aid to decision making in low-back pain patients. *Spine* 1979; 4:135.
66. Rosenberg NJ: Degenerative spondylolisthesis: Predisposing factors. *J Bone Joint Surg* 1975; 57:467.
67. Scham SM, Taylor TKF: Tension signs in lumbar disc prolapse. *Clin Orthop* 1971; 75:195.
68. Simons DG: Fibrositis/fibromyalgia: A form of myofascial trigger points? *Postgrad Med* 1982; 73:81.
69. Simons DG, Travell J: Myofascial origins of low back pain. *Postgrad Med* 1982; 73:81.
70. Sokoloff L: *The Biology of Degenerative Joint Disease.* Chicago, University of Chicago Press, 1969.
71. Southwick SM, White AA: Current concepts review. The use of psychological tests in the evaluation of low-back pain. *J Bone Joint Surg* 1983; 65:560.
72. Spangfort EV: The lumbar disc herniation: A computer aided analysis of 2,504 operations. *Acta Orthop Scand [Suppl]* 1972; 142:1.
73. Spitzer WO, LeBlanc FE, Dupuis M, et al: Scientific approach to the assessment and management of activity-related spinal disorders: A monograph for clinicians. Report of the Quebec Task Force on Spinal Disorders. *Spine* 1987; 12(suppl 7):S1–S59.

74. Stokes IAF, Frymoyer JW: Segmental motion and instability. *Spine* 1987; 12:688.

75. Svensson HO: *Low Back Pain in Relation to Other Diseases and Cardiovascular Risk Factors* (thesis). Goteborg University, Sweden, University of Goteborg, 1981.

76. Troup JDG: Driver's back pain and its prevention: A review of the postural, vibratory and muscular factors, together with the problem of transmitted road-shock. *Appl Ergonom* 1978; 9:207.

77. Troup JDG, Martin JW, Lloyd DCEF: Back pain in industry: A prospective survey. *Spine* 1981; 6:61.

78. Valkenburg HA, Haanen HCM: The epidemiology of low back pain, in White AA, Gordon SL (eds): *American Academy of Orthopaedic Surgeons Symposium on Idiopathic Low Back Pain*. St. Louis, CV Mosby, 1982.

79. Vallfors B: Acute, subacute and chronic low back pain: Clinical symptoms, absenteeism and working environment. *Scand J Rehab Med [Suppl]* 1985; 11:1.

80. Verbiest H: A radicular syndrome from developmental narrowing of the lumbar vertebral canal. *J Bone Joint Surg* 1954; 36:230.

81. Vernon-Roberts B: Pathology of intervertebral discs and apophyseal joints, in Jayson MI (ed): *The Lumbar Spine and Back Pain*. Edinburgh, Churchill Livingstone, 1987.

82. Weinstein J, LaMotte R, Rydevik B: Nerve: Future directions, in Frymoyer JW, Gordon SL (eds): *New Perspectives on Low Back Pain*. Chicago, American Academy of Orthopaedic Surgery, 1989.

83. White AWM: Low back pain in men receiving workmen's compensation: A follow-up study. *Can Med Assoc J* 1969; 101:61.

84. White AA III, Panjabi MM (eds): *Clinical Biomechanics of the Spine*. Philadelphia, Lippincott, 1978.

85. White AA III, McBride ME, Wiltse LL, et al: The management of patients with back pain and idiopathic vertebral sclerosis. *Spine* 1986; 11:607.

86. Wiesel SW: Personal communication, 1989.

87. Wiesel SW, Feffer HL, Rothman RH: Industrial low back pain: A prospective evaluation of a standardized diagnostic and treatment protocol. *Spine* 1984; 9:199.

88. Wiesel SW, Feffer HL, Borenstein DG: Evaluation and outcome of low-back pain of unknown etiology. *Spine* 1988; 13:679.

89. Willis TA: Anatomical variations and roentgenographic appearance of low back pain in relation to sciatic pain. *J Bone Joint Surg* 1941; 23:410–416.

90. Wiltse LL, Widell EH Jr, Jackson DW: Fatigue fracture: The basic lesion in isthmic spondylolisthesis. *J Bone Joint Surg* 1975; 57:11.

91. Wiltse LL, Newman PH, Macnab I: Classification of spondylolysis and spondylolisthesis. *Clin Orthop* 1976; 117:23.

92. Wright V: Psoriatic arthritis, in Kelley WN, Harris ED, Ruddy S, et al (eds): *Textbook of Rheumatology*. Philadelphia, Saunders, 1981.

4

Acute and Chronic Pain

Gordon Waddell, B.Sc., M.D.
John W. Frymoyer, M.D.

INTRODUCTION

"Pain, ache, discomfort—these are the common complaints of those who seek a doctor's help. Pain issues a warning with kindly intent. She calls to action and, pointing the way, brooks no delay. And thus the ancient cycle is served, from pain to cause, to treatment to cure."[53]

In this chapter we consider the various pain syndromes associated with low back disorders, the peripheral mechanisms of pain production (nociception), the neurologic pathways from the periphery to the brain, the cognitive and emotional aspects of pain, and the behavioral consequences of pain. We then look at how this basic information affects clinical assessment and management of low back pain sufferers.

GENERAL CHARACTERISTICS OF PAIN

Pain is only a symptom: it is not a disease and only a fickle diagnosis. Recognizing different pain syndromes is a necessary pragmatic step to clinical management, but often this only gives doctor and patient a convenient label for the problem. It is dangerous to allow such simplistic labels to mask the true clinical complexity of the problem or hinder better understanding of pain. To illustrate this danger we need only look at some of the simplistic surgical answers for low back pain that have been tried and failed.

Since the time of Descartes[11] pain has been regarded as a simple physiologic sensation or warning signal of tissue injury. To this day routine clinical practice often approaches pain in this way. It works well for most acute pain but has been much less successful for most chronic pain. Over the past generation there has been increasing recognition that pain is a much more complex neurophysiologic, psychologic, and clinical phenomenon. It involves stimulation of specialized peripheral nerve endings, termed nociceptors, transmission of electrical stimuli through the peripheral nerves and spinal cord, central processing and integration of the signal in the spinal cord and brain, and psychologic and behavioral outcomes. Pain has been defined by the International Association for the Study of Pain as "an unpleasant sensory and emotional experience associated with actual or potential tissue damage, or described in terms of such damage."[46] There are a number of important corollaries to this definition:

1. Pain is experienced, evaluated, and acted upon at a mental level. It is always subjective. The way that pain is dealt with and expressed varies with each individual's experience, attitudes, and beliefs about pain in general and each pain in particular.

2. All pain is real to the sufferer. It is illogical and unhelpful in clinical practice to make an artificial distinction between organic and nonorganic pain and, moreover, any attempt to do so destroys the doctor-patient relationship. Pragmatically, we physicians should simply accept that the back pain is real to the sufferer and direct our efforts to understanding what physical, psychologic, and social influences may cause it to become chronic or disabling.

3. Doctors think about pain, communicate about pain, and generally treat pain in terms of tissue damage or injury. But even if low back pain originated from tissue damage or dysfunction, it may sometimes continue long after tissue healing should have occurred and long after we are able to detect any objective physical abnormality. By that stage it is impossible to understand or explain the clinical syndrome in purely physical terms, and purely physical treatment is then unlikely to solve the problem.

4. Because pain is ultimately subjective, there is a major problem in communicating pain across the barriers of language between patient and doctor.

5. The pain experience is not only sensory but also motor, in the form of reflex muscle activity, pain behavior, and altered social function.

6. Pain is only one element of an illness and must be considered in its complete clinical context.

Most acute pain may be dealt with successfully by primarily physical treatment, as in the few patients with a clearly identifiable physical pathology for which a satisfactory treatment exists, such as an acute disk prolapse that fails to resolve naturally and requires surgery. As pain becomes chronic, however, and especially when it is associated with failed physical treatment, adopting a more comprehensive biopsychosocial approach to pain becomes necessary. The Glasgow Illness Model[69] includes physical, psychological, and social elements (Fig. 4.1). It is predicated on the assumption that most back pain has a physical origin, which implies peripheral nociception, at least initially. It also includes the recognition that psychological distress may considerably modify the subjective pain experience. Psychological distress may also lead to abnormal illness behavior, which modifies the clinical presentation and may confuse clinical assessment. All of these

A BIOPSYCHOSOCIAL CONCEPT OF ILLNESS

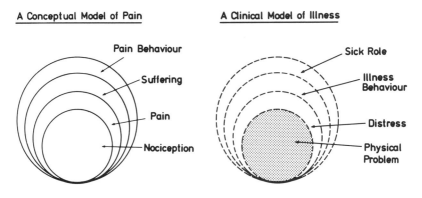

FIG 4.1.
Concepts of pain and illness: Loeser's conceptual model of pain and the Glasgow Illness Model—an operational clinical model of low back disability. (From Loeser JD: Concepts of pain, in Stanton-Hicks M, Boas R (eds): *Chronic Low Back Pain.* New York, Raven Press, 1982. Used by permission.)

physical, emotional, and behavioral phenomena may affect social function, leading to invalidity and the adoption of a "sick role." In a small minority of patients the end result may be magnification of the pain experience out of proportion to the original nociception. Such magnification may persist even when healing would be expected and peripheral nociception may have ceased.

CLINICAL LUMBAR PAIN SYNDROMES

Low back pain is typically located between the lower rib cage and the gluteal folds on the posterior aspect of the thighs. It is frequently associated with pain radiating into the thighs to the level of the knees and sometimes into the lower legs. Historically, this symptom complex was known as lumbago. Contunnius Dominicus[9] first recognized certain patterns of radiating leg pain. Radiating leg pain is often aching and badly localized and does not follow the classic nerve distributions. Contunnius distinguished this nondiscrete radiation of pain from the more localized true nervous sciatica. Currently, nondiscrete leg radiation is termed sclerotome pain. The most precise definition of true sciatica is pain radiating into the lower limb below the level of the knee in the distribution of a single nerve root, associated with other neurosensory changes such as numbness, tingling, or weakness.[17] Figure 4.2 shows the normal relationships of the lumbar spine nerve roots and Figure 4.3 the usual anatomy of a lumbar nerve root, which is divided into anterior and posterior primary rami. Most low back pain and sclerotome pain arises from posterior primary ramus innervated structures, whereas sciatica involves mechanical and chemical stimulation of the anterior primary ramus.

Sciatica usually radiates down one leg in the distribution of the L5 or S1 nerve root. In the case of the S1 nerve root, this involves the lateral border of the lower leg and foot, and in the case of the L5 root, the anterolateral aspect of the leg and dorsum of the foot. When a single nerve root is involved, the symptom may be described as a monoradiculopathy. If more than

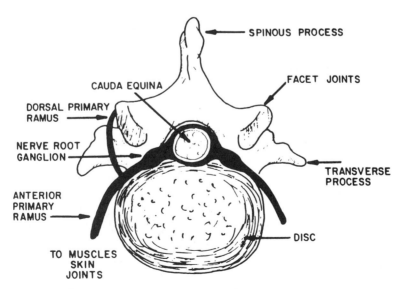

FIG 4.2.
Normal relationships of lumbar nerve roots.

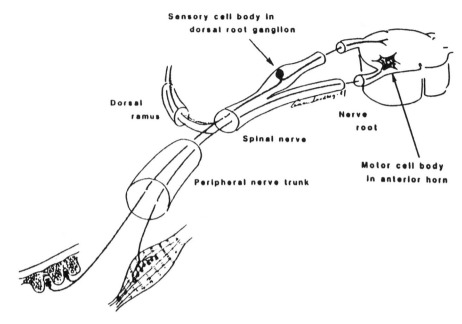

FIG 4.3.
Usual anatomy of lumbar nerve root. (From Rydevik B, Brown MD, Lundborg G: Pathoanatomy and pathophysiology of nerve root compression. *Spine* 9:7–15, 1984.)

one nerve root is involved, the condition is termed a polyradiculopathy, though it is then important to distinguish true objective neurology from nonanatomical and nonorganic illness behavior.[68] Either a mono- or a polyradiculopathy may also involve the lumbar nerve roots above the L5 and S1 levels, in which case the pain radiates into the anterior aspect of the thigh. Because the upper lumbar nerve roots (L2, L3, L4) form the femoral nerve, this type of pain is often called femoral neuritis.

Neurologic claudication is another variant of the peripheral manifestations of lumbar disease. In this condition pain is felt in the distribution of one or more lumbosacral nerve roots, though the pain is often less well localized than the sciatica or femoral neuritis associated with a disc prolapse. It is often accompanied by neurologic symptoms such as numbness or weakness. Multiple nerve roots may be involved in spinal stenosis, and so the condition is a common cause of a polyradiculopathy. The *sine qua non* of claudication is the production of leg pain or neurologic symptoms or both by walking and relief after stopping walking. Similar leg pain may also be produced by vascular claudication, but the pain is then usually localized to the muscles. Further useful differentiation is that relief of neurologic claudication often involves the need not only to stop walking but also to sit down for several minutes. The usual cause of neurologic claudication is diminished space within the bony canal of the spine, termed spinal stenosis. The characteristic relief of claudication by spinal flexion, (for example, when sitting), results from the anatomy of the lumbar spine, where the space available for the nerves increases in the flexed position.

A rare but catastrophic type of low back disease is the cauda equina syndrome. This condition may arise from a massive lumbar disc herniation, spinal stenosis, tumors, infections, injuries, or other neurologic diseases. It is often preceded or accompanied by symptoms of sciatica or neurologic claudication that may be bilateral. The clinical characteristics are as follows: (1) anesthesia in the distribution of the S2–S4 nerve roots, which supply the perineum in the distribution of a person sitting on a saddle, leading to the term saddle anesthesia; (2) disturbance of bladder and bowel control with urinary incontinence or retention and fecal incontinence. Any urinary disturbance in a patient with back pain constitutes an emergency and requires urgent investigation.

Pain in the low back or legs may also be referred from other organs and caused by many conditions that do not directly affect the lumbar spine or lumbosacral nerves. These include diseases of the pelvic organs such as prostatitis in the male, gynecologic disease in the female, and retroperitoneal conditions such as gastric and duodenal ulcers or tumors of the pancreas. Such referred pain is important in a complete differential diagnosis of low back pain.

THE PHYSICAL BASIS OF BACK PAIN: PERIPHERAL NOCICEPTION

A structure capable of giving rise to pain must be innervated by specialized nerve endings, which are collectively termed nociceptors.[29,77,79] Histologic criteria have been developed to identify nerve endings that have nociceptive properties. Most commonly these structures are arborizing, unmyelinated, free nerve endings. Other specialized nerve endings found in ligaments and joint capsules appear to be sensitive to mechanical stimuli and are termed mechanoreceptors.[78,79] To fulfill the experimental criteria for nociception, pain should be produced by chemical or mechanical stimuli of the structure, and relief of pain should be obtained by the injection of local anesthetic.

Nociception: Low Back Pain

The classic clinical experiments to identify the anatomic origins of low back pain were performed by Lewis and Kellgren[30] and later reproduced by other investigators.[23,33] In these experiments, structures thought to produce low back pain were injected with hypertonic saline, and the character and distribution of pain were observed. In later experiments the placement of the injections was guided by radiographic control. Relief of pain was then produced by the injection of local anesthetic. Similar results were also obtained by electric stimulation. Complementary to these studies have been the detailed anatomic investigations of Pedersen et al.,[52] Wyke,[78,79] Bogduk,[6] and Paris.[49] On the basis of these clinical and neuroanatomic studies the nociceptor innervated structures of the lumbar spine are thought to include the following (Fig. 4.4):

1. Facet joint capsules.
2. Ligaments — posterior longitudinal, interspinous, ligamentum flavum.
3. Intervertebral discs — peripheral annulus.
4. Vertebrae — vertebral periosteum, as well as nonciceptors accompanying blood vessels within the cancellous bone.
5. Dura Mater.
6. Muscle — Nociceptors are found in the region of blood vessels. It is uncertain if there are any within the muscle fibers themselves.

Noxious stimulation of most of these structures by hypertonic saline produces both low back pain and sclerotome radiation into the lower limb. The distribution of the pain depends on the specific lumbar level stimulated. Sciatica or claudication is not produced. Moreover,

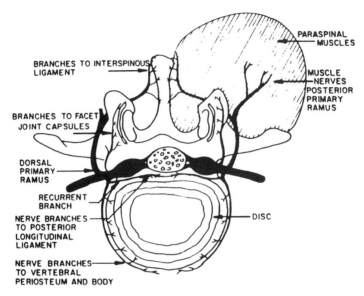

FIG 4.4.
Posterior primary ramus innervation.

the injection of muscles does not appear to produce typical pain distribution but rather results in local muscle tenderness and focal pain. Particularly interesting is the lumbar disk itself. There is little anatomic evidence that the normal disc is innervated except in its most peripheral annular fibers.[6,40,60] Degeneration causes disruption of the normal disk, which is sometimes associated with ingrowth of granulation or scar tissue, however, and the new blood vessels that accompany such granulation tissue are thought to contain nociceptors. This concept is central to "discogenic pain" as well as to the diagnostic use of pain provocation by diskography.[31,72,80]

As previously noted, what all of these structures that can produce low back pain have in common is an innervation by the posterior primary ramus of the lumbar nerve root (Fig. 4.4). This nerve arises adjacent to the dorsal root ganglion and typically innervates the spinal structures in several segments.[49] A recurrent branch returns into the nerve root canal to supply the posterior longitudinal ligaments, vertebral periosteum, and outer fibers of the annulus fibrosis. Some investigators have identified branches of the posterior primary rami that supply the outer annulus on its anterior and lateral aspects. Possible interconnections between these branches and sympathetic and parasympathetic nerves have been identified and may be important in chronic pain syndromes.

Another mechanism of low back pain production relevant to spinal degeneration is increased intraosseous pressure. As previously noted, nociceptors are identified adjacent to blood vessels. In the osteoarthritic spine and other degenerative joints such as the hip and knee, increased intraosseous pressure is recorded.[1] Theoretically, such increase in intraosseous pressure may be due to increased venous pressures, whose presence in degenerative diseases is demonstrable by larger and more tortuous veins. It is possible that these increased pressures might activate the nociceptors accompanying the smaller veins and lead to pain.

The most uncertain site of low back pain is muscle. This is surprising because the most common clinical diagnosis used to explain low back pain is "low back strain." As previously noted, local noxious stimuli in muscles do not produce typical radiation of low back pain, nor are nociceptors identified within muscle fibers. Furthermore, there is almost no evidence that injuries to the paraspinous muscle fibers actually occur except in direct major trauma. In peripheral muscles, magnetic resonance imaging has been a powerful tool to identify subtle injuries. The application of this technology to lumbar muscles may give new insights into this type of injury. A number of theories have evolved to explain the muscular aching and spasm that accompanies low back pain. One theory, supported by data from peripheral muscles, indicates that overuse causes diminished oxygen to be available to the muscles, and the accumulation of metabolites such as lactic acid follows. With disuse the possibility of these physiologic events is greater, whereas with training the possibility is reduced.[58] The metabolic by-products are presumed to stimulate a pain response. A second theory suggests that because the muscles of the spine are contained within a compartment, pressures may become elevated with subsequent reduction in muscle blood flow (Fig. 4.5).[8,26,64] (Clinical studies have yet to support this condition as a common cause of low back pain.[64]) A third theory suggests that muscle spasm and pain are the result of a yet to be determined reflex arc between nociceptor innervated structures of the functional spinal unit and the corresponding muscles. The paraspinal muscles have the unique property of being innervated by the posterior primary rami, whereas all other striated muscles in the human body are innervated by the anterior primary rami. Thus, it seems plausible that there are reflex pathways between the posterior primary ramus, nociceptor innervated structures of the spine, and the posterior primary ramus innervated muscles.

Sciatica

The production of sciatica involves both direct compression or tension and chemical stimulation of an anterior primary ramus either within the nerve root itself or at the dorsal root ganglion. The classic experiment was performed by Smyth and Wright,[61] who placed

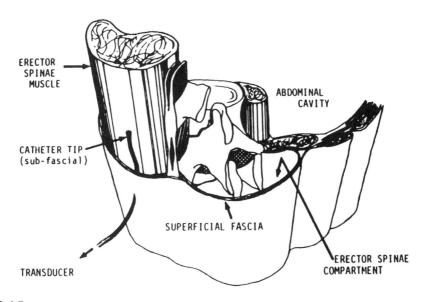

FIG 4.5.
Muscle compartment. (From Carr D, Gilbertson L, Frymoyer J, et al: Lumbar paraspinal compartment syndrome: A case report with physiologic and anatomic studies. *Spine* 1985:10:816–282.)

threads around the nerve roots of patients undergoing disc excision and applied traction on the threads after the patient was awake. They found that this only produced sciatica when traction was applied to a nerve root that had been compressed by a disc herniation and not when applied to normal nerve roots. This led to the hypothesis that simple compression or traction alone was insufficient to produce sciatica, and that some form of inflammation and inflammatory mediator must also be present. This theory has been suppported by the finding of alterations in pH and concentration of lactic acid in the vicinity of a nerve root compressed by a lumbar disc herniation.[47] It has also been demonstrated in animal experiments that nucleus pulposus material can produce an inflammatory response when placed in the epidural space.[34] Others have suggested that the dorsal root ganglion rather than the nerve itself may be compressed.[25]

When a nerve root or peripheral nerve is compressed, a series of events take place, depending on the magnitude and degree of compression. Elegant animal experiments performed by Rydevik[57] have shown that when alterations in nerve conduction occur, blood flow and transport of nutrients within the nerve are diminished, and edema forms. Continuous compression may lead to demyelination and nerve root degeneration. Such continued injury may also alter the excitability of the nerve, making it generate spontaneous impulses (ectopic generators) even after the compression is released (Fig. 4.6).[24,31] The dorsal root ganglion appears to be unusually active in the production of such spontaneous impulses. This may be one explanation for continued pain after decompression of a chronically compressed lumbar nerve root. Lastly, there is some evidence that the nerves themselves have a nerve supply that fulfills the criteria for nociception. These structures are termed nervi nervorum.

Neurologic Claudication

Unlike sciatica, neurologic claudication seems to be primarily a vascular event, although later degeneration of nerve roots within the cauda equina may also contribute to the

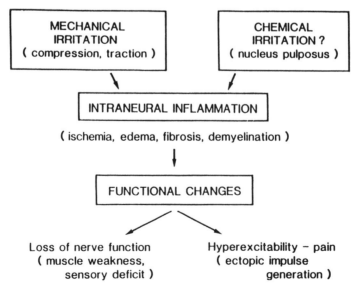

FIG 4.6.
Spontaneous nerve impulses. (Adapted from Rydevik B, Garfin SR: Nerve root compression syndromes, in Szabo R (ed): Nerve Compression Syndromes: Diagnosis and Treatment, New York, Slack Medical Publishers, in press.)

symptoms. Detailed anatomic studies have demonstrated the somewhat tenuous nature of the cauda equina's vascular supply.[10,13,50] This vasculature has the unusual characteristic of having significant arteriovenous anastomoses.[51] Thus, impaired blood flow may occur not only with exercise, which increases the demand on the arterial side, but may also result from increased venous pressure.[15,28,35] Aggravation of symptoms of neurogenic claudication is indeed sometimes observed in patients with right-sided heart failure and venous hypertension.

Studies of the anatomy of the spinal canal show that the amount of space available for the cauda equina is increased in flexion and reduced in extension due to the collapse of the ligamenta flava and greater impingement of the facets.[59] This explains the favored posture of spinal flexion and the need to sit down for relief of symptoms in patients with spinal stenosis and neurologic claudication.

CHEMICAL STIMULATION OF NOCICEPTORS: NONNEUROGENIC AND NEUROGENIC INFLAMMATORY MEDIATORS

As previously noted, the production of low back pain and sciatica involves mechanical stimuli. This is best understood in the lumbar nerve root and only beginning to be understood in the lumbar nerve root and in the posterior primary ramus innervated structures. It appears that chemical stimuli are also a requisite, at least in sciatica, but quite possibly in other structures such as joints. An extensive literature exists on chemicals termed nonneurogenic and neurogenic inflammatory mediators. It has been reviewed in depth by others.[22]

Nonneurogenic mediators are elaborated by circulating cells within the blood and released at the site of many types of injury. This group of chemicals includes bradykinin, serotonin, histamine, acetylcholine, prostaglandins E_1 and E_2, and leukotrienes. Histochemical analyses have revealed receptor sites for these substances located in some peripheral nociceptors and in the dorsal root ganglion. Such nonneurogenic inflammatory mediators are also found within degenerative joints and are thus possible mediators of pain.

Neurogenic inflammatory mediators are a group of special neuropeptides that are produced within the cells of the dorsal root ganglion. It is popularly believed that these chemicals may serve as neurotransmitters, although this theory remains unproved. These chemicals include substance P, somotostatin, cholecystokininlike molecule, vasoactive intestinal polypeptide, calcitonin gene-related peptide, gastrin-releasing peptide, dynorphin, enkephalin, galanin, and angiotensin II. Not all of these substances have been identified in the dorsal root ganglion of the lumbar spine, but their possible importance to the production of low back pain and sciatica are underscored by a number of important experiments. For one, substance P has been identified in peripheral joint degeneration, as well as in the cerebrospinal fluid of patients with arachnoiditis. Alterations of the concentration of some of these neurogenic inflammatory mediators are produced by vibration and discography, both of which are associated with the production of low back pain.

CENTRAL TRANSMISSION OF PERIPHERAL NOCICEPTION

When a peripheral nociceptor is activated by mechanical and chemical stimuli, it generates electrical impulses that pass into the central nervous system. Traditional physiology described the passage of these impulses via spinal pathways to special areas of the brain: in particular via the spinothalamic tract to the thalamus and hence to the somatosensory cortex (Fig. 4.7). This, however, is too easily envisaged as a kind of gigantic telephone exchange where pressing a particular peripheral button would ring a bell in the corresponding area of the cortex and bring the peripheral stimulus to conscious attention. This is clearly a gross oversimplification. The central nervous system — at both brain and spinal cord level — may be better compared with inserting a stimulus into an active computer network.

Both myelinated and unmyelinated afferent fibers in the ventral root make multiple connections in the dorsal horn of the spinal cord. The dorsal horn consists of complex grey matter organized in interconnected laminae of specialized cells (reviewed in detail by Wall).[71] Sensory information coming into the dorsal horn is projected spatially both by site of origin and by its sensory modality so that more distal receptors connect more medially and more proximal receptors laterally in the dorsal horn. Large afferent fibers connect ventrally and small afferent fibers more dorsally. There are extensive interconnections between the laminae. Not only does each lamina receive stimuli from the periphery and transmit stimuli centrally, the more central laminae receive and modify information from the more peripheral laminae. Activity in the laminae is further influenced by descending fibers from the brain and by the chemical milieu of the dorsal horn itself. Incoming signals from the periphery may thus be modified dramatically before central transmission to the brain. Efferent connections at cord level may also, at least theoretically, give rise to reflex muscle activity and segmental autonomic activity.

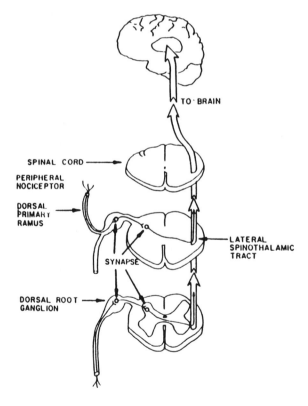

FIG 4.7.
Spinal pathways.

The cells of the dorsal horn give rise to a whole series of both monosynaptic and polysynaptic connections to the brain (reviewed in detail by Willis).[69] The spinothalamic tract is generally regarded as the most important pathway for transmitting painful stimuli to consciousness. A whole network of other polysynaptic tracts, however, pass from the spinal level through the reticular system to the brain. Sensory-discriminative information about pain may be transmitted mainly via the spinothalamic tract, but the other polysynaptic tracts may crucially modify or control the thresholds, intensity, and central effect of incoming pain signals.

The somatosensory cortex provides the final cortical representation for painful stimuli, but it cannot be regarded as the sole site where pain reaches consciousness. The somatocortex is richly connected to many midbrain nuclei and to other areas of the cortex. Midbrain activity contributes greatly to the autonomic and affective components of pain, whereas adjacent areas of the parietal cortex and the frontal cortex are involved in the interpretation, memory, and behavioral response to pain.

Although the detailed neural circuitry and neurophysiology of pain is beyond the scope of this chapter, a number of points are clinically relevant:

1. The complexity of pain transmission explains why surgical transection of a particular sensory tract is unlikely to provide long-term relief of pain. Selective section of the spinothalamic tract has been tried in the management of chronic pain conditions, but unfortunately pain soon recurs, and associated sensory disturbance may make it even more unpleasant. We emphasize that this kind of ablative surgery is rarely if ever indicated in the treatment of benign low back pain.

2. Incoming pain signals may be modulated at many levels before reaching the brain. Connections between the different pain pathways and with other afferent and efferent pathways enable neural activity in other parts of the central nervous system to influence the transmission of pain signals. One of the most intriguing and stimulating explanations for pain modulation is the gate control theory.[44] Leaving aside debate about the exact neural pathways and connections involved, it is now generally believed that nerve conduction of pain may be "gated" and either blocked or facilitated by other afferent and efferent stimuli. This kind of theoretical model offers an attractive explanation for the sometimes beneficial effects of counterirritation, acupuncture, and transcutaneous electric stimulation.

3. Pain transmission may also be modulated by chemical substances within the cerebrospinal fluid that have a morphinelike analgesic action[16] and are called endorphins, or endogenous opioid peptides. These substances appear to be elaborated in cells within the central nervous system, most prominently in the periaqueductal grey matter. Elevations of these substances are found in the cerebrospinal fluid after exercise, which is yet another mechanism by which low back pain might be modulated.

4. Incoming pain sensation may be modulated to some extent by psychological factors, whereas the affective component of pain and behavioral responses to pain are primarily psychological rather than physiologic in nature.

5. The central nervous system is not a set of fixed electric circuits but is plastic in nature. The neural networks themselves can change and may be altered by neural activity itself over time or by pathology. Chronic pain may involve functional changes in the neurologic pathways.

PAIN COGNITION

The cognitive experience of pain is clearly modified by psychologic phenomena. Some of the relevant modifiers of pain cognition include the following:

1. the setting of the pain experience
2. prior pain experience
3. age
4. ethnic and social background
5. psychologic status

Beecher[4] compared chronic pain in soldiers and civilians. He observed that soldiers injured on the battlefield frequently had few complaints of pain and often did not require morphine injections for relief. Civilians with comparable injuries usually complained of severe pain and more often required morphine. Based on these observations he suggested that the setting in which pain occurs markedly affects the cognition of the experience. For the soldier the injury represented a release from intolerable battlefield conditions, thus favorably modifying the pain experience. For the unskilled heavy laborer back pain may threaten to destroy his livelihood. Similarly, prior experience may modify favorably or unfavorably the current pain episode. In low back disease, as in other diseases, it is observed that the pain experience tends to increase as a function of repeated episodes. Pain is also modified by age and sex.[48,76] In general, diminished tolerance to certain painful stimuli may be demonstrated as a function of age and sex, with males generally more tolerant than females. Whether these differences are the result of anatomic, hormonal, or other factors is unclear. It has also been shown that specific ethnic groups have varying tolerance to pain.[75]

Pain, particularly as it becomes chronic, is associated with a variety of emotions. For many years it has been recognized that emotional or psychologic disturbances are both common and clinically important in patients with chronic low back pain and disability. From an extensive review of previous work and his own detailed clinical studies Sternbach[62] showed that the most important psychologic disturbances associated with pain were anxiety in the acute stage and depression in the chronic stage. Extensive studies of chronic low back pain and disability showed that the most important psychologic disturbances in chronic low back pain were somatic anxiety, increased bodily awareness, and depressive symptoms.[36,69] Frymoyer et al.[20] in a study of males aged 18 to 55, compared those who had never had low back pain and those with chronic disabling pain (Table 4.1). In all these studies the most common affective states associated with chronic low back pain and disability are anxiety (fear), depressive symptoms, focusing on bodily symptoms (somatic anxiety or somatization), feelings of hopelessness and helplessness (catastrophizing), and anger.

Not only do these emotional states modify the cognition of pain and the complaint of pain, but studies of patients with arthritis have shown that even the objective signs of disease often wax and wane as a function of the emotional state. During periods of depression and anxiety symptoms, and sometimes signs, worsen. It has also been recognized for many years that these emotional and psychologic disturbances are associated with poor outcomes from either medical or surgical treatment of low back pain. They both result from failed treatment and make treatment less successful.

For many years it was questioned whether these emotional disturbances were the cause or result of the pain experience. It was even suggested that there was a "pain-prone personality," although in 30 years there has been no scientific evidence to support this as an explanation of back pain, except in rare individuals or highly selected groups of patients. Patients who develop back pain and even those with chronic back pain and disability are generally normal people. Preexisting and unrelated psychologic distress may make people

TABLE 4.1
Comparison of Asymptomatic, Non-Disabling and Disabling Low Back Pain Patients*

	Asymptomatic	LBP Non-disabling*	LBP Disabling**
	n = 106	n = 193	n = 20
Unhappy	5.2	10.1	30.0
Hopeless	8.0	12.4	33.0
Worried	15.6	32.8	55.0
Scared	7.4	18.3	30.0
Nervous	11.2	26.5	36.8
Annoyed	32.3	54.3	55.0
Temper Outbursts	8.0	18.7	31.6
Lonely	21.1	23.5	35.0
Touchy	7.8	14.8	15.0
Hurt	4.2	8.6	15.0
Unsympathetic	9.1	13.9	50.0
Headaches	6.1	20.0	30.0
Sleep Disturbances	28.3	52.1	80.0
Dissatisfied with Medical Care	79.1	78.9	60.0
Feels Handicapped	0.0	5.3	50.0
Feels Miserable	6.1	23.1	60.0
Alcohol & Drug Abuse	7.1	7.0	15.0
Has Had Nervous Breakdown	3.0	1.1	10.5
Requires Psychiatric Help	8.9	8.2	15.8
Requires Counseling	8.6	12.8	35.0

*Non-disabling pain is defined as less than 7 days of work loss in the previous year because of back pain (many of the 193 had lost no time from work whatsoever.)
**Disabling is defined as greater than 7 days work loss in the past year.
*From Frymoyer JW, Pope MH, Clements JH, et al: Risk factors in low back pain. *J Bone Joint Surg* 1983;65:213. Used by permission.

more likely to report back pain or less able to cope (Boeing study),[5] but it has not proved possible to identify a personality type that is liable to develop back pain. On the contrary, there are now two good prospective studies that show that these psychologic disturbances appear to be secondary to the physical problem and improve or worsen with the success or failure of physical treatment.[63,70]

ACUTE AND CHRONIC PAIN

Acute and chronic pain are not only different in time scale but are fundamentally different in kind.[62,66] Acute and experimental pains usually bear a relatively straightforward relationship to peripheral stimulus, nociception, and tissue damage. There may be some understandable anxiety about the meaning and consequences of acute pain, although experimental pain by its very nature lacks the affective component of any clinical pain. But acute pain, acute disability, and acute illness behavior are generally proportionate to the physical findings. Appropriate pharmacologic, physical, and even surgical treatment directed to the underlying physical disorder are usually highly effective in relieving acute pain.

Chronic pain is a completely different clinical syndrome. Chronic pain, chronic disability, and chronic illness behavior become increasingly dissociated from the physical problem; there may indeed be very little objective evidence of any remaining nociceptive stimulus. Instead, chronic pain and disability become increasingly associated with emotional distress, depression, disease conviction, failure to cope, and adaptation to chronic invalidity. Chronic pain progressively becomes a self-sustaining condition that is resistant to traditional medical management. Purely physical treatment directed to a hypothetical but unidentified and possibly nonexistent nociceptive source is not only likely to be unsuccessful but may cause additional physical damage. Failed treatment may then reinforce and aggravate pain, distress, disability, and illness behavior. Pain clinics are now full of such patients who have undergone failed back surgery.

CLINICAL ASSESSMENT

Modern clinical practice emphasizes pain, and most doctors spend much of their working life treating pain. It has even been suggested that "the relief of pain is the primary social role of the physician."[14] Some research workers have also suggested that the patient's report of pain is the only possible measure of clinical severity. That is naive. Such statements either present pain as a deceptively simple clinical symptom or regard it as so complex that no one can even try to understand it except at the most pragmatic level. When we see the physiologic and psychologic complexity of pain phenomena, it should come as no surprise that the clinical assessment of pain is both difficult and all too often woefully inadequate.

Anatomic Pattern and Characteristics of Pain

The anatomic distribution of pain, its clinical characteristics, and its relationship to other symptoms form the basis of clinical diagnosis and the recognition of different pain syndromes.

Severity of pain, however, is of fundamental importance for making decisions about how much and what kind of treatment is required, for monitoring progress, and for judging final outcome of treatment and any residual impairment. Yet despite the fact that assessment of pain is a routine and basic part of clinical practice, it is given little attention, and it still needs to be greatly improved. Methods of assessing pain have been reviewed in detail by Main and Waddell.[38]

Pain Scale

The simplest, most widely used, and most useful clinical method of measuring the severity of pain is some form of visual analog scale (Table 4.2).[62] The patient is asked to put a mark on a 100-mm scale, and this is measured in millimeters from 0 to 100%. It is simple to administer and to score, and most patients find it easy to understand. Words may be used to anchor the line at either end, or numbers may be added below the line. A diagram of a thermometer may be used to clarify the concept of a scale (Fig. 4.8). The major difficulty is to interpret exactly what the pain scale measures. It is in no sense an absolute or objective

TABLE 4.2
The Short-Form McGill Pain Questionnaire*

Please tick which of these words describes your pain. Put the tick in the box which gives the intensity of that particular quality of your pain.

	None	Mild	Moderate	Severe
Throbbing	0) ———	1) ———	2) ———	3) ———
Shooting	0) ———	1) ———	2) ———	3) ———
Stabbing	0) ———	1) ———	2) ———	3) ———
Sharp	0) ———	1) ———	2) ———	3) ———
Cramping	0) ———	1) ———	2) ———	3) ———
Gnawing	0) ———	1) ———	2) ———	3) ———
Hot-burning	0) ———	1) ———	2) ———	3) ———
Aching	0) ———	1) ———	2) ———	3) ———
Heavy	0) ———	1) ———	2) ———	3) ———
Tender	0) ———	1) ———	2) ———	3) ———
Splitting	0) ———	1) ———	2) ———	3) ———
Tiring-exhausting	0) ———	1) ———	2) ———	3) ———
Sickening	0) ———	1) ———	2) ———	3) ———
Fearful	0) ———	1) ———	2) ———	3) ———
Punishing-cruel	0) ———	1) ———	2) ———	3) ———

Please put a mark on the scale to show how bad your *usual pain* has been *these days.*

No
pain ——————————————————————————— Worst
possible
pain

How bad is your pain now?

0	No pain	———
1	Mild	———
2	Discomforting	———
3	Distressing	———
4	Horrible	———
5	Excruciating	———

*From Melzack R: The short-form McGill Pain Questionnaire. *Pain* 1987; 30:191–197. Used by permission.

measure of pain, and it bears very little relationship to any physiologic or pathologic change. The patient's report of pain is influenced by nociceptive stimuli, physiologic phenomena, cognition, psychologic distress, pain behavior, and communication. With these qualifications it is obviously important not to overinterpret the pain scale but to accept it simply as a measure of how bad the patient tells the doctor the pain is.

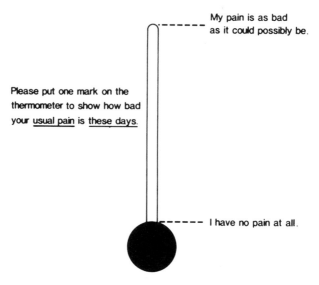

My pain is as bad
as it could possibly be.

Please put one mark on the
thermometer to show how bad
your <u>usual pain</u> is <u>these days.</u>

I have no pain at all.

FIG 4.8.
The pain scale. The scale should be exactly 100 mm long and the level marked by the patient is scored as a percentage.

Pain Ratings

Verbal rating scales are frequently used to describe the severity of pain (Table 4.2). It is difficult to define the exact severity of each adjective used, and the "steps" on the scale may not be equal.

The fundamental limitation of both a visual analog scale and the rating of severity is that no one-dimensional scale can adequately reflect the complexity of the pain experience. In particular, these scales fail to distinguish the sensory and affective components of the pain.

Pain Adjectives

The quality of the pain may be assessed to some extent by the patient's use of descriptive adjectives. The most widely used method is the McGill Pain Questionnaire,[41] which was originally administered as an interview but is now frequently given as a self-report questionnaire. Detailed scoring methods are available, but the adjectives may be broadly divided into those that describe the sensory qualities and those that describe the emotional or affective qualities of the pain. A shorter version of the McGill Pain Questionnaire has been developed[43]; it is more practical for routine use and is presently being tested in United Kingdom patients with low back pain (Table 4.2).

Pain Drawing

The pain drawing was developed specifically for back pain patients[55] (Fig. 4.9) and was designed to disentangle the sensory and emotional elements of the clinical presentation of pain. It is based on both the site and the nature of the pain. Patients willingly record their pain on an outline of the body, but the *way* in which they draw their pain reflects the affective component of their pain and their psychologic distress. The pain drawing is based

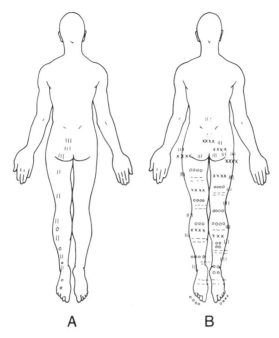

FIG 4.9.
The pain drawing provides information about both the physical and emotional aspects of the patient's pain. Patient A describes the anatomic pattern of pain and paresthesia from an S1 root lesion. Patient B with simple low back pain does not have a cauda equina lesion but is communicating distress.

on an important clinical concept, although further research has not supported the original complex scoring system. It is perhaps best regarded as a relatively crude screening test to alert the clinician to the possibility of psychologic factors being important in the clinical presentation of that patient's pain.

In the same way, inappropriate or behavioral descriptions of symptoms[68] and nonorganic or behavioral responses to examinations[67] may be distinguished from the standard physical symptoms and signs of disease (Table 4.3).

Overt Pain Behavior

Behavior is another indicator that someone is in pain. It is part of routine medical and nursing observation to assess whether patients behave as if they are in more or less pain than they tell us they have. Keefe and Block[27] provided a scientific basis for these clinical impressions when they described overt pain behavior in low back pain:

Guarding — Abnormally stiff, interrupted, or rigid movement while moving from one position to another.

Bracing — A stationary position in which a fully extended limb supports and maintains an abnormal distribution of weight.

Rubbing — Any contact between hand and back, that is, touching, rubbing, or holding the affected area of pain.

Grimacing — Obvious facial expression of pain, which may include furrowed

TABLE 4.3
A Comparison of the Symptoms and Signs of Physical Disease and Abnormal Illness Behavior in Chronic Low Back Pain*

	Physical Disease/ Normal Illness Behavior	Abnormal Illness Behavior
Symptoms		
Pain	Anatomic distribution	Whole leg pain
		Tailbone pain
Numbness	Dermatomal	Whole leg numbness
Weakness	Myotomal	Whole leg giving way
Time pattern	Varies with time and activity	Never free of pain
Response to treatment	Variable benefit	Intolerance of treatments
		Emergency admissions to hospital
Signs		
Tenderness	Anatomic distribution	Superficial
		Widespread nonanatomic
Axial loading	No lumbar pain	Lumbar pain
Simulated rotation	No lumbar pain	Lumbar pain
Straight leg raising	Limited on distraction	Improves with distraction
Sensory	Dermatomal	Regional
Motor	Myotomal	Regional, jerky, giving way

*From Waddell G, Bircher M, Finlayson D, et al: Symptoms and signs: Physical disease or illness behavior? *Brit Med J* 1984; 289:739. Used by permission.

brow, narrowed eyes, tightened lips, corners of mouth pulled back, and clenched teeth.

Sighing — Obvious exaggerated exhalation of air, usually accompanied by shoulders first rising and then falling; cheeks may be expanded.

Pain and Suffering: Psychologic Distress

Pain and suffering are inextricably linked, but the amount and quality of suffering varies greatly and is more closely related to the affective or emotional component of the pain than it is to the sensory or physical component. Suffering may indeed be better regarded and assessed in terms of psychologic distress rather than pain itself.

Historically, psychologic disturbances were first demonstrated by the Minnesota Multiphasic Personality Inventory (MMPI), which has been the most widely used psychologic questionnaire in back pain patients. The common MMPI disturbance associated with back pain and related to the outcome of treatment is the "neurotic triad."[2,74] The MMPI was originally developed as a screening instrument in psychiatric patients. Although loosely labeled "neurotic" and originally derived from psychiatric ideas of hypochondriasis, depression, and hysteria, these labels have never been clinically valid in back pain. Very few back pain patients are psychiatrically ill. They are generally not personality deficient, neurotic, hypochondriacal, or insane, but simply distressed by their physical problem. The psychologic disturbances associated with back pain are best regarded clinically as forms of current psychologic distress, a simple emotional reaction to pain and disability.

Although of great historical value, the MMPI is long, cumbersome, and poorly accepted by many patients. There are now very much shorter, better psychologic questionnaires that specifically measure current psychologic distress. Examples of simple, one-page questionnaires that are now well established in the clinical assessment of low back pain are depressive inventories by Beck et al.[3] or Zung[81] and the modified somatic perception questionnaire (MRPQ) by Main.[36]

Attitudes and Beliefs: Coping Strategies

Pain behavior and disability depend ultimately on the patient's attitudes and beliefs about pain. The earliest attempt to explore cognitive factors in back pain was the Illness Behavior Questionnaire by Pilowsky and Spence.[54] In the past few years, a number of better questionnaires have been developed that look specifically at cognitive factors and coping strategies.[39,56] At the moment these may best be regarded as research tools rather than as routine clinical instruments, but potentially they show great promise in helping us to understand why some patients cope with back pain and others become totally disabled.

MANAGEMENT OF PAIN

Here are some general principles of the clinical management of pain. More detailed descriptions specifically applicable to low back pain sufferers are discussed in later chapters.

Analgesics

One of the fundamental duties of the physician is to provide relief of pain. There are some qualifications to this statement, however: it is only one of the duties, and pain relief may be given only as far as reasonably possible. It is unrealistic to expect total abolition of pain, and it may be better for both patient and doctor to think in terms of controlling pain.

The standard and almost universal first line of controlling pain is analgesic medication. In the acute phase, analgesics are often underprescribed. In the first day or two of a single acute attack there should be no hesitation in providing adequate analgesia, including, if necessary, parenteral narcotics. In the chronic phase, however, analgesics, sedatives, and tranquilizers are badly overprescribed. Chronic analgesia abuse not only loses any symptomatic benefit with time but may lead to serious problems.

It is important that analgesics be prescribed regularly on a fixed dose-time regime for a fixed duration rather than on a prn basis. This not only gives better relief of pain but also reduces drug dependency.[19]

Reinforcement of Pain Behavior

Behavioral psychologists have looked at the relationship between chronic pain and disability and suggested that pain behaviors may be powerfully influenced and modified by their consequences.[19] Exercise to the limit of pain tolerance is strongly influenced by conscious feedback of how much exercise has been done: in the absence of such feedback chronic pain patients perform the same amount of exercise as normal pain-free people. The exercise tolerance of chronic pain patients is also markedly improved by verbal praise and encouragement from a physiotherapist. Patients with chronic backache almost universally report lower levels of activity. But careful observation shows that subjective reports of pain are largely unrelated to activity levels: observed pain behavior is in fact inversely proportional to the amount of exercise performed. In a very elegant clinical experiment, Fordyce et al.[19] compared traditional medical treatment with a behavioral approach to acute low back pain. Traditional treatment was rest, analgesics, and activity on a prn basis, where the patient was advised to "let pain be your guide." This was compared with a fixed regime of incremented activity based on tissue healing times. At the one-year follow-up, patients treated on the traditional basis reported that disability had actually increased. Patients treated on the rehabilitation regime had returned to preonset levels of activity. Dolce et al.[12] independently confirmed the value of a fixed exercise quota. They showed increased exercise tolerance, increased self-estimate of exercise capability, and decreased anxiety about the effects of exercise.

Pain behavior and disability may be powerfully modified by how relatives, co-workers, employers, health professionals, and physicians react to the patient's pain. The patient's own attitudes and beliefs about pain and about what the patient should or should not do about it are also shaped by the medical information received and, at least potentially, might be influenced by education.

Pain Clinic Principles

This topic is included in Chapter 10. It is instructive here to look generally at how pain clinics manage chronic symptoms. The goal of pain management programs is rehabilitative rather than curative. The goal is to control pain and its effects rather than to abolish it; to increase functional activities; and to reduce illness behavior. It is instructive to compare the goals and methods of traditional medicine, back schools, and pain management programs (Table 4.4).[37]

TABLE 4.4
The Goals of Treatment for Acute versus Chronic LBP*

	Disease Acute	Illness Chronic
GOALS	TREATMENT	REHABILITATION
Pain reduction	major	major
Disability and mobility	minor†	major
Reduce distress	minor†	major
Reduce illness behavior	iatrogenic†	major
Reduce invalidity and sick role	iatrogenic†	major
Educational	minor†	major
PATIENT'S ROLE	PASSIVE	ACTIVE

*From Main CJ, Parker H: The evaluation and outcome of pain management programs for chronic low back pain, in Roland R, Jenner R (eds): *Back Pain: New Approaches to Rehabilitation and Education.* Manchester, England, University Press, 1989. Used by permission.
†Tragically, this is often true. These should, however, be part of good medicine.

Clinical Management of Pain

Many of these concepts about pain clearly raise questions about our current medical management of back pain. Much acute back pain may be treated satisfactorily on a largely physical basis. When physical therapy fails, however, and as back pain becomes chronic, it becomes increasingly essential to understand and manage pain according to a biopsychosocial model rather than a disease model. Symptomatic treatment of pain alone is then no longer enough: pain is only one element of the total illness.

Physicians may agree in principle with the need to treat people rather than spines. To make this a practical reality it must be recognized that low back pain is only a symptom, and low back disability should be considered an illness rather than a disease. In theory, the physical, psychologic, and social aspects of illness should be considered. To put this into practice pain and disability must be distinguished from each other, the symptoms and signs of distress and illness behavior must be distinguished from those of physical disease, and treatment must be directed to restoration of function as well as the relief of pain. Paradoxically, such an approach may actually lead to better relief of pain than the results that traditional medicine is currently producing.

BIBLIOGRAPHY

1. Arnoldi CC: Intravertebral pressures in patients with lumbar pain: A preliminary communication. *Acta Orthop Scand* 1972; 43:109.
2. Beals RK, Hickman NW: Industrial injuries of the back and extremities. *J Bone Joint Surg* 1972; 54:1593–1611.
3. Beck AT, Ward CH, Mendelson MM, et al: An inventory for measuring depression. *Arch Gen Psychiatry* 1961; 4:561–571.
4. Beecher HK: Relationship of significance of wound to pain experienced. *J Amer Med Assoc* 1956; 161:1609–1613.
5. Bigos SJ, Battié MC: Surveillance of back problems in industry, in N.M. Hadler (ed.) *Clinical Concepts in Regional Musculoskeletal Illness*. Orlando, Fla, Grune & Stratton, 1987.
6. Bogduk N, Tynan W, Wilson A: The nerve supply to the human lumbar intervertebral discs. *J Anat* 1981; 132:139.
7. Burstein R, Cliffer KD, Giesler GJ Jr: Direct somatosensory projections from the spinal cord to the hypothalamus and telencephalon. *J Neurosci* 1987; 7:4159.
8. Carr D, Gilbertson L, Frymoyer J, et al: Lumbar paraspinal compartment syndrome: A case report with physiologic and anatomic studies. *Spine* 1985; 10:816–820.
9. Contunnius D: *De Ischiade Nervosa Commentarius. Neapoli Apud Frat Simonios. (A Treatise on the Nervous Sciatica or Nervous Hip Gout)*. English trans 1775, London, Wilkie, 1764.
10. Crock HV, Yoshizawa H: The Blood Supply of the Vertebral Column and Spinal Cord in Man. New York, Springer-Verlag, 1977.
11. Descartes R: *L'homme*. (1644) Foster M (trans). New York, Cambridge University Press, 1901.
12. Dolce JJ, Crocker MF, Moletteire C, et al: Exercise quotas, anticipatory concern and self-efficacy expectancies in chronic pain: A preliminary report. *Pain* 1986; 24:365–372.
13. Dommisse GF: *The Arteries and Veins of the Human Spinal Cord fom Birth*. Edinburgh, Churchill Livingstone, 1975.
14. Engel GL: Psychogenic pain and the pain prone patient. *Amer J Med* 1959; 26:899–918.
15. Evans JG: Neurogenic intermittent claudication. *Br Med J* 1964; 2:985.
16. Fields H: Endogenous mechanisms of pain modulation, in White AA III, Gordon S: *American Academy of Orthopaedic Surgeons Symposium on Idiopathic Low Back Pain*. St Louis, CV Mosby, 1982.

17. Foerster O: The dermatomes in man. *Brain* 56:1, 1933.

18. Fordyce WE: Behavioral methods for chronic pain and illness. CV Mosby, St Louis, 1976.

19. Fordyce WE, Brockway JA, Bergman JA, et al: Acute back pain: A control group comparison of behavioral vs traditional management methods. *J Behav Med* 1986; 9:127–140.

20. Frymoyer JW, Pope MH, Clements JH, et al: Risk factors in low-back pain. *J Bone Joint Surg* 1983; 65:213.

21. Frymoyer JW, Rosen JC, Clements J, et al: Psychologic factors in low-back-pain disability. *Clin Orthop* 1985; 195:178–184.

22. Frymoyer JW, Gordon SL (eds): *New Perspectives on Low Back Pain*. Park Ridge, Ill, American Academy of Orthopaedic Surgeons, 1989.

23. Hirsch C, Ingelmark B-E, Miller M: The anatomical basis for low back pain: Studies on the presence of sensory nerve endings in ligamentous, capsular and intervertebral disc structures in the human lumbar spine. *Acta Orthop Scand* 1963; 33:1.

24. Holt S, Yates PO: Cervical spondylosis and nerve root lesions: Incidence at routine necropsy. *J Bone Joint Surg* 1966; 48:407.

25. Howe JF, Loeser JD, Calvin WH: Mechanosensitivity of dorsal root ganglia and chronically injured axons: A physiological basis for the radicular pain of nerve root compression. *Pain* 1977; 3:25.

26. Jokl P: Muscle and low back pain, in White AA III, Gordon SL, (eds): *American Academy of Orthopaedic Surgeons Symposium on Idiopathic Low Back Pain*. St Louis, CV Mosby, 1982.

27. Keefe FJ, Block AR: Development of an observation method for assessing pain behavior in chronic low back pain patients. *Behavior Therapy* 1982; 13:363–375.

28. LaBan MM: "Vespers curse" night pain: The bane of Hypnos. *Arch Phys Med Rehab* 1984; 65:501.

29. LaMotte RH: Nociceptors in skin, joint, muscle and bone, in White AA III, Gordon SL (eds): *American Academy of Orthopaedic Surgeons Symposium on Idiopathic Low Back Pain*. St Louis, CV Mosby, 1982.

30. Lewis T, Kellgren JH: Observations relating to referred pain, visceromotor reflexes and other associated phenomena. *Clin Sci* 1939; 4:47.

31. Lindblom K, Rexed B: Spinal nerve injury in dorso-lateral protrusions of lumbar disks. *J Neurosurg* 1948; 5:413.

32. Loeser JD: Concepts of pain, in Stanton-Hicks M, Boas R (eds): *Chronic Low Back Pain*. New York, Raven Press, 1982.

33. McCall IW, Park WM, O'Brien JP: Induced pain referral from posterior lumbar elements in normal subjects. *Spine* 1979; 4:441.

34. McCarron RF, Wimpee MW, Hudkins PG, et al: The inflammatory effect of nucleus pulposus: A possible element in the pathogenesis of low-back pain. *Spine* 1987; 12:760–764.

35. Madsen JR, Heros RC: Spinal arteriovenous malformations and neurogenic claudication. *J Neurosurg* 1988; 57:793.

36. Main CJ: The modified somatic perception questionnaire. *J Psychosomatic Res* 1983; 27:503–514.

37. Main CJ, Parker H: The evaluation and outcome of pain management programs for chronic low back pain, in Roland R, Jenner JR (eds): *Back Pain: New Approaches to Rehabilitation and Education*. Manchester, U.K. University Press, 1989.

38. Main CJ, Waddell G: The assessment of pain. *Clin Rehab* in press.

39. Main CJ, Wood PLR, Parker H, et al: The pain locus of control questionnaire. *Pain*, Submitted for publication.

40. Malinsky J: The ontogenetic development of nerve terminations in the intervertebral discs of man. *Acta Anat* 1959; 38:96.

41. Melzack R: *The Puzzle of Pain*. New York, Basic Books, 1973.

42. Melzack R: The McGill Pain Questionnaire: Major properties and scoring methods. *Pain* 1975; 1:277–299.
43. Melzack R: The short-form McGill Pain Questionnaire. *Pain* 1987; 30:191–197.
44. Melzack R, Wall PD: Gate control theory of pain, in Soulairac A, Cahn J, Charpentier J, (eds): *Pain,* New York, Academic Press, 1968.
45. Melzack R, Wall PD: Psychophysiology of pain. *Int Anesthesiol Clin* 1970; 8:3.
46. Merskey R: Pain terms: A list with definitions and notes on usage. *Pain* 1979; 6:249–252.
47. Nachemson A: Intradiscal measurements of pH in patients with lumbar rhizopathies. *Acta Orthop Scand* 1969; 40:23.
48. Notermans SLH, Tophoff MMWA: Sex differences in pain tolerance and pain appreciation. *Psych Neurol Neurochir* 1967; 70:23–29.
49. Paris SV: Anatomy as related to function and pain. *Orthop Clin N Am* 1983; 14:475.
50. Parke WW, Gammell K, Rothman RH: Arterial vascularization of the cauda equina. *J Bone Joint Surg* 1981; 63:53.
51. Parke WW, Watanabe R: The intrinsic vasculature of the lumbosacral spinal nerve roots. *Spine* 1985; 10:508.
52. Pedersen HE, Blunck CFJ, Gardner E: The anatomy of the lumbosacral posterior rami and meningeal branches of the spinal nerves (sinuvertebral nerves) with an experimental study of their functions. *J Bone Joint Surg* 1956; 38:377.
53. Penfield W: Foreword, in White J, Sweet WH (eds): *Pain and the Neurosurgeon.* Springfield, Ill, CC Thomas, 1969.
54. Pilowsky I, Spence ND: *Manual for the Illness Behavior Questionnaire (IBQ),* ed 2, Adelaide, University of Adelaide, 1983.
55. Ransford AO, Cairns D, Mooney V: The pain drawing as an aid to the psychological evaluation of patients with low back pain. 1976; *Spine* 1:127.
56. Rosensteil AK, Keefe FJ: The use of coping strategies in chronic low back pain: Relationships to patient characteristics and current adjustment. *Pain* 1983; 17:33–44.
57. Rydevik, B. Nerve, in Frymoyer J, Gordon G (eds): *New Perspectives in Low Back Pain.* Park Ridge, Ill, American Academy of Orthopaedic Surgeons, pp. 35-130, 1989.
58. Saltin B, Gollnick PD: Skeletal muscle adaptability: Significance for metabolism and performance, in Peachey LD, Adrian RH, Geiger SR, (eds): *Handbook of Physiology,* sec 10, *Skeletal Muscle.* Bethesda, Md, American Physiological Society, 1983.
59. Schonstrom N: *The Narrow Lumbar Spinal Canal and the Size of the Cauda Equina in Man.* Goteborg, Sweden, Dept of Orthopaedics, Gothenburg University, Sahlgren Hospital, 1988.
60. Shinohara H: A study on lumbar disc lesions: Significance of histology of free nerve endings in lumbar discs. *J Jpn Orthop Assoc* 1970; 44:553.
61. Smyth MJ, Wright V: Sciatica and the intervertebral disc: An experimental study. *J Bone Joint Surg* 1958; 40:1401.
62. Sternbach RA: *Pain Patients: Traits and Treatment.* New York, Academic Press, 1974.
63. Sternbach RA, Timmermans G: Personality changes associated with reduction of pain. *Pain* 1975; 1:177–181.
64. Styf J: Pressure in the erector spinae muscle during exercise. *Spine* 1987; 12:675.
65. Styf J, Lysell E: Chronic compartment syndrome in the erector spinae muscle. *Spine* 1987; 12:680.
66. Waddell G: A new clinical model for the treatment of low back pain. *Spine* 1987; 12:632–644.
67. Waddell G, McCulloch JA, Kummel EG, et al: Non-organic physical signs in low back pain. *Spine* 1980; 5:117–125.
68. Waddell G, Bircher M, Finlayson D, et al: Symptoms and signs: Physical disease or illness behavior? *Brit Med J* 1984; 289:739.
69. Waddell G, Main CJ, Morris EW, et al: Chronic low back pain, psychological distress and illness behavior. *Spine* 1984; 9:209–213.

70. Waddell G, Morris EW, DiPaola M, et al: A concept of illness tested as an improved basis for surgical decisions in low back disorders. *Spine* 1986; 11:712.

71. Wall PD: The dorsal horn, in Wall PD, Melzack R (eds): *Textbook of Pain*. Edinburgh, Churchill Livingstone, 1984.

72. Walsh TR, Weinstein JN, Spratt KF, et al: Lumbar discography: A controlled, prospective study of normal volunteers to determine the false-positive rate. Presented to the International Society for the Study of the Lumbar Spine, Kyoto, 1989.

73. Willis WD: The origin and destination of pathways involved in pain transmission, in Wall PD, Melzack R (eds): *Textbook of Pain*. Edinburgh, Churchill Livingstone, 1984.

74. Wiltse LL, Rocchio PD: Pre-operative psychological tests as predictions of success of chemonucleolysis in the treatment of the low back syndrome. *J Bone Joint Surg* 1975; 57:478–483.

75. Wolff BB, Langley S: Cultural factors and the response to pain: A review, in Weisenberg M (ed): *Pain: Cultural and Experimental Perspectives*. St. Louis, CV Mosby, 1975.

76. Woodrow KM, Friedman GD, Seiglamb AB, et al: Pain tolerances: Differences according to age, sex and race. *Psychosom Med* 1972; 34:548–556.

77. Wyke BD: Neurological aspects of low back pain, in *The Lumbar Spine and Back Pain*, ed 1. London, Pitman, 1976.

78. Wyke BD: The neurology of low back pain, in *The Lumbar Spine and Back Pain*, ed 2. London, Pitman, 1980.

79. Wyke BD: Receptor systems in lumbosacral tissues in relation to the production of low back pain, White AA III, Gordon SL (eds): in *American Association of Orthopaedic Surgery Symposium on Idiopathic Low Back Pain*. St. Louis, CV Mosby, 1982.

80. Yoshizawa H, O'Brien JP, Smith WT, et al: Neuropathology of intervertebral disc removed for low back pain. *J Pathol* 1980; 132:95.

81. Zung WWK: A self-rated depression scale. *Arch Gen Psychiatr* 1965; 32:63–70.

5

Epidemiology and Cost

Gunnar B.J. Andersson, M.D., Ph.D.
Malcolm H. Pope, Dr. Med. Sc., Ph.D.
John W. Frymoyer, M.D.
Stover Snook, Ph.D.

INTRODUCTION

Epidemiology is derived form the Greek: *epi* = on; *demos* = people; *logos* = study. It is often defined as the study of epidemics, which was its initial main purpose. This conjures up in the imagination quarantine signs and the plague. In fact, in the view of many authorities, low back pain (LBP) has become epidemic in the twentieth century. For example, disabling low back episodes increased 26% in the United States from 1974 to 1978, while the population increased only 7%. Modern epidemiology, however, is not only descriptive in nature, it also includes studies of intervention and etiology. Epidemiology offers at least three insights critical to understanding back pain: first, it provides information on the magnitude of the problem and the resultant demand on medical and social resources (descriptive epidemiology), which is necessary to appropriate health resource allocations. Second, it provides information on the natural history, which is important to patient counseling about prognosis, and provides a standard for determination of treatment effects. Third, epidemiology offers the ability to determine associations between pain and individual and external factors (such as work-related factors). This allows risk factors to be identified and eliminated or modified.

Despite the increasing magnitude of the low back problem, epidemiologic research on LBP is in its infancy compared to the epidemiologic efforts for other diseases such as cancer, infection, and cardiovascular malfunction. Perhaps this is because LBP carries a negligible risk of mortality and therefore has been of less public concern. Epidemiologic research in LBP has been, and still is, often hampered by methodologic problems in definition, classification, and diagnosis (as discussed in Chapter 3). Objective evidence of existing low back pain is often lacking, and people's recall of previous episodes is poor. The intermittent nature of low back pain complicates prevalence studies, and studies of disability due to LBP are influenced by legal and socioeconomic factors. Methodologic problems also exist in the quantifying of physical exposures that might be of etiologic importance, such as loads applied to the spine over time.

In general, data for epidemiologic studies may be obtained from official health registers or by retrospective, prospective, or cross-sectional surveys of general populations or of specific industrial populations. Such data are useful in defining the magnitude of the problem. They may also be useful in planning health care facilities and other medical and social programs, including preventive programs. Data of this kind also partially define the natural history of LBP episodes and may help in identifying environmental or individual factors that may cause or contribute to LBP and disability caused by LBP. These data are also useful in defining prevention strategies. Care must be taken when interpreting these data, however. As mentioned above, there is no consensus on classification and diagnosis, making it difficult to rely on insurance and hospital data.[82] Sickness absence and disability data are heavily influenced by work conditions and the legal and socioeconomic situation, and there is a poor correlation between tissue injury and disability.

Data from workers' compensation claims are affected by inherent biases[1]: (a) all workers are not always covered by worker compensation programs; (b) the claims data are mainly administrative and therefore, while accurate on absence and cost, lack validity on diagnosis; (c) all workers with back pain do not file a claim, and many do not stay away from work.

In spite of these difficulties, epidemiology has provided invaluable information useful for prevention, treatment, and rehabilitation of workers with occupational low back pain.

Because epidemiology is the source of much of our knowledge regarding LBP, this section is divided into three chapters. The first defines the magnitude of the problem in society and industry and its cost, the second discusses the role of the workplace, the third covers the individual risk factors for LBP.

THE MAGNITUDE OF THE PROBLEM

The magnitude of any health problem is measured by prevalence and incidence. In a prevalence study, the presence of LBP and other important variables are determined at one point in time (point prevalence) or during one period of time (period prevalence) for each member of the population studied or for a representative sample. Incidence may be defined as the number of people who develop LBP over a specified time period, such as their lifetimes (lifetime incidence, which is synonymous with lifetime prevalence) or a single year (annual incidence). In short, prevalence means all cases of LBP, whereas incidence means all new cases of LBP. Table 5.1 presents the prevalence and incidence of LBP, as

TABLE 5.1
Prevalence and Lifetime Incidence of LBP as Determined by Several Studies*

Study	Lifetime Incidence (%)	Prevalence (%) Point	Prevalence (%) Period	Study Group N	Study Group Age	Study Group Sex	Comment
Biering-Sorensen	62.6	12.0	—	449	30–60	M	
(1982)	61.4	15.2	—	479	30–60	F	
Hirsch et al. (1969)	48.8	—	—	692	15–72	F	
Hult (1954)	60.0	—	—	1193	25–59	M	Industrial
Frymoyer et al. (1983)	69.9	—	—	1221	28–55	M	
Nagi et al. (1973)	—	18.0	—	1135	18–64	MF	
Svensson & Andersson	61	—	31	716	40–47	M	1-month period
(1988; 1982)	67	—	35	1640	38–64	F	1-month period
Valkenburg & Haanen	51.4	22.2	—	3091	20–	M	
(1982)	57.8	30.2	—	3493	20–	F	
Magora & Taustein (1969)	—	12.9	—	3316	—	MF	8 work group
Gyntelberg (1974)	—	—	25		40–59	M	1-year period

*The sources of these data are the individual studies, cited in the bibliography by author and year.

determined by several studies. The prevalence rates vary from a low of 12.0% to a high of 35.0%. Some authors report a higher prevalence in females, but others could not demonstrate a difference. The lifetime incidence rates are higher and range from 48.8% to 69.9%. Frymoyer et al.[26] determined the lifetime incidence of LBP in 18- to 55-year-old males and subdivided the symptoms by their intensity. They found that 66.4% of this population had experienced some form of back pain. Of those who had experienced LBP, 46.3% had moderate LBP, and 23.5% had LBP that they rated as severe. The data presented in Table 5.1 have been gathered from retrospective, cross-sectional, and some prospective studies performed in the United States, Great Britain, Scandinavia, and the Netherlands. These studies allow estimates of the frequency of occurrence of LBP and its impact on society.

NATIONAL STUDIES

Information obtained from different countries is considered separately because the differing socioeconomic factors of these populations may influence the results. This is particularly true for disability data, which are significantly determined by local legal, social, and economic factors.

United States

There are 2.5 million low back-injured and about 4.8 million low back-disabled adults in the United States. Between 10 and 17% of adults have a back pain episode each year.[21,24] LBP is the diagnosis in 10% of all chronic health conditions.[38,39]

Other epidemiologic data demonstrate the importance of LBP.[9] Impairments of the back are the most frequent cause of activity limitation in persons under age 64. In subjects aged 25 to 44, LBP is the most common cause of a decrease in work capacity. An average of 28.6 days per 100 workers was lost each year, and there was an average of 9 days of confinement to bed. The rate of physician visits is second only to heart problems among chronic conditions, and back pain is the fifth-ranking reason for hospitalization. Each year 258,000 lumbar spine operations are performed, making back problems the third-ranking reason for surgical procedures.

United Kingdom

Benn and Wood[12] found that the number of sickness absence episodes per 1,000 persons was 11 for women and 22.6 for men. Wood[80] later attempted to calculate the impact of back problems on medical and social services (Table 5.2). Other surveys have shown that 25% of all working men are affected by low back disorders each year.[29] Annually, one man out of 25 workers changes his job because of a back condition. In 1979, 79,000 persons were chronically disabled.[30]

Estimating the British population at 50 million, these statistics indicate that chronic low back disability was less prevalent there than in the United States. This difference is due to short-term disability and may be the result of recording practices. On any given day, 0.05% of the work force has been chronically disabled for more than six months by a back problem,[81] which is closer to the United States figures. Wood and Badley[82] estimate that one-third of all musculoskeletal complaints in 1978 were back related, with 2.1% of the population reporting sick to work. The average absence period was 32.6 days.

TABLE 5.2
The Back Patient's Need for Medical and Social
Services (Expressed as Rates per 1,000 Persons of
Both Sexes at Risk per Year)*

	No. of subjects per 1,000 per Year
Handicapped/pension	2.0
General practitioner	20.0 (58 visits)
Referrals	9.0
Admissions	1.0
Operations	0.1
Spinal braces/corsets	7.0

*From Benn RT, Wood PHN: Pain in the back: An attempt to
estimate the size of the problem. *Rheum Rehabil* 1975;14:121.
Used by permission.

Scandinavia

In a 10-year period from 1961 to 1971, 12.5% of all annual sickness absence days were related to low back disorders. This means that 1% of all workdays were lost annually because of low back conditions.[31] The average sickness absence period was 36 days, which is quite similar to the 28.6 days for the United States and the 32.6 days for Great Britain reported in different studies. Forty percent of the low back-affected workers were disabled for less than one week, while 9.9% were disabled for more than six months. No other disease category was responsible for a greater number of days lost from work. The number of sickness absence periods in 1970 was 10 per 100 men and 6 per 100 women.[7] More recent data (from 1983) show that 10.9% of sickness absence was due to LBP.[57] LBP accounts for many cases of early retirement and disability pensions. In any given year, 25% of all new pension cases resulted from a chronic low back condition. This amounts to 12,500 new retirements per annum.

During 1983 and 1984, a prospective Swedish study analyzed all patients who were sicklisted for LBP in a district of Gothenburg containing 49,000 subjects from 20 to 65 years of age.[45] A total of 7,526 sickness absence episodes for LBP were reported over an 18-month period. Fifty-seven percent of patients recovered in 1 week, 90% in 6 weeks, and 95% after 12 weeks. At the end of a year 1.2% remained work disabled. Those with sciatica were out of work for longer periods of time than were patients who had back pain only. Recurrent pain and disability occurred in 12% over the 18-month period of observation.

Data from Finland is similar, with a prevalence of self-reported chronic back pain of 3.6% in 1964; 7.1% in 1976.[41]

Canada

Lee et al.[47] analyzed data on musculoskeletal complaints based on the 1978 to 1979 Canada Health Survey. A prevalence of 4.4% with "serious back and spine problems" was calculated. The total number of disability days exceeded 21 million, and the average sickness absence period was 21.4 days.

CROSS-SECTIONAL STUDIES

A cross-sectional epidemiologic study is one in which a population is studied at a single point in time in an attempt to evaluate all members of that population. In the past few years several cross-sectional studies have been performed. Again, because of possible influences resulting from socioeconomic conditions, these studies have been arranged by country.

UNITED STATES

Frymoyer et al.[25,26] performed a retrospective and cross-sectional analysis of 1,221 males 18 to 55 years of age who had enrolled in a family practice facility from 1975 to 1978. Almost 70% had had LBP (Table 5.1). When the data from that study were extrapolated to the 50 million working American males in the age group 18 to 55, it was calculated that 38.5 million workdays are lost annually. Patients with severe LBP had significantly more leg complaints, sought more medical care and treatment for LBP, and had lost more time from work for this reason when compared to subjects with no or moderate LBP. Sciatica-like symptoms were present in 28.9% of the males with moderate LBP and 54.5% of the males with severe LBP. Objective reports of numbness were present in 14.0% of the males with moderate LBP and 37.4% of those with severe LBP, while weakness was reported by 17.9% of those with moderate LBP and 44.0% with severe LBP. Table 5.3 shows the utilization of health care services. It is clear that a very high percentage of individuals with severe LBP required care from health care practitioners and that a variety of medical treatments was also required.

TABLE 5.3
Type of Health Care Services and Treatment Utilized by Men with Low Back Pain

	Percent Moderate (n = 565)	Percent Severe (n = 288)
Health care practitioner		
Family physician	30.5	66.7
Orthopedic surgeon	8.8	32.3
Neurosurgeon	2.7	9.5
Osteopath	7.0	23.8
Chiropractor	12.7	27.5
Physiotherapist	3.8	16.1
Other	5.0	12.1
Treatment		
Bed rest	35.1	72.8
Muscle relaxant	17.1	52.6
Prescription pain medication	21.1	58.0
Physiotherapy	9.5	23.9
Back support	11.3	37.4
Other nonsurgical treatment	12.6	27.4
Lumbar spine surgery	2.0	10.5

*From Frymoyer JW, Pope MH, Costanza MC, et al: Epidemiological studies of low back pain. *Spine* 1980;419–23. Used by permission.

Kelsey[37] sampled 20- to 64-year-olds residing in the New Haven (Connecticut) area who had lumbar x-rays taken over a two-year period for suspected herniated nucleus pulposus. She divided the sample into those with surgically confirmed herniated discs and those who had probable or possible herniated discs based on clinical signs and symptoms. She was able to define a variety of risk factors related to the diagnosis of herniated lumbar disc, as discussed further in Chapter 6.

Kelsey et al.[40] later performed another case-control study in Connecticut from 1979 to 1981 with minor methodologic modifications. The study population was 20- to 64-year-old women and men who had had x-rays and myelograms at various health centers in New Haven and Hartford. As in the previous study, they were divided into those with surgically confirmed disc herniations and those with probable or possible disc herniations. A control group of nonback patients admitted for in-hospital services was matched for sex and age. A number of possible risk factors were studied and odds ratios determined (see Chapter 6).

In 1973, Nagi, Riley, and Newby determined the prevalence rates of persistent back pain of persons between 18 and 64 years residing in Columbus, Ohio.[51] A random sample of 1,135 subjects was studied, of whom 203 (18%) reported "often being bothered with pain in the back." Of those with back problems, 62% had had a spine radiograph; 26% had worn a back support; and 4% had had back operations. The 4% who underwent surgery corresponds to the observation of Frymoyer et al.[25] that 3% of their population had had back operations.

Scandinavia

Hirsch, Jonsson, and Lewin[33] interviewed 692 women (15 to 72 years of age) from three census districts in Göteborg, Sweden, selected at random to represent the adult Swedish female population. The lifetime incidence of LBP was found in 48.8% of all women and increased with age up to 55 years, after which no further increase was noted. Svensson and Andersson[10,65-69] studied a randomized sample of 940 40- to 47-year-old men in Göteborg, Sweden. Seven hundred sixteen men were personally interviewed, and information about the remaining 234 was obtained from the Swedish National Health Insurance Office. Over their entire working lifetimes 96% of the men had been off work at some time for some disease or injury, 74% because of disease or injury to the locomotor system. Thirty-three percent of sickness absence episodes were spine related, but these constituted 47% of all sickness absence days. Total disability existed in 3.6% of the participants, and 4% had been off work more than 3 months because of LBP in the 3 years preceding the study. Forty percent had sciatica, 40% had consulted a physician, 3.5% had been admitted to a hospital, and 0.8% had been operated on because of their LBP.

The same study design was later used to survey 1,640 38- to 64-year-old women in Göteborg, Sweden.[70,71] Of these, 19% had been off work because of LBP in the preceding three-year period, 3.5% for 3 months or longer. About 2.6% of 38- to- 49-year-old women had significant work disability, whereas the corresponding percentage among 50- to 64-year-olds was 5.9. Horal[34] and Westrin[78,79] studied a random sample of subjects who in 1964 had been sicklisted for LBP by physicians in Göteborg, Sweden. They were compared to a control group matched with respect to sex, age, and sickness benefit but not previously sicklisted for LBP. Of the total group, Horal studied 212 pairs of probands and controls, and shortly thereafter Westrin studied 214 (78% of the base material). Table 5.4 shows that 95% of the probands had had LBP in the preceding 3 to 4 years and that 52% had ongoing pain at the time of the interview. In the control group, the corresponding figures were 49% and 27%, respectively. This means that once LBP is experienced, it is more likely to recur.

TABLE 5.4
LBP in Subjects Sicklisted for LBP (Probands) and in Controls*

	Probands (%)	Controls (%)
LBP previous 3–4 years	95	49
Thereof:		
Duration more than 1 week	83	21
Medication	73	6
Physiotherapy	47	3
Brace	18	1
LBP at examination	53	27

*From Westrin CG: Low back sicklisting. A nosological and medical insurance investigation. *Scand J Soc Med (suppl)* 1973;7:1.

Biering-Sorensen[13] sampled 82% of all 30- to 60-year-old inhabitants in Glostrup, Denmark. There were 449 men and 479 women. An extensive questionnaire of low back problems was administered along with objective measurements of spine function. Twelve months after the examination 99% of the study population completed a follow-up questionnaire on LBP occurring in the intervening period. The lifetime prevalence/incidence of LBP appears in Figure 5.1 along with the one-year period and point prevalence data. In general, increasing age was associated with increasing episodes of LBP. Work absence at some time was reported by 22.5% of those who had LBP, 10% had needed some job adjustment, and 63% had changed their jobs because of this symptom. Of those who had experienced LBP, 60% had consulted a physician, 25% a specialist, and 15% a chiropractor.[15] About 30% had had radiographs taken of the lumbar spine, 4.5% had been admitted to a hospital, and 1% had been operated on because of LBP.

Heliovaara et al. (1987)[32a] determined the prevalence rate of sciatica and its impact on Finnish society based on a sample of 8,000 persons representative of the Finnish population aged 30 or over. Sciatica was present in 5.3% of men and 3.7% of women. In both sexes the prevalence rates were higher in the 45- to 64-year-old group. The prevalence of definite herniated disks was 1.9% for men and 1.3% for women, whereas 0.2% of both sexes had a probable herniated nucleus pulposus (HNP). Low back syndrome other than sciatica was present in 12.5% of men and 17% of women. Disability due to lumbar disc syndrome (LDS) was estimated at 3.5% in men, 4.5% in women.

Israel

Magora and Taustein[49] performed geoethnic, psychosocial, economic, and occupational investigations on 3,316 individuals taken at random. Present and past LBP was determined. Four hundred twenty-nine (12.9%) were found to suffer from LBP at the time of the survey (point prevalence), and 92% (394) of those had pain on and off from 6 months to 11 years or more before the investigation. The majority of the subjects with LBP did not take sick leave (57.8%) and, of those who did, 29.4% had absence periods from 1 to 10 days.

The Netherlands

Valkenburg and Haanen[74] reported on a study of 3,091 men and 3,493 women 20 years of age and older performed in 1975 through 1978 in the Dutch city of Zoetermeer. A

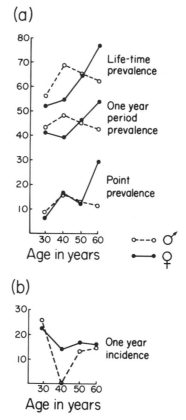

FIG 5.1.
Lifetime incidence, one-year prevalence of low back pain. (Adapted from Biering-Sorensen[13].)

questionnaire, physical examination, and radiographs were obtained. The prevalence of LBP in men and women increased slightly with age up to 65 years, and thereafter decreased (Table 5.5). Disc prolapse, defined by clinical signs and symptoms, was found in 1.9% of men and 2.2% of women. Considerable disability was attributed to LBP: 85% had recurrences; 30% had LBP for more than 3 months, and 30% had become bedridden at some point by their symptoms. Nearly half of the men and one-third of the women reported that they had been unfit to work because of LBP at some time, and 8% of the men as well as 4% of the women had changed their jobs because of LBP. Twenty-eight percent of the men and 42 percent of the women had consulted a physician for LBP.

THE INDUSTRIAL PROBLEM

Numerous reports focus particularly on the prevalence of low back pain in the workplace. Much of these data are difficult to evaluate because the work environment is highly selective.[5,8,62] Again, data are presented by country.

TABLE 5.5
Age- and Sex-Specific Prevalence Rates of LBP in the EPOZ Study*

Prevalence	Frequency in Age Groups (0/0%)							
	20	25	35	45	55	65	75	All
Men								
Lifetime	51.7	50.6	53.8	53.0	53.8	41.8	32.6	51.3
Point	22.2	19.5	20.7	23.5	23.0	26.6	17.0	15.2
Women								
Lifetime	46.0	56.1	61.1	64.9	60.0	52.7	46.4	57.8
Point	30.2	23.6	26.0	31.4	32.6	34.4	33.4	28.4

*From Valkenburg HA, Haanen HCM: The epidemiology of low back pain, in White AA III, Gordon SL (eds): *Symposium on Idiopathic Low Back Pain.* St. Louis, Mosby, 1982. Used by permission.

United States

Rowe[58,60] followed the employees at a plant in New York over a 10-year period (1956 to 1965). LBP was second to upper respiratory illness in terms of length of sickness absence period. From 35% (sitting workers) to 47% (workers with physically heavy work) of the employees had made visits to the medical department because of LBP during the study period. The yearly sickness absence per worker (all workers included) was estimated to be four hours. Recurrences were frequent, occurring in about 85%. Snook[62] has compiled data from the Liberty Mutual Insurance Company indicating annual rates of LBP for individual workers ranging from less than 1% to over 15%. Kelsey and White[39] estimates that about 2% of all employees in the United States have a compensable back injury each year.

Back problems account for 19% of all workers' compensation claims in the United States,[43] resulting in 400,000 such claims in 1978. Data from the Bureau of Labor Statistics Supplementary Data Systems were used to calculate the 1979 incidence rate of "back sprains/strains" for 26 states. The average incidence rate was 0.75%, with large interstate differences ranging from 0.15% (New Mexico) to 2.08% (Washington). Males produced 76% of all claims, and the highest rates occurred in 20- to 24-year-olds. The male-to-female risk ratio in that age group (20 to 24) was 3.0 and then decreased to 1.4 in the 55- to 64-year-old age group.

Spengler et al.[64] analyzed retrospectively work-related injuries among 31,200 employees at the Boeing Company over a 15-month period during 1979 and 1980. Nine hundred back injuries were reported (19% of all workers' compensation claims). The back injuries were responsible for 41% of the total cost. Ten percent of back injuries were responsible for 79% of the cost. Material handling was the most common cause.[17] Mechanics, maintenance and transportation employees, and clerks had the highest injury rates (3.8, 3.1, and 2.7 per 100 workers, respectively). Most injuries occurred in workers 25 years of age and younger, but those injuries were typically more benign than injuries occurring in the older population.

Canada

Abenhaim and Suissa[1] studied the one-year incidence of work-related LBP in the Province of Quebec. The incidence of low back disability resulting in work absence was 1.4% in 1981. Of those disabled, 74% were off work for less than 1 month, and 7.4% were off work for 6 months or longer and were therefore responsible for 75% of all sickness absence days. Ten percent of the absentees accounted for 75% of the total direct cost.[2] The recurrence rate at 1 year was 20%, rising to 36.3% at 3 years. Men had a higher risk of recurrence than women, and 25- to 44-year-old subjects had the highest recurrence rate.

United Kingdom

In a British survey of 2,685 male postal workers, Anderson[4] found that 23% had LBP. Seven percent of the total population were referred to the hospital for their complaint, and 2% were admitted because of LBP. The annual absenteeism from work for LBP is 70 weeks per 100 men employed, which is a very high figure.[5] Afacan[3] surveyed the medical records of 12 collieries of the National Coal Board. The study group comprised 12,125 men, 9,414 of whom were underground workers. Over one year (February 1976 through January 1977) 14.8% of the total work force was absent from work because of back injuries. The number of new sickness absences was 19.1 for every 100 men employed.

Anderson[6] analyzed cross-sectional data of 2,684 men. The prevalence of musculoskeletal complaints was 15%, whereas 25% had had musculoskeletal pain in the previous year. A cohort of 1,249 subjects with mixed jobs within a dockyard were followed for 2 years. The incidence rate of back pain was 4.5%, and 8.9% of those affected at the start had at least one episode of sickness absence due to LBP over the 2 years. In another study, Lloyd et al.[48] surveyed 359 miners and 181 office workers at a Scottish colliery. Sixty-nine percent of the miners had had LBP at some time in life, 137 (35%) during the 3 months preceding the survey. The corresponding figures for the office workers were a lifetime prevalence of 58% and a 3-month prevalence of 26%. Work loss in the 3-month period preceding the survey had occurred in 32% of miners with back pain and 14% of office workers.

Scandinavia

The prevalence of back pain in various Scandinavian industries has been reported by several investigators. Hult[35] found that 60% of a sample of Swedish males with various jobs (1,193 persons) had had back pain at some time. Four percent had been off work more than 6 months because of these symptoms, and 11% had had disability for between 3 weeks and 6 months. In the Swedish building industry Östlund[55] found that 22% had lost work time because of LBP during the preceding year, and 33.5% had received sickness allowance because of back pain at some time. Corresponding figures from the forestry industry showed an incidence of 37.5% and a prevalence of 18%.[73] A Danish study of LBP among males aged 40 to 59 report that 25% of all had LBP in the previous year, 8% severe enough to warrant bedrest or absence from work.[28]

Biering-Sorensen[16] reported the national Danish statistics on work-related injuries. Particularly high accident rates were reported for hospital work, home nursing, and patient treatment, which accounted for 42% of all injuries from 1979 to 1981.

A sample of 295 male Finnish concrete reinforcement workers were interviewed about musculoskeletal symptoms and radiologically examined.[76,77] The lifetime prevalence of LBP was 80%. In a later study based on a new sample, sciatica was significantly more common in concrete reinforcement workers than in a reference group of house painters, while "nonspecific" back pain was equally common in the two groups.[56] In a Danish study from the construction industry, Damlund et al.[22,23] found a one-year prevalence of 65% among construction workers, compared to 53% among warehouse workers.

A survey of a random sample of 764 Finnish female nurses and 453 nursing aides revealed that symptomatic sciatica and disabling sciatica had affected nursing aides significantly more often than it did qualified nurses.[75]

Other Countries

As reported previously in this chapter, Magora and Taustein[49] found prevalence rates from 6.4 to 21.6 per 100 males and females in their survey of 3,316 Israeli workers in 8 different jobs. Ikata,[36] in a study of 1,110 Japanese workers in 10 jobs, reported a sciatica prevalence rate between 5.2 and 22.4%.

COSTS

It is difficult to determine accurately the cost of work-related low back pain (LBP) because of the many variables involved. In the United States, for example, payments for direct costs of LBP comes from many sources, such as workers' compensation insurance (including federal, state, and private insurers), group and individual health insurance plans, and social security benefits. These direct costs typically include wage loss and wage replacement, medical care, temporary and permanent disability, rehabilitation expenses, and death benefits. The amount of workers' compensation payments, if any, vary according to state law, the personnel policies of the employer, and the inflationary cycles of the economy. The form of payment may be a lump sum, an annuity, or investments in rehabilitation or retraining. The requests for payments are influenced by labor negotiations, plant closings, and the general state of the economy. Finally, there are the indirect costs associated with production losses and personal suffering. These costs include loss of production, new hires, training, supervision, administration, and legal expenses.

Most of the cost information that does exist for LBP in the United States comes from the various systems of workers' compensation. Consequently, this chapter concentrates on compensation costs. It should be recognized, however, that these costs are only part of the total cost. All workers are not covered by compensation insurance, and all back injuries do not qualify for compensation payments.

Compensation Costs

Total Compensation Costs in the United States. —In a survey of 9 states that publish detailed workers' compensation statistics, back injuries averaged 21% of all compensable work injuries, ranging from 15% in Kansas to 24% in California.[11] This figure is similar to the 19.3% reported by Klein, Jensen, and Sanderson,[42] and the 22% reported by Leavitt, Johnston, and Beyer more than 10 years earlier.[44] The cost of compensable back injuries in the same 9 states, however, averaged 33% of compensation and medical costs for all occupational injuries, ranging from 26% in New York to 42% in Kansas. This figure is supported by the National Council on Compensation Insurance,[11,52] which has also estimated the cost of back injuries to be 33% of all compensation costs. Spengler et al.[64] found back injuries to be responsible for 41% of the total workers' compensation costs at the Boeing factory, which may reflect the nature of the work. In 1978, the Social Security Administration reported that the total cost of occupational injuries was $8 billion. One estimate of the total compensation costs for back pain in 1978 may be obtained by taking 33% of $8 billion—$2.7 billion.

The cost (and incidence) of back injuries in the state of California were recently estimated by Clark[20] and extrapolated to the whole country. In 1988, there were 100,540 back injuries, about 0.83 per 100 workers. These injuries respresented about 23% of all workers' compensation injuries in California and an estimated 34% of costs. Total direct costs for all injuries were $4.53 billion. This translates to $1.54 billion for back injuries alone. Extrapolated to the nation as a whole, these costs would be $13.4 billion. Indirect costs have been estimated by the National Security Council as equal to direct costs, which brings the total cost of back injuries in the United States to $26.8 billion.

Clark illustrates the difficulty in making these estimates by using other data to calculate cost. The workers' compensation insurance premiums and premium equivalents for 1988 was $9.36 billion in California or about $81 billion for the whole country. If 34% of these claims are related to back injuries, the direct cost to employers would be $27.5 billion or, assuming a 10% insurance profit, $24.75 billion. Adding $13.4 billion in indirect cost, the total bill is $38.15 billion.

Another indirect cost to industry comes from back pain that has resulted from nonwork-related injuries but that interferes with work. Clark[20] estimates the indirect cost of these injuries at $13.4 billion. This means that the total cost of low back pain to industry in 1988 in the United States may be estimated at between $26.8 billion and $56 billion. These figures are reasonably close to a 1983 estimate by the National Safety Council[54] of $31.4 million.

Another estimate of total compensation costs can be derived from the experience of the Liberty Mutual Insurance Company. Liberty Mutual has been the largest underwriter of workers' compensation insurance in the United States for almost 50 years. The company reported that in 1980 they paid $217,441,000 for compensable back pain; almost $1 million each working day.[11] Liberty Mutual represents about 9% of the insured workers' compensation market. The entire industry represents about 52% of the market, with the balance consisting of 35% for state and federal funds and 13% for self-insurers. Assuming that other insurance carriers have had the same experience as Liberty Mutual, the total annual workers' compensation costs for back pain in the United States may be estimated at $4.6 billion.

Cost per Case of Back Pain. —Table 5.6 summarizes some of the estimates of the cost per case of compensable back pain. The effects of inflation are quite evident in this data. The estimate by Leavitt, Johnston, and Beyer[44] is based upon 100 disability cases of back pain occurring in 1967. Snook's estimate is based upon 191 cases occurring in 1976.[61] Antonakes[11] based his estimate on 1978 data from the Social Security Administration and the National Safety Council. The estimate attributed to Klein, Jensen, and Sanderson[42] covers all forms of back injuries, based on reported workers' compensation claims closed

TABLE 5.6

Cost per Case of Compensable Back Pain

Year	Source	Mean Cost	Median Cost
1967	Leavitt, Johnston, & Beyer (1971)	$2,911	$404
1976	Snook (1980)	4,500	563
1978	Antonakes (1981)	6,600	—
1979	Klein, Jensen, & Sanderson (1983)	5,081	—
1979	National Council on Compensation Insurance (1983)	5,500	—

during 1979 in 5 states. The estimate from the National Council on Compensation Insurance[52] is based on first, second, and third reportings of Massachusetts cases beginning in 1979. Based on this information, Snook[63] concluded that the 1986 mean compensable back pain was about $6,000 per case, and the median cost was $750.

Two of the references in Table 5.6 show median cost per case in addition to the mean cost.[44,61] The median is the dollar value that 50 percent of the back pain cases were equal to or less than. The large discrepancy between the mean and the median indicates that back pain costs are not normally distributed. A few high-cost cases account for most of the cost. Twenty-five percent of cases were responsible for 90% of cost in the study by Leavitt et al.[44] Snook[61] found also that 25% of the cases accounted for 90% of the cost. Spengler et al.[64] reports that 10% of back injuries were responsible for 79% of cost, and Abenhaim and Suissa[1] that 10% were responsible for 75% of direct costs. The high-cost cases were characterized by greater degrees of hospitalization, surgery, litigation, and psychologic impairment.

Leavitt, Johnston, and Beyer[44] reported that medical costs accounted for only one-third of the total costs, and disability payments accounted for the remaining two-thirds (see Table 5.7). It is interesting to note that hospital costs accounted for one-third of the medical dollar in spite of the fact that only 30% of the injured were hospitalized. Physician fees also comprised one-third of the medical dollar. Two-thirds of the disability dollars went for permanent disability, with one-third for temporary disability. Antonakes[11] presented data to show that as the duration of disability for back pain increases the cost rises at an accelerating rate. Most of the added expense is for permanent partial and permanent total disability. Costs increase dramatically when surgery is performed, which in most states is accompanied by payment for permanent partial disability. For example, permanent partial payments as a result of laminectomies generally range from 10 to 25% of permanent total disability.

Cats-Baril and Frymoyer[18] used data collected in the 1982 to 1984 National Health and Nutrition Examination Survey (NHANES) II U.S. National Survey to study the influence of demographic and socioeconomic factors on low back disability. Disability prevalence increased with increasing age, with a rapid increase in the 45- to 55-year age range. The prevalence of disability was four times higher in the lowest income category compared to the highest. Disability was five times as common among those with a maximum

TABLE 5.7
Percentage of Costs by Type of Treatment and Compensation*

Back Pain Costs	%	%
Medical Costs		33
Physicians' fees	11	
Hospital costs (not including drugs or physical therapy)	11	
Diagnostic tests	4	
Physical therapy	3	
Drugs	2	
Appliances	2	
Disability		67
Temporary	22	
Permanent	45	
Total Costs		100

*Adapted from Leavitt, Johnston, Beyer[44]

eighth-grade education compared to a college education and was higher among divorced and widowed individuals. Disability was also more common in jobs where the work environment was described as unpleasant.

Clark[20] analyzed the legal costs in California. All workers' compensation litigation cost $1.3 billion in 1988. Forty-six percent of this was related to back injuries, or $0.6 billion. For the United States as a whole, this means $5.2 billion in legal costs for worker's compensation low back injuries.

The results of an assessment of more recent workers' compensation costs are summarized in Tables 5.8 and 5.9.[42] The tables are based on cost data for cases closed in 1979 in five states: Arkansas, Delaware, North Carolina, New York, and Virginia. Table 5.8 shows medical care payments for back injuries according to the nature of the injury. These figures do not include the cost of medical care provided by the employer's in-house medical personnel.

Table 5.9 lists the payments to partially indemnify workers who lost wages because of a work-related back injury. Those injuries reported as dislocated backs obviously involved the most prolonged period of disability, having an average wage indemnification cost of close to $20,000 per case.

Other Costs

According to the National Safety Council,[53] workers' compensation costs for medical care and wage indemnification represent only a portion of the total costs of occupational injuries. Some of the less obvious costs associated with occupational LBP include:

1. Medical treatment and rehabilitation provided at a plant dispensary.
2. Wages paid to other workers during the time their work was interrupted because of the injury of their co-worker.
3. Wages paid to the injured worker between the time of injury and the time when workers' compensation payments began (usually called the waiting period).
4. Wages paid to the supervisor for time spent assisting the injured, investigating the incident, preparing a report, and training a replacement employee.
5. Cost for paying full wages to a replacement worker during the learning period, when work output is lower than it would have been if the experienced worker had not been injured.

TABLE 5.8
Mean Medical Costs for Workers' Compensation Claims Closed During 1979 in Five States for Back Injuries*

Nature of Injury	Number of Reported Cases with Cost Data	Mean Cost per Case
Inflamed joint	200	$4,689
Dislocation	762	3,533
Fracture	344	1,888
Strain/sprain	11,740	470
Laceration	24	425
Contusion	578	303
TOTAL	13,648	$ 731

*From Klein BP, Jensen RC, Sanderson LM: Assessment of workers' compensation claims for back strains/sprains. *J Occup Med* 1984;26:443–448.

TABLE 5.9

Mean Indemnity Compensation Costs for Workers' Compensation Claims Closed During 1979 in Five States for Back Injuries*

Nature of Injury	Number of Reported Cases with Cost Data	Mean Cost per Case
Dislocation	2,905	$19,536
Inflamed joint	235	7,120
Fracture	848	6,710
Nerve involvement	132	5,045
Strain/sprain	33,794	3,063
Laceration	40	2,712
Contusion	1,101	1,439
Burn/scald	23	891
TOTAL	39,079	$ 4,351

*From Klein BP, Jensen RC, Sanderson LM: Assessment of workers' compensation claims for back strains/sprains. *J Occup Med* 1984;26:443–448.

6. Wages paid to clerks and others to prepare and process compensation application forms.

Such costs are often difficult to quantify. One British report estimates that back pain costs the community more than $300 million a year in lost productivity: the equivalent of the output of a British town of 120,000 people.[27] The community also loses tax revenue and community service, for example, litigation of compensation claims contributes to the overloading of the legal system.

In a study of 1,230 males Frymoyer et al.[26] were able to extrapolate that the total annual cost for work loss in this group was $11 billion. Eighty-five percent of the subjects had had no costs because of work loss, 13% incurred a cost of $4 billion, and 1.7% (the chronic group) accounted for $8 billion (75%) of the total. The most pertinent finding in Leavitt's study was that high-cost cases involved "lag time."[45] Time was lost by delays from first examination to first referral, date of injury to last day worked, delays in hospitalization, and delays in the performance of surgery. If surgery were mentioned but never performed, the patients tended to fall into a high-cost group. The high-cost group also had an average of 5.2 referrals, compared to an average of 1.6 referrals for the other lower-cost group. It is important to emphasize that the actual cost of any physician's consultation is negligible compared to the costs attendant on delays, with continued work loss. As the duration of disability increased, the chance of successful restoration of function became progessively smaller. McGill[50] found that patients whose symptoms continued and who were disabled for longer than 6 months had a 50% chance of successful rehabilitation; at 1 year this figure was reduced to 20%, and at 2 years the chances for successful rehabilitation were virtually nil.

SUMMARY

In spite of varying socioeconomic conditions among countries, there are a surprising number of similarities. Several problems exist in the validity and reliability of LBP data. For one, the main difficulty in using the national statistics is that they are based on reported information and may not truly reflect the problem. Second, classification systems vary, so that data retrieval becomes difficult, and erroneous diagnoses may be given. Third, there is a tendency to overreport severe LBP in comparison to milder forms. Social and personal factors enter the tendency to report sick. Svensson[65] found that men who had been sicklisted for LBP on average had 30% more sickness absence episodes and 70% more sickness absence days than men who had not been sicklisted because of LBP.

The reproducibility of autoanamnestic information concerning LBP has recently been estimated by Biering-Sorensen.[14] In 6- and 12-month follow-up studies he analyzed a general population of 30-, 40-, 50-, and 60-year-old men and women and a population of 20- to 68-year old male hospital porters. At an interval of about 6 months, the question of ever having had LBP was answered yes or no in a ratio of approximately 2:1, and 84% answered consistently on the two occasions. Affirmative or negative answers concerning previous lumbar spinal x-ray examination were contradicted at a one-year interval by 11%. After six months, two-fifths of the subjects reproduced their statement of age at onset of LBP within one year. The cumulative incidence curves of LBP estimated by age at onset varied systematically between the 30-year-olds and 60-year-olds, suggesting forgetful behavior. The annual risk of first-time experience of LBP was seemingly about fourfold higher during the follow-up year than during the seven preceding years.

Westrin[79] and Horal[34] studied the same group of subjects on different occasions. Most interviews took place on the same day. The concordance between the two interviewers regarding lifetime incidence was about 87%. Svensson and Andersson[66] compared their interview data to insurance data. Twenty-seven percent of men who stated that they had never had LBP in their lives had in fact been sicklisted for LBP. This means that any data on frequency of LBP must be handled with caution.

Payments to those suffering from LBP come from many sources. This complicates our determination of the total cost. This chapter has concentrated on compensation costs, which are only one small part of the total societal cost of LBP. Back injuries average 21% of all compensable work injuries but average 33% of the cost. The total compensation costs for LBP are estimated to be $4.6–13.4 billion and the cost per case, $6,000, but 25% of the cases account for 90% of the cost. As the duration of disability increases, the total costs accelerate. Medical costs account for 33% of the total cost, and disability payments make up the remainder. The total cost for low back pain to industry in 1988 is estimated between $26.8 and $56 billion.

BIBLIOGRAPHY

1. Abenhaim LL, Suissa S: Importance and economic burden of occupational back pain: A study of 2500 cases representative of Quebec. *J Occup Med* 1987; 29:670–674.
2. Abenhaim L, Suissa S, Rossignoi M: Risk of recurrence of occupational back pain over three year follow-up. *Brit J Ind Med* 1988; 45:829–833.
3. Afacan AS: Sickness absence due to back lesions in coal miners. *J Soc Occup Med* 1982; 32:26.
4. Anderson JA: Rheumatism in industry: A review. *Br J Ind Med* 1971; 28:103.
5. Anderson JAD: Back pain and occupation, in Jayson M, (ed): *The Lumbar Spine and Back Pain,* ed. 2. London, Pitman, 1980, pp 57–82.
6. Anderson JAD: Epidemiological aspects of back pain. *J Soc Occup Med* 1986; 36:90–94.
7. Andersson G, Svensson HO: Prevalence of low-back pain, (in Swedish). *Social Planerings - och Rational iseringsinstitut Rapport* 1979; 22:11.
8. Andersson GBJ: Epidemiologic aspects of low back pain in industry. *Spine* 1981; 6:53.
9. Andersson GBJ: The epidemiology of spinal disorders, in Frymoyer JW (ed): *The Adult Spine: Principles and Practice.* New York, Raven Press, 1990.
10. Andersson GBJ, Svensson HO, Oden A: The intensity of work recovery in low back pain. *Spine* 1983; 8:880–884.

11. Antonakes JA: Claims costs of back pain. *Best's Review* September, 1981.
12. Benn RT, Wood PHN: Pain in the back: An attempt to estimate the size of the problem. *Rheum Rehab* 1975; 14:121.
13. Biering-Sorensen F: Low back trouble in a general population of 30-, 40-, 50-, and 60-year-old men and women. Study design, representativeness, and basic results. *Dan Med Bull* 1982; 29:289.
14. Biering-Sorensen F: A prospective study of low back pain in a general population, I: Occurrence, recurrence and aetiology. *Scand J Rehab Med* 1983a; 15:71.
15. Biering-Sorensen F: A prospective study of low back pain in a general population, III: Medical service-work consequence. *Scand J Rehab Med* 1983b; 15:89.
16. Biering-Sorensen F: Risk of back trouble in individual occupations in Denmark. *Ergonomics* 1985; 28:51–60.
17. Bigos SJ, Spengler DM, Martin NA, et al: Back injuries in industry: A retrospective study, III: Employee-related factors. *Spine* 1986; 3:252–256.
18. Cats-Baril WJ, Frymoyer JW: Demographic factors associated with the prevalence of disability. Submitted for publication, 1989.
19. Chöler U, Larsson R, Nachemson A, et al: *Back Pain* (in Swedish). Report 188, *Social Planerings - och Rational iseringsinstitut Rapport,* Stockholm, 1985.
20. Clark WL: *Occupational Low Back Pain* (unpublished manuscript).
21. Cunningham LS, Kelsey JL: Epidemiology of musculoskeletal impairments and associated disability. *Am J Public Health* 1984; 74:574–579.
22. Damlund M, Goth S, Hasle P, et al: Low back pain and early retirement among Danish semi-skilled construction workers. *Scand J Work Environ Health* 1982; 8:100–104.
23. Damlund M, Goth S, Hasle P, et al: Low back strain in Danish semi-skilled construction work. *Applied Ergonomics* 1986; 17:31–39.
24. Deyo RA, Tsui-Wu Y-J: Descriptive epidemiology of low-back pain and its related medical care in the United States. *Spine* 1987; 12:264–268.
25. Frymoyer JW, Pope MH, Costanza MC, et al: Epidemiologic studies of low-back pain. *Spine* 1980; 5:419.
26. Frymoyer JW, Pope MH, Clements JH, et al: Risk factors in low back pain. *J Bone Joint Surg* 1983; 65:213.
27. Great Britain Department of Health and Social Security: *Working Group on Back Pain,* London, Her Majesty's Stationery Office, 1979.
28. Gyntelberg F: One year incidence of low back pain among male residents of Copenhagen aged 40–59. *Dan Med Bull* 1974; 21:30.
29. Haber LD: Disabling effects of chronic disease and impairment. *J Chronic Dis* 1971; 24:469.
30. Harris AI: *Handicapped and Impaired in Great Britain, Part 1.* London, Office of Population Censuses and Surveys, Social Survey Division, Her Majesty's Stationery Office, 1971.
31. Helander E: Back pain and work disability, (in Swedish). *Socialmed Tidskr* 1973; 50:398.
32. Heliovaara M: *Epidemiology of Sciatica and Herniated Lumbar Intervertebral Disc.* Helsinki, Finland, Research Institute for Social Security, 1988; pp 1–147.
32a. Heliovaara M, Knekt P, Aroma A: Incidence and risk factors of herniated lumbar disc or sciatica leading to hospitalization. *J Chron Dis* 1987; 3:251–285.
33. Hirsch C, Jonsson B, Lewin T: Low-back symptoms in a Swedish female population. *Clin Orthop* 1969; 63:171.
34. Horal J: The clinical appearance of low back pain disorders in the city of Gothenburg, Sweden. Comparisons of incapacitated probands and matched controls. *Acta Orthop Scand [suppl]* 1969; 118:1.
35. Hult L: Cervical, dorsal, and lumbar spinal syndromes. *Acta Orthop Scand [suppl]* 1954; 17:1.
36. Ikata T: Statistical and dynamic studies of lesions due to overloading on the spine. *Shikoku Acta Med* 1965; 40:262.

37. Kelsey JL: An epidemiological study of acute herniated lumbar intervertebral discs. *Rheumatol Rehabil* 1975; 14:144.

38. Kelsey JL, Pastides H, Bigbee GE Jr: *Musculoskeletal Disorders: Their Frequency of Occurrence and Their Impact on the Population of the United States.* New York, Prodist, 1978.

39. Kelsey JL, White AA III: Epidemiology and impact on low back pain. *Spine* 1980; 5:133.

40. Kelsey JL, Githens PB, White AA III, et al: An epidemiologic study of lifting and twisting on the job and risk for acute prolapsed lumbar intervertebral disc. *J Orthop Res* 1984; 2:61–66.

41. Klaukka T, Sievers K, Takala J: Epidemiology of rheumatic diseases in Finland in 1967–76. *Scand J Rheumatol [suppl]* 1982; 47:5–15.

42. Klein BP, Jensen RC, Sanderson LM: Assessment of worker's compensation claims for back strains/sprains. *J Occup Med* 1984; 26:443–448.

43. Klein BP, Jensen RC, Sanderson LM: Assessment of worker's compensation claims for back strains/sprains. *J Occup Med* 1984; 26:443–448.

44. Leavitt SS, Johnston TL, Beyer RD: The process of recovery: Patterns in industrial back injury. Part 1: Costs and other quantitative measures of effort. *Ind Med Surg* 1971a; 40:7.

45. Leavitt SS, Johnston TL, Beyer RD: The process of recovery: Patterns in industrial back injury. Part 2: Predicting outcomes from early case data. *Ind Med* 1971b; 40 (9):7.

46. Leavitt SS, Johnston TL, Beyer RD: The process of recovery: Patterns in industrial back injury. Part 4: Mapping the health care process. *Ind Med Surg* 1972; 41:5.

47. Lee P, Helewa A, Smythe HA, et al: Epidemiology of musculoskeletal disorders (complaints) and related disability in Canada. *J Rheumatol* 1985; 12:1169–1173.

48. Lloyd MH, Gould S, Soutar CA: Epidemiologic study of back pain in miners and office workers. *Spine* 1986; 11:136–140.

49. Magora A, Taustein I: An investigation of the problem of sick-leave in the patient suffering from low back pain. *Ind Med Surg* 1969; 38:398.

50. McGill CM: Industrial back problems. A control program. *J Occ Med* 1968; 10:174.

51. Nagi SZ, Riley LE, Newby LG: A social epidemiology of back pain in a general population. *J Chron Dis* 1973; 26:769.

52. National Council on Compensation Insurance: Detailed claim information, lower back injuries, state of Massachusetts, breakdown by class code. Unpublished data. New York, National Council on Compensation Insurance, 1983.

53. National Safety Council: *Accident Prevention Manual for Industrial Operations,* ed 7. Chicago, National Safety Council, 1974; pp 162–169.

54. National Safety Council: in Antonakes JA (ed): Cost of back pain, *Best's Review* Sept 1981.

55. Östlund EW: Personal communication. 1975.

56. Riihimäki H: Back pain and heavy physical work: A comparative study of concrete reinforcement workers and maintenance house painters. *Br J Ind Med* 1985; 42:226.

57. Riksförsakringsverket: Statistical Information Is-1. Stockholm, 1987–1988.

58. Rowe ML: Preliminary statistical study of low back pain. *J Occup Med* 1963; 5:336.

59. Rowe ML: Disc surgery and chronic low back pain. *J Occup Med* 1965; 7:196.

60. Rowe ML: Low back pain in industry. A position paper. *J Occup Med* 1969; 11:161.

61. Snook SH: Unpublished data. Hopkinton, Mass, Liberty Mutual Insurance Co, 1980.

62. Snook SH: Low back pain in industry, in White AA III, Gordon SL (eds): *Symposium on Idiopathic Low Back Pain.* St Louis, Mosby, 1982, pp 23–28.

63. Snook SH, Webster BS: The cost of disability. *Clin Orthop* 1987; 221:77–84.

64. Spengler DM, Bigos SJ, Martin NA, et al: Back injuries in industry: A retrospective study. I: Overview and cost analysis. *Spine* 1986; 11:241–245.

65. Svensson H-O: *Low Back Pain in Forty to Forty-Seven Year Old Men: A Retrospective Cross-Sectional Study.* (thesis). Goteborg, Sweden, Univ of Goteborg, 1981.

66. Svensson H-O, Andersson GBJ: Low back pain in 40–47 year old men. I: Frequency of occurrence and impact on medical services. *Scand J Rehabil Med* 1982; 14:47.

67. Svensson H-O: Low-back pain in 40–47 year old men: Some socioeconomic factors and previous sickness absence. *Scand J Rehabil Med* 1982; 14:54–59.
68. Svensson H-O, Andersson GBJ: Low back pain in 40–47 year old men. Work history and work environment factors. *Spine* 1983; 8:272.
69. Svensson HO, Vedin A, Wilhelmsson C, et al: Low back pain in relation to other diseases and cardiovascular risk factors. *Spine* 1983; 8:277.
70. Svensson H-O, Andersson GBJ, Johansson S, et al: A retrospective study of low back pain in 38- to 64-year-old women. Frequency and occurrence and impact on medical services. *Spine* 1988; 13:548–552.
71. Svensson HO, Andersson GBJ: The relationship of low-back pain, work history, work environment, and stress: A retrospective cross-sectional study of 38- to 64-year-old women. *Spine* 1989; 14:517–522.
72. Taylor PJ: Personal factors associated with sickness absence. A study of 194 men with contrasting sickness absence experience in a refinery population. *Brit J Ind Med* 1968; 25:106.
73. Tufvesson B: unpublished data. Stockholm, Swedish Work Environment Fund, 1973.
74. Valkenburg HA, Haanen HCM: The epidemiology of low back pain, in White AA III, Gordon SL (eds): *Symposium on Idiopathic Low Back Pain.* St Louis, Mosby, 1982, pp 9–22.
75. Videman T, Numminen T, Tola S, et al: Low back pain in nurses and some loading factors of work. *Spine* 1984; 9:400–404.
76. Wickström G, Hanninen K, Lehtinen M, et al: Previous back syndromes and present back symptoms in concrete reinforcement workers. *Scand J Work Environ Health [suppl]* 1978; 1:20–28.
77. Wiikeri M, Numni J, Riihimäki H, et al: Radiologically detectable lumbar disc degeneration in concrete reinforcement workers. *Scand J Work Environ Health [suppl 1]* 1978; 4:47.
78. Westrin CG: *Sicklisting Because of Low Back Pain. A Nosologic and Medical Insurance Investigation.* (thesis in Swedish). Göteborg, Sweden, Univ of Goteborg, 1970.
79. Westrin CG: Low back sicklisting. A nosological and medical insurance investigation. *Scand J Soc Med [suppl]* 1973; 7:1.
80. Wood PHN: Epidemiology of back pain. The lumbar spine and back pain, in Jayson M (ed): *The Lumbar Spine and Back Pain.* London, Pitman, 1976, pp 13–17.
81. Wood PHN, Badley EM: Epidemiology of back pain, in Jayson M (ed): *The Lumbar Spine and Back Pain,* ed 2. London, Pitman, 1980, pp 29–55.
82. Wood PHN, Badley EM: Epidemiology of back pain, in Jayson M (ed): *The Lumbar Spine and Back Pain.* London, Churchill Livingstone, 1987, pp 1–15.

PART II

Etiology

6

The Workplace

Malcolm H. Pope, Dr. Med. Sc., Ph.D.
Gunnar B.J. Andersson, M.D., Ph.D.
Don B. Chaffin, Ph.D.

INTRODUCTION

Chapter 5 detailed the magnitude of low back pain (LBP) in terms of suffering, work loss, and cost. In this chapter we consider the role of the workplace in the causality of LBP. This is extremely important because the greatest potential for LBP prevention exists in the workplace. A number of subsections consider the general relationship of LBP to physical and psychologic factors in the workplace as well as to the work environment in general. Emphasis is placed on physical work factors, specifically on work posture, lifting, pulling, pushing, and cyclic loading.

It is difficult to determine the relationship between occupational factors and low back pain because (1) low back pain is not easily defined, (2) sickness absence data are influenced not only by pain but also by physical and psychologic work factors, social factors, and the insurance system, (3) the healthy worker effect may bias data, (4) exposure is difficult to determine, and (5) there is poor relationship between tissue injury and disability. Most studies are case-control studies and, as such, do not prove causality. Modern epidemiology calculates odds ratios (risk ratios) for various factors of interest by comparing the number of exposed subjects who develop back pain to the number of nonexposed with back pain. Only a few studies have used this technique.

PHYSICAL WORK FACTORS

A few words on present injury models are useful in the discussion of the importance of specific physical work factors. A musculoskeletal injury may be triggered by a direct trauma, a single overexertion, or frequent or sustained loading. The strengths of the various tissues are influenced by such factors as age, fatigue, and concomitant disease and thus the loading level at which an injury occurs may vary greatly. In the case of direct trauma, several structures may be hurt at the same time. For example, a blow to the back may fracture vertebral bodies and at the same time cause muscular, ligamentous, and neurologic damage. In single overexertion injuries, such as from a single heavy lift, the injury usually occurs at one site only. For example, a fissure may occur in an intervertebral disc or a muscle may rupture. Repetitive loading may cause fatigue failure. Again, failure usually occurs at one location. It is important to remember here that tissue heals if given sufficient time. For example, a fatigue failure bone crack may not propagate to fracture if rest periods allow healing to occur. Temporal factors, as well as healing properties, are therefore critical to such failure. It should also be remembered that a fatigue failure injury may not become obvious until complete failure occurs and that the final event may be trivial and could occur outside the workplace.

Another mechanism of injury is sustained static loading of tissues. Interference with the circulation of blood in a muscle, and thereby with oxygen supply and removal of breakdown products, occur at contraction levels as low as 10% of maximum contraction (Chapter 2). Strong contractions rapidly become fatiguing and painful, and secondary changes may occur in the muscle. Tendons are similarly influenced by sustained tension and may necrotize, in part setting the stage for a total failure at much lower load levels than otherwise.

Heavy exertions during work are common in the United States and elsewhere. The National Institutes for Occupational Safety and Health (NIOSH[68]) have stated that approximately one-third of the U.S. workforce is currently required to exert significant strength as part of their jobs. One researcher presented the following U.S. statistics[47]:

1. Overexertion was claimed as the cause of LBP by over 60% of LBP patients.
2. Overexertion injuries of all types occur in about 500,000 workers per year (that is, in about 1 in 24 workers each year).
3. Overexertion injuries account for about one-fourth of all reported occupational injuries, with some industires reporting that over half of the total reported injuries are caused by overexertion.
4. Approximately two-thirds of overexertion injury claims involved lifting loads, and about 20% involved pushing or pulling loads.
5. Less than one-third of the patients with LBP from overexertion and with significant time loss from work eventually returned to their previous jobs.

Overexertion is also a problem in other industrial countries. Troup and Edwards[85] reviewed British statistics and found that 50,000 work injuries were caused by overexertion in 1979. Sixty-seven percent were the result of "lifting, carrying, etc.," and another 19% from pulling and pushing. Sixty-one percent of all injuries affected the back. Similar data may be found for Canada,[1,82] while data from Sweden indicates even higher injury rates.[10,67]

In a British survey of 2,685 men, Anderson[4] found that 30% had backache, 76% of whom (23% of all men) had pain in the lumbar region. Anderson also reported that 22% of the low back pain sufferers were referred to the hospital, and 6% were admitted for treatment (that is, 7% and 2% of the total population respectively). The annual rate of absenteeism from work in Great Britain is calculated to be 70 weeks per 100 male employees. Hult[43] found that 60% of 1,193 Swedish workers had had back pain at some time, with a mean yearly work absence rate of 2.93 days per 100 men. Magora and Taustein[64] found prevalence rates of 6.4 and 21.6 per 100 men and women in a survey of 3,316 Israeli workers in eight different jobs, whereas Ikata,[27] in a study of 1,110 Japanese workers in 10 jobs, reported sciatica in 5.2 to 22.4%.

Other studies indicating high prevalence rates in industrial populations include those by Wikstrom,[92] Wiikeri et al.,[91] and Riihimaki[73] among Finnish concrete reinforcement workers and Damlund et al.[32] among Danish construction workers. Videman et al.[87] found high injury rates among Finnish nurses and nursing aides, and Biering-Sorensen[14] reported similar high rates among Danish health care workers.

Despite these impressive statistics, it is often difficult to relate the workplace to the complaint of LBP in a specific worker. Rowe[76] found that only 20% of industrial LBP sufferers had recognizable trauma at the onset of symptoms. Brown[18,19] and Magora[63] have indicated that specific lifting or bending episodes account for approximately one-third of the work-related cases. Brown[19] found that another third of the cases are attributable to some other specific occupational event, and one-third have no remembered incident or work demand. Magora[63] showed that the most expensive injuries for industry are those for which there is a traumatic event associated with the onset. These events are generally identified as suddenly applied loads, slips, and falls. In a recent study of 8,000 people, Frymoyer et al.[34,35] showed that the workplace environment was related to LBP, although other factors such as personal life-style, psychologic stress, and driving were also implicated. In a separate case-control study of this population, Damlund et al.[30] indentified differences between people with and without LBP in specific lifting postures, in requirements for pushing and pulling objects, and in repetitive load-bearing requirements.

Brown,[18] Chaffin,[22] Hult,[43] Magora,[62,63] Rowe,[76] Snook,[79] and Andersson[7] have all shown some relationship between LBP and physically demanding work. Magora[63] showed that LBP sufferers are found in sedentary as well as physically demanding occupations. Video display terminal (VDT) users are particularly at risk because of the constrained postures inherent in their tasks.[54]

LIFTING

From an epidemiological perspective, the NIOSH guide[68] cites studies revealing that musculoskeletal injury rates (that is, number of injuries per worker-hours on job) and severity rates (that is, number of hours lost because of injury per worker-hours on job) increase significantly when:

1. Heavy objects are lifted.
2. The object is bulky or cannot be held close to the body while lifting.
3. The object is lifted from the floor.
4. The object is frequently lifted.

A revision of the 1981 lifting guide[68] is currently underway. It will include the same job risk factors mentioned above with the addition of asymmetry as a factor in loading of the spine while lifting. In the new NIOSH guide asymmetry is related to the degree of lateral deviation of the load away from the midsagittal plane, thus requiring some amount of twisting of the torso while lifting. Snook et al.[79,80] and Chaffin et al.[21,22] have separately identified means of determining the lifting capacity of a worker and developed guidelines. These are discussed in Chapters 12 to 14[79,80] (Chaffin et al.[21,22]). Magora[63] and Andersson, Ortengren and Schultz[6] found that when a worker exceeds his capacity, symptomatic LBP is more likely to occur. These data also suggest that the specific method of lifting may be relevant to low back complaints. Bergquist-Ullman and Larson[13] found a strong relationship between LBP caused by lifting and the duration of sickness absence.

Chaffin and Park[21] found that over a one-year period LBP was three times greater in workers who were less strong than their jobs required. This was validated in a later study (Chaffin et al.[23]). Snook, Campanelli, and Hart[80] concluded that the proper design of lifting tasks could reduce the incidence of LBP by up to one-third, but simply training workers in good lifting technique was ineffective. ("Good" lifting technique is usually defined as an erect back and squat lift posture.) Damlund et al.[30] found significant differences between pain groups (severe, moderate, or no LBP) in the way they lifted. The severe LBP group tended to lift with much more bending of the legs, whereas those without LBP tended to use various lifting techniques, depending upon the specific work situation. Lifting instructions had been given to 70% of the no-pain group, to 82.6% of the moderate-pain group, and to 92.6% of the high-pain group. Perhaps the clinical lifting instructions were faulty. Hultman, Nordin, and Ortengren[44] have shown that training must be carefully done and properly monitored to be effective. Chaffin et al.[25] stated that a short training program does have beneficial, albeit minor, effects on lifting posture. Training is no substitute, however, for poor ergonomics that restrict the choice of posture. Both theoretical and laboratory research suggest that this may be true. In a theoretical analysis Roozbazar[74] found that the bent knee 'lifting method produced less mechanical stress on the spine, but only if intraabdominal pressure (IAP) was included. In many postures IAP does not have a major role in spinal support (Gilbertson, Krag, and Pope[36]). Figure 6.1 demonstrates that the bent-leg lift may increase the moment and the disc load. Extensive investigations, particularly by the group in Gothenburg,[5,8,66] have demonstrated the relationship between various lifting postures and increased or decreased intradiscal pressures. The moment (the product of the weight and the distance from the spinal axis) rather than the lifting method has been found to be most important in affecting these pressures. A recent biomechanical study by Anderson and Chaffin[3] of five different lifting methods disclosed that the squat lift, when performed in a way that permits the object to move close to the body (between the knees), does reduce the load moment on the back compared to a stoop-lift posture. This study revealed that such a lifting technique is facilitated by having the person lift with the hands placed on opposite diagonal corners of the object being lifted. Obviously, such squat lifting is only effective when the object is small enough to fit between the knees (Chapter 2).

Long-term physiologic changes accompanied heavy lifting. Hult[43] showed the long-term heavy lifting was related to osteophyte formation. One proposed mechanism, for osteophytic formation relates to the annular bulging that occurs in lifting or bending. Fibers

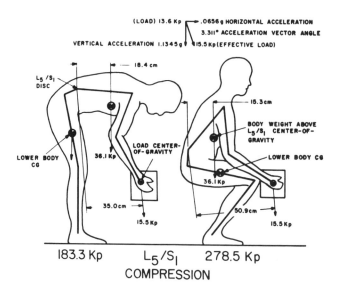

FIG 6.1.
Mathematical model showing that the bent-knee lifting method may produce a greater moment and disc load than does lifting with the back.

of the annulus attached at the disc margins are placed under tension, stimulating new bone formation at that site.[60] These osteophytes actually increase the cross-sectional area of vertebrae and may reduce disc stresses later. In that light, the osteophyte may be a physiologic adaptation to the requirement for lifting.[60] Large osteophytes, however, can interfere with motion and create stenosis.

Several investigations indicate an increase in sickness absence because of LBP as well as an increase in low back symptoms in jobs generally considered to be physically heavy. Some of those papers are summarized by Andersson[7] and in Chapters 2 and 11 of this volume. A few are discussed here. In the previously mentioned study by Hult[43] the frequency of LBP was 64.4% in subjects with physically heavy work and 52.7% in other types of work. Severe back pain was present in 6.8% of those with light physical work and 10.6% of those with heavy physical work. Differences were more pronounced when work absence was considered: 43.5% (heavy) compared to 25.5% (light) had been off work because of back pain. Lawrence[55] studied 362 workers in four jobs. LBP was found in 41% of those working in physically heavy jobs, 38.68% in miners, and 29% in subjects with light physical work. In his study of sciatica Ikata[45] reported a point of prevalence of 22.4% in heavy jobs, 5.2% in light. Magora[61] found LBP in 21.6% of subjects with heavy industrial work and 10.4% in bank employees. Klein, Jensen, and Sanderson[51] found the highest incidence rates of back sprain among workers in physically heavy jobs. Lloyd, Gauld, and Souter[57] compared miners and office workers. The lifetime prevalence of LBP was 69% and 58%, respectively.

A large study of 55 industrial jobs comprised of almost 3,000 different manual tasks was conducted by Herrin, Jaraiedi, and Anderson.[41] Various physical job stress indices were used to rank the manual exertion requirements of these jobs. The rankings were then statistically compared to both two-year retrospective medical reports and one-year prospective medical reports from the 6,900 workers on the study jobs. The resulting analyses disclosed that if the peak L5–S1 disc compression forces (predicted by the models discussed in Chapter 12) were greater than 1,500 pounds, then both musculoskeletal and overexertion medical problems were almost twice as severe. Also, if the strength requirements of the task were such that only 10% of the population could be expected to perform the most strenuous tasks (as judged by both a psychophysical and biomechanical strength analysis) the incident rates of (1) back problems were about 2.5 times greater, (2) musculoskeletal problems were about 4 times greater, and (3) overexertion injuries were almost 5 times greater, compared to the rates associated with jobs that over 90% of the population could perform.

Snook[81] found that a worker was three times more susceptible to compensable low back injury if exposed to excessive manual handling tasks. Unskilled laborers had the highest prevalence rate for disc prolapse and lumbago in the Dutch study by Valkenburg and Haanen.[86] Svensson and Andersson[83] found that heavy physical work was strongly associated with the occurrence of LBP, and the highest prevalence of LBP in their cross-sectional study was in men with professions involving physically heavy work. Chaffin and Park[21] conducted a longitudinal study that showed a threefold increase of LBP in those with isometric strength less than that required on the job. In her first study Kelsey[48] found no indication that workers with disc herniations did more lifting on the job than workers without low back pain. In a subsequent study, however, frequent lifting was a risk factor for disc herniation, and the risk increased with the heaviness of the lifts and the greater frequency with which they were performed. Twisting while lifting increased the risk further.[50] Thus, the odds ratio for frequent lifting of heavy weights while twisting was 3.4. Other investigators have concluded that physically heavy work is not associated with back pain.[16,72] The bulk of reported studies, however, clearly point in the direction of heavy physical work being a risk factor. Whether this is true for LBP causation or only for disability is presently unclear.

PULLING AND PUSHING

There is relatively little information regarding pushing and pulling activities and their role in work-related LBP. In one recent study (Damkot et al.[30]), a measure of pushing exposure was derived by multiplying the weight of pushed objects by the number of pushing efforts required each day. Significant differences were found between the LBP group and controls in the frequency of pushing activities. The controls averaged 326 weight-day units, and the severe LBP respondents averaged 1,612 weight-day units. There was also a tendency for increased severity of LBP for those with increased pulling requirements. In a theoretical analysis White and Panjabi[90] have shown that high disc loads accompany these activities. A biomechanical study by Chaffin, Andres, and Garg[24] disclosed that freely chosen postures during pushing and pulling on an isometric load cell resulted in an L5–S1 disc compression force predicted to be slightly greater than that used as a basis for the NIOSH action limit (that is, 730 pounds or 3,300 N), when the load is positioned at about 26 inches (66 cm) from the floor. Much lower compression forces and low back moments resulted when the load cell was raised to about waist height or slightly above the shoulders. In the latter posture, arm strengths seemed to limit the push and pull forces, thus protecting the back from high moments.

CYCLIC VIBRATIONAL LOADING

Many jobs expose the worker to small but repetitive loadings. In this section a distinction is made between loads derived from voluntary acts and those due to vibration. There are a variety of epidemiologic studies confirming the relationship between vehicular use and the severity of low back complaints.[26–28,33,42,49,75,78] Typically, vehicular stresses involve vibration, and vibration occurs most commonly in vehicles. Vibration may be applied to the spine in many ways. Kelsey[48] found that truck drivers were four times more likely than others to have had a disc herniation. In commuters traveling more than 20 miles per day, she found two to four times as many low back complaints and twice the incidence of herniated nucleus pulposus compared with a less frequent driving population. In a later study of significant difference in odds ratio was found between brands of cars. Buckle et al.,[20] Frymoyer, Pope, and Costanza,[34] Backman,[11] Damlund et al.,[32] and Biering-Sorensen and Thomsen[15] all report an association between driving and low back pain. Also, those who drive tractors or trucks had two to four times as many low back complaints as those who do not.[38,52,93] Pope, Wilder, and Frymoyer[70] analyzed vibration and found that many vehicles vibrate at a fundamental frequency similar to the body's natural frequency. The vibration levels of many vehicles are shown in Table 6.1, which gives the average frequency weighted acceleration meter second^2 and a time acceleration multiple (ms2 hr). The latter was computed by estimating working time per day. Obviously, this can vary enormously by time of year. The average tractor driver probably has a daily exposure that exceeds 8 hours at certain seasons but averages less than 4 hours over the year. True exposure data is needed to move toward dose-response curves. Nevertheless, the prevailing weight of evidence suggests a link between vibration and low back pain and pathologic changes to the spine.

International Organization for Standardization (ISO) standards for vibration are reproduced in Figure 6.2, along with typical vehicle vibration levels. It may be seen that many

TABLE 6.1

Vibration Exposure in Certain Vehicles

Rating	Vehicle/Environment	Freq Verified Acceleration (ms^{-2})	Time Exposure Per Day (hrs.)	Time Acceleration Multiple $(ms^{-2}$ hr.)
1.	Older military truck	2.6	6	15.6
2.	Tank	2.5	5	12.5
3.	Wheel loader	1.45	8	11.6
4.	Wheel dozer	1.4	8	11.2
5.	Grader	1.27	8	10.2
6.	Forklift	1.2	8	9.6
7.	Ship Crew	1.27	12	9.24
		.6	12	
8.	Ship Crew	2.1	12	8.4
		.6	12	
9.	Truck, building site	1.05	8	8.4
10.	Roller	1.	8	8.0
11.	Agricultural tractor	.82	8	6.76
12.	Crawler levelers	.8	8	6.4
13.	Newer military truck	1.05	7	6.3
14.	Excavator	.7	8	5.6
15.	Truck, road	.55	8	4.4
16.	Buses	.6	7	4.2
17.	Forging equipment	3.5	8	4.0
18.	Bridge crane	.45	8	3.6
19.	Locomotives	.45	8	3.6
20.	Car	.47	6	2.8
21.	Track crane	.15	8	1.2

1. 24 hour exposure included 12 hour in crews quarters partly in supine position and working time on bridge (vertical) standing.
2. As above but working time in other parts of ship (vertical) standing exposure.
3. Vertical standing exposure. Many investigators have investigated the response of the seated human subject to vibration and impact.

Adapted from Frymoyer JW, Pope MH, Costanza MC: Epidemiologic Studies of low-back pain. Spine 1980; 5:419.

vehicles exceed those standards. Studies of the effects of vibration on seated individuals demonstrate a mechanism by which LBP may occur (Chapter 2). Measuring the transmission of vibration through the body, reveals that certain frequencies are accompanied by enhanced transmission and greater energy absorption. These particular frequencies are a function of the material properties of the spine and its supportive structures. This phenomenon of enhanced transmission and energy absorption is termed resonance and represents a frequency at which there are potential destructive forces.

Figure 6.3 demonstrates measurements of transmission through the spinal column of individuals subjected to vibration in the seated posture. Note the enhanced transmission that occurs at 4 to 6 Hz and 9 to 11 Hz. Direct measurements of many vehicles reveal the dominant frequency of those vehicles to be in the 4 to 6 Hz range. In many occupations (for example, train workers) both side-to-side and fore-aft vibrations are also important.

The implication of these observations is that vehicle operators are being exposed to vibration at the resonating frequencies of their spines. It remains to be established that this effect can be responsible for spinal degeneration, but it is a convenient explanation for the greater prevalence of degenerative lesions in vehicle drivers.

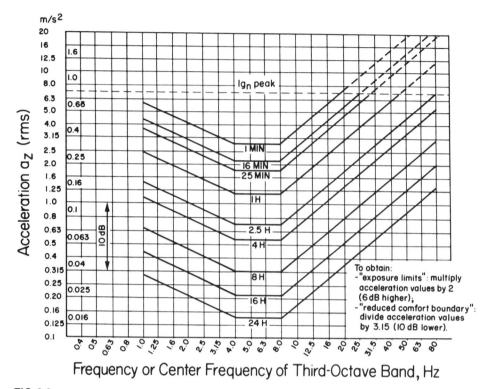

FIG 6.2.
International Organization for Standardization (ISO) standards for vibration and typical vehicular vibration levels.

Evidence also exists that vibration affects other spinal structures. Exposure to vibration leads to fatigue of the paraspinal muscles as measured by frequency shifts of the electromyography. These observations suggest that the muscles become more vulnerable and less capable of load bearing after vibration. Damlund et al.[30] stated that exposure to vehicular vibration, lifting, pulling and pushing, and vehicle-driving tasks probably combine as important risk factors for LBP. Thus, truck drivers may have a reduced capacity for material handling (Mital et al.[65]). Pope, Wilder, and Frymoyer[70] showed that cyclic loading may result in ligament fatigue and disc herniations (see Chapter 3). Workers using hand-held vibrating machinery (particularly chainsaws) are observed to have accelerated osteoporosis as well as carpal and phalangeal degenerative lesions.

Repetitive lifting imposes an entirely different stress on the tissues than vibration. Magora[61] found that repetitive lifting (5 kg or more for an average of at least 10 times per hour of the working day) was found to be related to low back pain when combined with poor technique in lifting. These data have also been confirmed by Kelsey et al.[50] for risk of disc herniation. Frymoyer et al.[35] identified repetitive heavy lifting and the use of jackhammers or machine tools as risk factors for severe low back pain. Luttmann, Laurig, and Gencoglu[58] compared the incidence of spine problems of people engaged in heavy handling and packing work to a control group not so involved. The authors showed the incidence to be significantly increased in the heavy manual handling group. Chaffin and Park[21] found increased risk of back pain in persons performing "more than 150 lifts per day." In a study on handling and transport of dustbins Luttman and colleagues[58] reported that lifting of the dustbins occurs at a rate of approximately 75 per workday. The peak compressive load on the L5–S1 segment of the lumbar spine was estimated at 6 to 8 kilo Newton (kN).[46] In the construction industry, lifting rates between one and three per minute are often reported (Luttmann and Jager [59]).

As stated earlier, mechanical damage of the spinal structure may be caused by a single overload or by mechanical fatigue after a number of load cycles. Hardy et al.,[40] for example, caused fatigue fracture of lumbar vertebrae in compression after 200 to 1,200,000 cycles. Liu et al.[56] tested motion segments in which a cyclic axial load was applied between 37 and 80% of the ultimate compressive strength of vertebral bodies. The authors noted a compression fracture below 2,000 load cycles in specimens loaded at between 60 and 80% of the mean ultimate compressive strength. Hansson, Keller, and Spengler[39] also tested lumbar motion segments under cyclic axial compressive load. The load varied between 60 and 100% of the ultimate compressive strength. Failure generally occurred between 1 and 950 cycles. Brinckmann et al.[17] tested lumbar motion segments under axial cyclic compressive load at 0.25 Hz. The load magnitude varied between 20 and 70% of the ultimate compressive strength. The probability that a motion segment would be fractured increased with increasing relative load and increasing number of load cycles. Fracture usually occurred in the end plates, but the annulus was not damaged. Liu et al.[56] investigated the effect of cyclic torsional loads on the behavior of intact lumbar intervertebral joints. Specimens that exceeded a motion range of more than $+/-1.5$ degrees failed in fatigue. Failure occurred in the end plates, facets, laminae, and capsular ligaments between 50 and 10,000 cycles. Adams and Hutton[2] cycled motion segments in axial compression and bending. The load ranged between 800 and 6,000 N at 0.67 Hz. The number of cycles

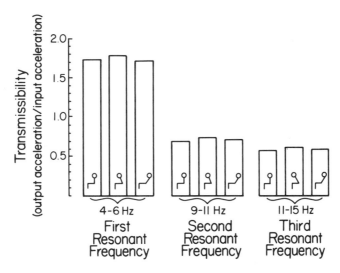

FIG 6.3.
Measurements of transmission through the spinal column of seated individuals. Transmissibility is a measure of the enhancement of the vibrational input. In this case, the vertical acceleration of the head (output acceleration) is divided by the vertical acceleration of the seat (input acceleration) to obtain the transmissibility in three seated postures.

to failure varied between approximately 2,000 and 20,000. The failure most commonly observed was an end-plate fracture, but some specimens showed a gradual disc prolapse.

In summary, there is a clear epidemiologic relationship between cyclic loading and low back pain. Spinal load moments must be reduced if loads are handled frequently or if vibration is present. It also seems clear from in vitro experiments employing cyclic loading that the safety margin between fatigue strength of vertebral bodies under axial load and in vivo loading levels is small.

POSTURE

Posture is defined as the overall positioning of the body. Several studies indicate an increased risk of low back pain in subjects who perform work in a predominantly sitting posture.[43,53,55,61,69] These studies also show an increase in back symptomology in subjects with preexisting LBP when they are required to sit for prolonged periods. Kelsey[48] found that men who spend more than half their workday in a car have a threefold increased risk of disc herniation. Whether this is caused by sitting posture or by vibration is difficult to establish in these studies. Other studies did not find seating duration to be a risk factor for LBP.[13,83,89] This may be true because sitting work is often physically lighter than production-line work. Regardless, it is important to change work posture often. Postural fatigue and sickness absence have been found to decrease when postural changes are frequent.[37,53,61]

Nachemson and Elfstrom[66] and Andersson[5] have extensively evaluated seating postures by electromyographic and intradiskal pressure methods (see Chapter 2). Their work may explain why both sedentary and other workers develop LBP. The disc pressure in a poorly designed seat is similar to that created in a worker bending 20 degrees forward. In any posture, lifting a load raises the disc pressure and muscle forces. Their work has identified optimal seating postures and seat design factors, which are discussed in Chapter 8.

Corlett and Bishop[29] have reported that other postural factors are related to muscular fatigue and LBP in the workplace. Damlund et al.[30] found significant differences in the incidence of LBP as a function of stretching versus reaching demands. Forty percent of the group without LBP and 36% of the moderate LBP group were required to stretch and reach, whereas 59% of the severe LBP group had these job requirements. Furthermore, those with severe LBP were more likely to reach out with their arms fully extended than were the other two groups.

Asymmetric postures have been associated with high disc loads.[77] This is particularly true in torsional loadings,[71] where high levels of antagonistic muscle activity lead to high muscle loads and large disc loads.

PSYCHOLOGIC WORK FACTORS

Of psychologic work factors, monotony at work and work dissatisfaction have been found to increase the risk of LBP. Monotony was primarily related to LBP in the study by Svensson and Andersson,[83] and Bergquist-Ullman and Larsson[13] found that workers with monotonous jobs requiring little concentration had a longer sickness absence following LBP than did others. Several researchers have found diminished work satisfaction to be related to an increased risk of LBP.[62,88] According to Taylor,[84] sickness absence is increased in subjects with work dissatisfaction, regardless of diagnosis. In prospective studies, Bigos et al.[16] concluded that psychologic work factors were more important than physical work factors as risk indicators for back injuries at the Boeing factory. Battié et al.[12] in prospective studies at the Boeing factory concluded that psychologic work factors were more important than physical work factors as risk indicators for back injuries.

SUMMARY

Injuries leading to LBP can occur by direct trauma, overexertion, or repetitive trauma. Overexertion is claimed as the cause of injury by 60% of LBP patients. Of these patients with overexertion injuries, 66% implicated lifting and 20% pushing or pulling. It is, however, difficult to relate the workplace to a specific worker's complaint of LBP, and LBP is found quite often in those with sedentary occupations.

Incidence, severity, and potential disability are all related to the demands on the individual in the workplace. Among the factors implicated are the requirements for lifting (particularly when compared to the worker's lifting capacity), pushing and pulling, posture, and cyclic loading. Injury and severity rates increase when load moment increases and when loads are lifted frequently. Decreasing the moment is more important than adopting a specific lifting style. Drivers of heavy vehicles have two to four times the average incidence of serious LBP. This is probably due to the cyclic loading environment. Many vehicles excite the spine's natural frequency, leading to muscle fatigue and tissue strain. Identifying these risk factors is the first step in developing the prevention strategies discussed in Chapter 13.

BIBLIOGRAPHY

1. Abenhaim LL, Suissa S: Importance and economic burden of occupational back pain: A study of 2500 cases representative of Quebec. *J Occup Med* 1987; 29:670-674.
2. Adams MA, Hutton WC: Gradual disc prolapse. *Spine* 1985; 10:524.
3. Anderson CK, Chaffin DB: A biomechanical evaluation of five lifting techniques. *Applied Ergonomics* 1986; 17:2.
4. Anderson JAD: Rheumatism in industry. A review. *Br J Ind Med* 1971; 28:103.
5. Andersson GBJ: On myoelectric back muscle activity and lumbar disc pressure in sitting postures (thesis). Gothenburg, Sweden, Univ Goteborg, 1974.
6. Andersson GBJ, Ortengren R, Schultz A: Analysis and measurement of the loads on the lumbar spine during work at a table. *J Biomech* 1980; 13:513.
7. Andersson GBJ: Epidemiologic aspects of low back pain in industry. *Spine* 1981; 6:53.
8. Andersson GBJ, Ortengren R, Nachemson A: Quantitative studies of back loads in lifting. *Spine* 1976; 1:178.
9. Andersson GBJ, Svensson HO, Oden A: The intensity of work recovery in low back pain. *Spine* 1983; 8:880–884.
10. Andersson GBJ: *Epidemiology of Spinal Disorders*. Frymoyer JF (ed): New York: Raven Press, 1990.
11. Backman A-L: Health survey of professional drivers. *Scand J Work Environ Health* 1983; 9:30–35.
12. Battié MC, Bigos SJ, Fisher L, et al: Isometric lifting strength as a predictor of industrial back complaints. *Spine* 1989; 14:851–856.
13. Bergquist-Ullman M, Larsson U: Acute low back pain in industry. A controlled prospective study with special reference to therapy and confounding factors. *Acta Orthop Scand [suppl]* 1977; 170:1.

14. Biering-Sorensen F: Risk of back trouble in individual occupations in Denmark. *Ergonomics* 1985; 28:51–60.
15. Biering-Sorensen F, Thomsen C: Medical, social and occupational history as risk indicators for low back trouble in a general population. *Spine* 1986; 11:720–725.
16. Bigos SJ, Battié MC, Fisher LD, et al: A longitudinal prospective study of acute industrial back problems: The influence of work perceptions and psychosocial factors. *Spine* 1990; in press.
17. Brinckmann P, Johannleweling N, Hilweg D, et al: Fatigue fracture of human lumbar vertebrae. *Clin Biomech* 1987; 2:94.
18. Brown JR: Lifting as an industrial hazard. *J Am Indus Hygiene Assoc* 1973; 34:292.
19. Brown JR: Factors contributing to the development of low-back pain in industrial workers. *J Am Indus Hygiene Assoc* 1975; 36:26.
20. Buckle PW, Kember PA, Wood AD, et al: Factors influencing occupational back pain in Bedfordshire. *Spine* 1980; 5:254.
21. Chaffin DB, Park KYS: Longitudinal study of low back pain as associated with occupational weight lifting factors. *J Am Indus Hygiene Assoc* 1973; 34:513.
22. Chaffin DB: Human strength capability and low back pain. *J Occup Med* 1974; 16:248.
23. Chaffin DB, Herrin GD, Keyserling WM, et al: A method for evaluating the biomechanical stresses resulting from manual materials handling jobs. *J Am Indus Hygiene Assoc* 1977; 38:662.
24. Chaffin DB, Andres RO, Garg A: Volitional postures during maximal push/pull exertions in the sagittal plane. *Human Factors* 1983; 25:541.
25. Chaffin DB, Gallay LS, Woolley CB, et al: An evaluation of the effect of a training program on worker lifting postures. *Int J Indus Ergon* 1986; 1:127.
26. Christ W, Dupuis H: Uber die Beanspruchung der Wirbelsaule unter dem Einfluss sinusformiger und stochastischer Schwingungen. *Int Z Angew Physiol Einschl Arbeitsphysiol* 1966; 22:258–278.
27. Christ W: Beanspruchung und Leistungsfahigkeit des Menschen bei underbrochener und Langzeit-Exposition mit stochastischen Schwingungen *VDI Ber* 1973; 11:1–85.
28. Christ W: Belastung durch mechanische Schwingungen und mogliche Gestunheitsschadigungen im Bereich der Wirbelsaule. *Fortschr Med* 1974; 92:705–708.
29. Corlett EN, Bishop RP: A technique for assessing postural discomfort. *Ergonomics* 1976; 19:175.
30. Damkot DK, Pope MH, Lord J, et al: The relationship between work history, work environment and low back pain in males. *Spine* 1982; 9:395.
31. Damkot DK, Pope MH, Lord J, et al: The relationship between work history, work environment and low back pain in men. *Spine* 1984; 9:395–399.
32. Damlund M, Goth S. Hasle P, et al: Low back pain and early retirement among Danish semi-skilled construction workers. *Scand J Work Environ Health* 1982; 8:100–104.
33. Dupuis H, Zerlett F: The Effects of Whole Body Vibration. Heidelberg, Germany Springer-Verlag, 1986.
34. Frymoyer JW, Pope MH, Costanza MC: Epidemiologic studies of low-back pain. *Spine* 1980; 5:419.
35. Frymoyer JW, Pope MH, Clements JH, et al: Risk factors in low-back pain: An epidemiologic study. *J Bone Joint Surg* 1983; 65:213.
36. Gilbertson LG, Krag MH, Pope MH: Investigation of the effect of intra-abdominal pressure on the load bearing of the spine. *Trans Orthop Res Soc* 1983; 8:177.
37. Griffing JP: The occupational back, in *Modern Occupational Medicine*, Philadelphia, Lea & Febinger, 1960; 219:227.
38. Gruber GJ: *Relationships Between Whole-Body Vibration and Morbidity Patterns Among Interstate Truck Drivers*. U.S. Department of Health, Education and Welfare, Publication No 77-167, 1976.

39. Hansson TH, Keller TS, Spengler DM: Mechanical behavior of the human lumbar spine. II: Fatigue strength during dynamic compressive loading. *J Orthop Res* 1987; 5:479.

40. Hardy WG, Lissner HR, Webster JE, et al: Repeated loading tests of the lumbar spine. *Surgical Forum* 1958; 9:690.

41. Herrin GD, Jaraiedi M, Anderson CK: Prediction of overexertion injuries using biomechanical and psychophysical models. *J Am Indus Hygiene Assoc* 1986; 47:322.

42. Hulshof CTJ, Veldhuijzen van Zanten OBA: Whole body vibration and low back pain—a review of epidemiological studies. *Int Arch Occup Environ Health* 1987; 59:205–220.

43. Hult L: Cervical, dorsal and lumbar spinal syndromes. *Acta Orthop Scand [suppl]* 1954; 17:1.

44. Hultman G, Nordin M, Ortengren R: The influence of an educational program on trunk flexion in janitors. *Applied Ergonomics* 1984; 15:127.

45. Ikata T: Statistical and dynamic studies of lesions due to overloading on the spine. *Shikoku Acta Med* 1965; 40:262.

46. Jager M, Luttmann A: Biomechanical model calculations of spinal stress for different working postures in various workload situations, in Corlett N, Wilson J, Manenica I (eds): *The Ergonomics of Working Postures: Models, Methods and Cases.* London, Taylor and Francis, 1986.

47. Jensen RC: Epidemiology of work-related back pain. *Topics in Acute Care and Trauma Rehab* 1988; 2:1.

48. Kelsey, JL: An epidemiological study of acute herniated lumbar intervertebral discs. *Rheum Rehab* 1975; 14:144.

49. Kelsey JL, Hardy RJ: Driving of motor vehicles as a risk factor for auto herniated lumbar intervertebral disc. *Am J Epidemiol* 1975; 102:63–73.

50. Kelsey JL, Githens PB, White AA III, et al: An epidemiologic study of lifting and twisting on the job and risk for acute prolapsed lumbar intervertebral disk. *J Orthop Research* 1984; 2:61–66.

51. Klein BP, Jensen RC, Sanderson LM: Assessment of workers' compensation claims for back strains/sprains. *J Occup Med* 1984; 2:443–448.

52. Kristen H, Lukeschitsch G, Ramach W: Untersuchung der Lendenwirbelsaule bei Kleinlasttransportarbeitern. *Arb Med Soz Med Prav Med* 1981; 61:226–229.

53. Kroemer KH, Robinette JC: Ergonomics in the design of office furniture. *Indus Med Surg* 1969; 38:115.

54. LaVille A: Postural reactions related to activities on VDU, in Grandjean E, Vigliania E (eds): *Ergonomic Aspects of Visual Display Terminals.* London, Taylor and Francis, 1980.

55. Lawrence JS: Rheumatism in coal miners: Occupational factors. *Brit J Industr Med* 1955; 12:149.

56. Liu YK, Goel VK, Dejong A, et al: Torsional fatigue of the lumbar intervertebral joints. *Spine* 1985; 10:894.

57. Lloyd DCEF, Gauld S, Souter CA: Epidemiologic study of back pain in miners and office workers. *Spine* 1986; 11:136–140.

58. Luttmann A, Laurig W, Gencoglu M: Ermittlung von Reviergrossen bei der Hausmullabfuhr unter Berucksichtigung der Beanspruchung der Beschaftigten. *Zentralblatt fur Arbeitsmedizin, Arbeitsschutz, Prophylaxe und Ergonomie* 1983; 33:49.

59. Luttmann A, Jager M: Ermittlung und Beurteilung von Korperhaltungen bei Maurertatigkeiten, in Laurig W, Gerhard L, Luttmann A, et al: *Untersuchungen zum Gesundheitsrisiko beim Heben und Umsetzen schwerer Lastsen.* Dortmund, Schriftenreihe der Bundesanstalt fur Arbeitsschutz Fb Nr 409, 1985.

60. Macnab I: The traction spur: An indicator of segmental instability. *J Bone Joint Surg* 1971; 53:663.

61. Magora A: Investigation of the relation between low back pain and occupation. *Indus Med* 1972; 41:5–9.

62. Magora A: Investigation of the relation between low back pain and occupation. IV: Physical requirements: bending, rotation, reaching and sudden maximal effort. *Scand J Rehab Med* 1973; 5:186.

63. Magora A: Investigation of the relation between low back pain and occupation. VI: Medical history and symptoms, *Scand J Rehab Med* 1974; 6:81–88.

64. Magora A, Taustein J: An investigation of the problem of sick leave in the patient suffering from low back pain. *Indus Med Surg* 1969; 38:398–408.

65. Mital MA, Ayoub MM, Asfour SS, et al: Relationhip between lifting capacity and injury in occupations requiring lifting, *Proceedings of the 15th Annual Meeting of the Human Factors Society* 1971, p 469.

66. Nachemson AL, Elfstrom G: Intravital dynamic pressure measurements in lumbar discs: A study of common movements, maneuvers and exercises. *Scand J Rehab Med [suppl 1]* 1970; 2:1.

67. Nachemson A: Report to the Swedish Department of Economy (manuscript in Swedish). 1989.

68. NIOSH (National Institute for Occupational Health and Safety): *A Work Practices Guide for Manual Lifting.* Cincinnati, Ohio, Technical Report No 81–122, 1981.

69. Partridge RE, Anderson JA: Back pain in industrial workers. *Proceedings of the International Rheumatology Congress at Prague, Czechoslovakia,* Abstract 284. 1969.

70. Pope MH, Wilder DG, Frymoyer JW: Vibration as an aetiologic factor in low back pain. Presented at the American Academy of Orthopaedic Surgery meeting. *I Mech E Proceedings* 1980; C121/80:43.

71. Pope MH, Svensson M, Broman H, et al: Mounting of the transducers in measurement of segmental motion of the spine. *J Biomech* 1986; 19:675–677.

72. Porter RW: Does hard work prevent disc protrusion? *Clin Biomech* 1987; 2:196–198.

73. Riihimaki H: Back pain and heavy physical work: A comparative study of concrete reinforcement workers and maintenance house painters. *Br J Ind Med* 1985; 42:226–232.

74. Roozbazar A: Biomechanics of lifting, R.C. Nelson and C.A. Morehouse (eds.) in *Biomechanics IV,* Univ Park Press, Baltimore; 1974, 37–43.

75. Rosegger R, Rosegger S: Arbeitsmedizinische Erkenntnisse beim Schlepperfahren. *Arch Landtechn* 1960; 2:3–65.

76. Rowe ML: Preliminary statistical study of low back pain. *J Occup Med* 1973; 5:336.

77. Schultz AB, Andersson GBJ, Ortengren R, et al: Analyses and quantitative myoelectric measurements of loads on the lumbar spine when holding weights in standing postures. *Spine* 1982; 7:390.

78. Seidel H, Heide R: Long-term effects of whole-body vibration: A critical survey of the literature. *Int Arch Occup Environ Health* 1986; 58:1–26.

79. Snook SH: The design of manual handling tasks. *Ergonomics* 1978a; 21:963.

80. Snook SH, Campanelli RA, Hart JW: A study of three preventive approaches to low back injury. *J Occup Med* 1978b; 20:478.

81. Snook SH: Low back pain in industry, in White AA III, Gordon SL (eds): *Symposium on Idiopathic Low Back Pain.* St Louis, CV Mosby, 1982.

82. Spitzer WO, LeBlanc FE, Dupuis M, et al: Scientific approach to the assessment and management of activity-related spinal disorders: A monography for clinicians. Report of the Quebec Task Force on spinal disorders. *Spine* 1987; 12(suppl 7): S1–S59.

83. Svensson HO, Andersson GBJ: Low back pain in 40–47-year-old men: Work history and work environment factors. *Spine* 1983; 8:272.

84. Taylor PJ: Sickness absence resistance. *Trans Soc Occup Med* 1968; 18:96–100.

85. Troup JDG, Edwards FC: *Manual Handling and Lifting.* London, Health and Safety Executive. Her Majesty's Stationery Office, 1985.

86. Valkenburg HA, Haanen HCM: The epidemiology of low back pain, in White AA III, Gordon SL: (eds): *Symposium on Low Back Pain.* St Louis, CV Mosby, 1982.

87. Videman T, Nurminen T, Tola S, et al: Low back pain in nurses and some loading factors of work. *Spine* 1984; 9:400.

88. Westrin CG: Low back sick-listing: A nosological and medical insurance investigation. *Acta Soc Med Scand* 1970; 23:127.

89. Westrin CG: Low back sick-listing: A nosological and medical insurance investigation. *Scand J Soc Med [suppl]* 1973; 7:1.

90. White AA, Panjabi MM: *Clinical Biomechanics of the Spine*. Philadelphia, JB Lippincott, 1978.

91. Wiikeri M, Nummi J, Riihimaki H, et al: Radiologically detectable lumbar disc degeneration in concrete reinforcement workers. *Scand J Work Environ Health* 1978; 4(suppl 1):47–53.

92. Wikstrom G: Effect of work on degenerative back disease: A review. *Scand J Work Environ Health* 1978; 4(suppl 1):1–12.

93. Wilder DC, Woodworth BB, Frymoyer JW, et al: Vibration and the human spine. *Spine* 1982; 7:243–254.

7

The Patient

Gunnar B.J. Andersson, M.D., Ph.D.
Malcolm H. Pope, Dr. Med. Sc., Ph.D.

It is important to understand which individual characteristics increase the risk for low back pain (LBP) and influence the disability from a LBP episode. Epidemiologic surveys provide the greatest insight. This chapter summarizes some of the current knowledge on individual factors and LBP. This knowledge is far from complete and frequently contradictory. Most studies are of a case-control design and, as such, are limited in terms of allowable conclusions. In many surveys there is poor definition of LBP, and the individual characteristics are often poorly (if at all) quantified. Furthermore, the statistical analyses are often univariate, so that any association found may be secondary. Associations are often expressed as p-values rather than odds ratios or risk ratios. Factors considered in this chapter include age, sex, body characteristics (anthropometry), posture, spinal mobility, muscle strength and physical fitness, and psychosocial characteristics. A sample of retrospective study findings of selected factors are given in Table 7.1.[4] Further discussion of risk factors appears in Chapter 13.

AGE

Age influences both the prevalence and incidence of LBP and of disc herniations. Although data on LBP in general lacks precision, data on the age at which disc surgery is performed are quite accurate.

The first attack of LBP usually occurs early in life.[6,8,102] Hirsch, Jonsson, and Lewin,[37] for example, found that 18% of a cross-sectional group of l5- to 24-year-old women had back pain. A comparable finding was identified in males by Hult[42] and Horal.[39] The maximum period of symptoms appears to be in the age range of 35 to 55 years, a point discussed in Chapter 4. Biering-Sorensen found that the lifetime incidence, one-year prevalence, and point prevalence increased consistently with increasing age in females. In males, the highest rates were found at age 40 and did not increase thereafter, in contrast to females, in whom a substantial increase occurred with advancing age. These differences may be caused by increasing osteoporosis in women as they get older or the tendency for men to place less physical demands on their backs after the age of 40. Hirsch, Jonsson, and Lewin,[37] on the other hand, found a gradual increase in the number of females with low back disorders until age 55. Thereafter, the incidence did not increase. Similar findings are reported from the Dutch study of Valkenburg and Haanen.[108] Svensson et al.[104] did not find significant differences between age groups when studying 38- to 65-year-old women in Göteborg, Sweden.

Most patients who have operations for disc herniations are between 35 and 45. Spangfort[98] found the mean age at operation in Sweden to be 40.8 years (41.0 years for

TABLE 7.1
A Sample of Retrospective Study Findings of Selected Individual Physical Factors Associated with Back Problems*†

	Back Pain		Herniated Disc	
	Associated	Not Associated	Associated	Not Associated
Standing ht.	Merriam et al. 1983 Lawrence et al. 1955 Tauber J, 1970 Mellin G, 1987	Pederson et al. 1975 Hult L, 1954(a) Hult L, 1954(b) Mellin G, 1987 Fairbank et al. 1984 Hirsch et al. 1969 Pope et al. 1985	Rowe ML, 1965 Kelsey JL, 1975	Kelsey JL, 1975
Sitting ht.	Merrian et al. 1983 Lawrence et al. 1955 Fairbank et al. 1984 Burwell et al. 1981	Hult L, 1954(a) Hult L, 1954(b)		
Weight	Pederson et al. 1975 Fairbank et al. 1984 Mellin G, 1987	Pederson et al. 1975 Merriam et al. 1983 Hult L, 1954(a) Hult L, 1954(b) Mellin G, 1987 Hirsch et al. 1969 Pope et al. 1984		Rowe ML, 1965 Kelsey JL, 1975
Relative wt.		Hult L, 1954(b) Pope et al. 1984		Kelsey JL, 1975
Posture		Hult L, 1954(a) Hult L, 1954(b) Pope et al. 1985		
Leg length inequality	Giles et al. 1981 Rush et al. 1946	Fisk et al. 1975 Rush et al. 1946 Hult L, 1954(a) Hult L, 1954(b) Fairbank et al. 1984 Pope et al. 1985		
Spinal mobility	Howell DW, 1984 Pope et al. 1985 Pearcy et al. 1985	Sweetman BJ, 1974 Tanz SS, 1953		
Strength	McNeil et al. 1980	Nachemson et al. 1969		
Smoking	Frymoyer et al. 1980 Frymoyer et al. 1983 Svensson et al. 1983		Kelsey JL, 1975	

*From Battié MC: *The Reliability of Physical Factors as Predictors of the Occurrence of Back Pain Reports*. Goteborg, Sweden, Acad Avhandling, 1989. Used by permission.
†Some citings appear as both "associated" and "not associated" due to differences between genders.

women, 40.7 for men). These data are shown in Figure 7.1. Spangfort's data are highly consistent with all previous reports for disc surgery from all parts of the world. It is interesting that the lumbar level involved in herniations was also age related. As seen in Figure 7.2, the incidence of L5–S1 herniations is low in juveniles, increases up to about age 35, and then decreases constantly with age, whereas the reverse pattern was found for

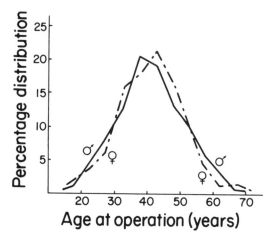

FIG 7.1.

The distribution in age groups by sex. From Spangfort EV: The lumbar disc herniation. *Acta Orthop Scand [suppl]* 1972; 142:1.

L4–L5 herniations. The incidence of lumbar herniations at the L2–L3 and L3–L4 levels increased with age (Fig. 7.3). This pattern is consistent with the evolution of disc degeneration, which starts at the L5–S1 level and then moves upward to higher lumbar interspaces. Spangfort's data are quite similar to those obtained in other countries.[36,41] The operation data are also consistent with data by Kelsey and Ostfeld[52] and Valkenburg and Haanen,[108] who studied subjects with clinically diagnosed herniated lumbar discs and in whom operations were not always performed.

GENDER

LBP seems as frequent in females as in males.[39,101,108] When the work situation is taken into account, however, the pattern changes. Magora[62] found that 35% of women in physically heavy jobs had LBP, as compared to 19.1% of males. In Sweden, women with

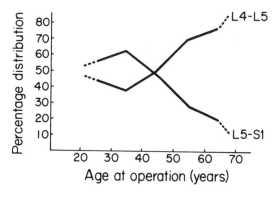

FIG 7.2.

The level of herniation in patients with complete herniations, by age at operation (percentage distribution). From Spangfort EV: The lumbar disc herniation. *Acta Orthop Scand [suppl]* 1972; 142:1.

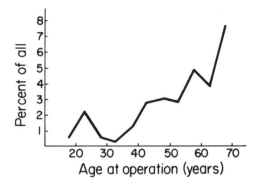

FIG 7.3.
The incidence of high lumbar herniations (above L4–L5 level), by age at operation. From Spangfort EV: The lumbar disc herniation. *Acta Orthop Scand [suppl]* 1972; 142:1.

physically heavy work have higher absence rates than do men performing the same jobs. Strength factors could be the reason for these differences. For example, mismatches between the requirements for lifting and lifting capacity may occur more often with females. Operations for disc herniations seem to be performed about twice as often in males as in females.[15,52,61,98,111] Valkenburg and Haanen,[108] on the other hand, found clinical signs of disc prolapse overall to be equal for both sexes (1.9% of males and 2.2% of females). In contrast, Table 7.2 shows that males employed as unskilled labor have a much higher risk of both prolapse and lumbago than females in similar employment.

ANTHROPOMETRY

Anthropometric data are conflicting but generally indicate that there is no strong correlation between height, weight, body build and LBP.[20,37,39,42,92,93,102] Tall people, however, have been found to have a higher than average risk of back pain in some

TABLE 7.2
Percentage of the EPOZ Population (Epidemiological Preventive Organization Zoetermeer, The Netherlands) with Clinical Diagnoses of Disc Prolapse and Lumbago*

Occupation	Men		Women	
	Disc Prolapse	Lumbago	Disc Prolapse	Lumbago
Unskilled labor	5.9	5.9	2.7	4.0
Skilled labor	2.1	3.3	2.3	4.0
Low-level employees	1.5	4.0	1.0	5.5
Intermediate level employees	0.3	3.2	0.9	4.7
Higher level employees	1.3	4.2	2.5	0.0
Self-employed	2.2	3.7	0.0	4.4
Unemployed†	2.6	4.9	2.6	5.6

*Adapted from Valkenburg HA, Haanen HCM: The epidemiology of low back pain, in White AA III, Gordon SL (eds): *Symposium on Idiopathic Low Back Pain.* St. Louis, Mosby, 1982. Used by permission.
†House-wives and pensioneers

studies.[34,60,70,105] Sitting height was found to be positively correlated by Merriam et al.,[70] Lawrence,[58] Fairbank et al.,[26] and Burwell and Fraser.[16] Ikata found sciatica to occur more frequently in the very obese,[45] but others have not confirmed this association[43,85] (see Tables 7.1 and 7.3).

Westrin[112] studied several anthropometric factors in addition to height and weight, such as lengths of tibia and femur and widths of femoral condyli and malleoli. None of these factors was related to risk of LBP. Biering-Sorensen[9] measured the femoral epicondylar width, the leg length, and the length of the upper part of the body and also calculated the so-called Röhrer's index[3] (weight in grams × 100 [height in meters]). None of these measurements had prognostic value either for the the first-time experience or for the recurrence of LBP. In a prospective study Battié found that in those without previous back problems no anthropometric measures were associated with low back pain. In those with previous problems taller men were at a slightly higher risk, as were women of higher weight or greater obesity. Heliovaara[36] found body height to be predictive of herniated nucleus pulposus (HNP) in both women and men. In tall men, the relative risk was 2.3; in tall women 3.7, compared to subjects who were at least 10 cm shorter. Riihimäki[88] found a weak correlation (risk ratio [RR] 1.7) between tallness and the lifetime prevalence of sciatica.

POSTURE

Postural deformities such as scoliosis, kyphosis, hypo- or hyperlordosis, and leg length discrepancy do not seem to predispose to LBP.[38,39,42,64,97] Scoliosis has frequently been suggested as a cause of LBP, but no hard evidence of a true association with LBP has emerged.[22,73,75] Some evidence indicates that back pain may be more prevalent when the Cobb angle of scoliosis is greater than 80 degrees, particularly when the curve involves the lumbar spine.[14,55] Kostuik and Bentivoglio[56] reviewed 5,000 intravenous pyelograms in adults over the age of 20. An increase in prevalence of back pain was found with increase in the magnitude of scoliotic curvatures. The prevalence of pain was not related to age.

The degree of lordosis or kyphosis was unrelated to LBP in studies by Hult,[42,43] Horal,[39] and Rowe.[93] Magora[64] found flattening of the spine (that is, decreased lordosis) in patients with LBP. Because loss of the lumbar lordosis was frequently accompanied by muscle

TABLE 7.3
Association of Anthropometric Variables with Low Back Pain*

| | Males with Low Back Pain | | | | | |
| | None (n = 106) | | Moderate (n = 144) | | Severe (n = 71) | | |
	Mean	SD†	Mean	SD†	Mean	SD†	Significance
Height (inches)	69.50	2.70	69.90	2.70	69.9	2.70	NS
Weight (pounds)	172.00	25.70	176.70	27.4	178.70	30.20	NS
Davenport index	0.03	0.005	0.03	0.0005	0.03	0.0005	NS

*From Pope MH, Bevins T, Wilder DG, and Frymoyer JW: The relationship between anthropometric, postural, muscular and mobility characteristics of males, ages 18–55. *Spine* 1985;10:644.
†SD = standard deviation

spasm, he concluded that the loss of lordosis caused pain rather than pain causing the lack of lordosis.

The possible association between LBP and leg length discrepancies has been the subject of several studies and much controversy. Leg length discrepancy is quite common and appears to be related to an increase of LBP in studies by Rush and Steiner[94] and Giles and Taylor.[33] Other studies have shown no correlation.[9,12,39,42,64,85,92] One of the major problems in determining the value of the leg length data is the poor accuracy of different measurement methods (including radiography).

SPINE MOBILITY

Spine motions are reduced in most subjects with back pain (Magora[64]; Pope et al.[86]). Although all motions are restricted, flexion is usually most severely affected. Bergquist-Ullman and Larsson[6] did not find decreased lumbar flexion to have any influence on the duration of a LBP episode, nor did it influence the risk of recurrence. Biering-Sorensen[9] found that reduced flexibility of the back was more pronounced in subjects who experienced recurrence of LBP in the year following examination. Battié[4] found no flexibility measures to be related to future low back pain reports. Among patients with a previous LBP history, the relatively rare finding of LBP occuring with straight leg raising was highly correlated with future LBP episodes.

MUSCLE STRENGTH

Measurements of trunk strength have been used to determine if there are differences between subjects with and without LBP. Clinical observations led Rowe[91] and Bergquist-Ullman and Larsson[6] to conclude that abdominal and spinal extensor muscle strength was decreased in patients with LBP. Many other investigators[2,3,7,35,69,74,76,77,78,80] have established that patients with LBP have lower mean trunk strength than do healthy subjects. Some investigators have found the extensors to be comparatively more influenced (weaker) than the flexors,[95] while others have identified LBP sufferers to have relatively greater extensor strength.[9,84] None of the preceding studies clarifies whether a muscle weakness or imbalance is primary or secondary to LBP. Chaffin, Keyserling, and Herrin[21,54] have used preemployment strength-testing procedures and found that the risk of a back injury increases threefold when the job requirement exceeds the strength capability on an isometric simulation of the job. In a prospective study Battié,[4] however, found that isometric trunk strength had no relationship to future low back pain reports. In the same study subjects with previous back pain were more likely to have future episodes if they had asymmetric extensor digitorum brevis bulk. The use of strength testing for preemployment purposes is discussed in Chapter 13.

PHYSICAL FITNESS

Is a physically fit individual less likely to have LBP than an unphysically fit person? Cady et al.[17] concluded from a study of Los Angeles fire fighters that physical fitness and conditioning have significant preventive effects on back injuries. A similar finding has been reported by Imrie[46] in his study of Toronto ambulance medics. Conversely, Battié,[4] in a prospective study, found no relationship between aerobic capacity and future episodes of low back pain. Dehlin et al.[24] compared physical training of nursing aides to ergonomic counseling and a control group. The physical training group did improve their conditioning and did perceive their work as less stressful. The incidence of low back problems nonetheless remained the same in all groups, but the training group recovered faster from their episodes.

Svensson and Andersson[102] found that subjects with LBP had greater physical activity at work than did those without LBP and less physical activity during their leisure time. This may be because LBP prevented or made physical activities less appealing. Bergquist-Ullman and Larsson[6] found no difference in the rates of recovery from acute LBP episodes with improved physical fitness.

Another measure of physical fitness is participation in other activities such as sports. Frymoyer et al.[31] found no difference between occurrences of LBP and a variety of sporting activities including tennis, football, baseball, downhill skiing, snowmobiling, and basketball (Table 7.4). Cross-country skiing and jogging were associated with complaints of moderate, nondisabling LBP. This particular relationship is discussed further by Frymoyer, Pope, and Kristiansen.[30] Some sports have been associated with specific structural diagnoses. Kelsey and Ostfeld[52] found that insufficient physical exercise and participation in some sports (baseball, golf, and bowling) were marginally associated with the risk for the development of a prolapsed lumbar disc. Bowlers, gymnasts, American interior football linemen, javelin throwers, and backpackers are all at increased risk for spondylolisthesis, as discussed in Chapters 1 and 3.

RADIOGRAPHIC FACTORS

The relationship between the occurrence of disc degeneration and low back pain is controversial. It is obvious from many different studies that disc degeneration per se is not symptomatic and is part of a general age process (Fig. 7.4). Back pain, however, appears to be more frequent in subjects with severe degenerative changes involving several discs.[11,18,42,60,61,65,91,92,93,107,114] In moderate or light degeneration the situation is less clear, and most literature reports that the correlation is negative.[37,39,42,44,65,99] There is evidence that disc degeneration is more frequent in individuals with heavy manual work,[42,48,61] although the nature of the stress inducing the degenerative changes is not clear.[18,50] Controversy exists in this respect, however. Magora and Schwartz[65] compared 372 subjects with back pain to 217 matched controls. They found no clear relationship between occupation and the occurrence either of degenerative changes of the disc or of the apophyseal joints. Evans, Jobe, and Siebert[25] used MRI techniques to compare 38 ambulating and 21 sedentary employees of a U.S. company. Disc degeneration was found to be significantly more frequent among sedentary than among ambulating females, whereas in the men there was no difference between the groups. This study is small, but it points to an interesting new possibility of studying the influence of work on disc degeneration.

Riihimäki et al.[89] studied the relationship of mechanical loading and lumbar disc degeneration in 216 concrete reinforcement workers and 201 house painters. Disc space narrowing occurred 10 years earlier and spondylosis five years earlier in the concrete workers. The risk for disc degeneration was 1.8, for spondylosis, 1.6. Earlier back accidents were found to increase the risk of disc degeneration significantly in a univariate analysis but not in a multivariate.

TABLE 7.4
Risk Factors in Low Back Pain*

Factors		
Risk Factors	Associated with LBP	Unassociated
Constitutional	Age Physical fitness Abdominal muscle strength Flexor/extensor balance Muscular insufficiency	Sex Weight Height Davenport index
Postural-structural	Severe scoliosis Some congenital abnormalities Narrowed spinal canal	Lordosis

Radiographic	Only specific structural abnormalities,
	   i.e., spondylolysis, fractures,
	   multilevel degenerative disk
	   disease, spondyloarthropathies
		Disk space narrowing
		Schmorl's nodes
		Spina bifida
		Osteophytes

Environmental	Smoking	

Occupational	Heavy lifting
	Vibration (vehicles and nonvehicles)
	Requirements for heavy, physical
	   lifting activity, prolonged sitting,
	   and other body postures	

Recreational	Golfing, tennis, football, gymnastics, jogging, cross-country skiing	Snowmobiling Downhill skiing Ice hockey Baseball, other sports
Psychosocial	Anxiety Depression Hypochondriasis Somatization	Psychoses and most neuroses
Other	Work dissatisfaction Multiple births in the female Some familia clustering	

*From Frymoyer JW: Helping your patients avoid low back pain. *J Musculoskeletal Med* 1984;1:65–74. Used by permission.

Videman, Numminen, and Troup[109] obtained careful occupational, recreational, and back pain histories from the relatives of 86 individuals who came to autopsy, all diseased before age 65. A history of back injury was related to the occurence of symmetric disc degeneration, annular ruptures, and vertebral osteophytosis. Symmetric disc degeneration was associated with sedentary work, and vertebral osteophytosis with "heavy" work. Obesity does not appear to be related to degenerative disc disease,[59] nor does generalized osteoarthritis.[48]

A large number of studies have been carried out to the purpose of establishing if a relationship exists between skeletal defects, congenital or acquired, and LBP. Further information on this topic appears in Chapters 3 and 11. Thus, only a short summary of some aspects is given here, as we interpret them from the current back literature. The prevalence of each defect is so small that studies are difficult to perform. Ninety-eight percent of the

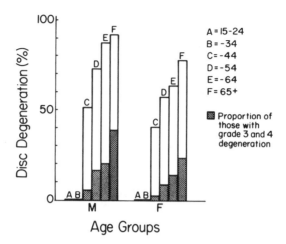

FIG 7.4.
Prevalence of radiographic disc degeneration in Great Britain. (From Lawrence JS: Disc degeneration: Its frequency and relationship to symptoms. *Ann Rheum Dis* 1969; 28:121. Used by permission.)

defects are located in the L4, L5, and upper sacral segments.[1,72] As with disc degeneration, it has been clearly established that several defects do not necessarily give rise to pain.[39,42,57,87,91,99] Some are associated with an increased risk of back pain, however.

Low back pain appears to be more common in subjects with spondylolisthesis,[27,39,42,53,67,116] but several reports indicate the opposite.[57,91,99] Scheuermann's disease and severe lumbar scoliosis are conditions in which an increased risk has often been claimed, but the association has not been clearly established.[97]

Sacralization or the presence of a lumbosacral transitional vertebra are other abnormalities in association with which an increased prevalence of back pain has sometimes been established,[79,106] but other studies have failed to confirm a positive correlation. Spina bifida occulta appears not to be more frequent in low back sufferers than in healthy controls.

Advanced osteoporosis with fractures of a macro or micro type is known to be painful. Studies of young or moderately old populations have not indicated that osteoporosis is more common in subjects with low back symptoms than in subjects without.[11,39,57]

PSYCHOLOGIC FACTORS AND PSYCHIATRIC PROBLEMS

An important consideration in any disease is the mental health of the patient as well as the psychologic adaptation to the disease process. This is certainly true in low back disease. In a comparison of back pain patients and controls, Westrin[112,113] found severe mental health problems to be no more common in the LBP group than in the controls. Psychologic factors, on the other hand, were much more common in the LBP group. A poorer intellectual capacity, less ability to establish emotional contacts, and a less sociophilic attitude were characteristics of the back pain sufferer. Several studies indicate that psychologic tests may be used as predictors of treatment and rehabilitation outcome. The most widely used test is the Minnesota Multiphasic Personality Inventory (MMPI). When the MMPI scores are elevated in hysteria, hypochondriasis, somatization, and depression, there is less likelihood of good recovery from chemonucleolysis[117] or after operative treatment for lumbar disc disease.[115] Workers' compensation recipients with such psychologic symptoms have a longer period of unemployment and less potential for reemployment.[5] After a back injury, psychologic distress is also associated with a greater restriction of the range of spinal motion.[86]

What characterizes these individuals with "poor adjustment"? Much of the research into psychological factors in LBP has divided the population into the "organic" pain patient and the "functional" pain patient.[19,23] The organic pain patient is usually defined as one with anatomic findings that could reasonably cause the symptoms reported; the patient copes well with the pain and has an appropriate degree of disability commensurate with symptoms. In contrast, the functional LBP patient exaggerates pain reports, often abuses alcohol or medications, and frequently does not respond appropriately to treatment. Physical findings are often exaggerated, a point discussed in more detail in Chapter 9. Obviously, there are problems with this dichotomy. Patients do not neatly fall into "organic" or "inorganic" categories. The present diagnostic tools do not permit physicians to diagnose accurately 50% of the population. The nonorganic or so-called functional patient is assumed to have created the pain out of a psychologic disturbance.[82] The lack of response to treatment, often after multiple unsuccessful surgeries,[71] probably causes a transformation into the chronic LBP patient, characterized by dependency and depression.[100] Since this patient population is so difficult to manage, attempts have been made to discriminate between the good and the poor surgical candidate.[13,32,47,51,81,110,117] Similarly, attempts have been made to predict the appropriately disabled from the inappropriately disabled,[62,96] the good medical management risk[68] and the good risk for acupuncture.[40] Methods used have included the MMPI, the Cornell Medical Index,[117] and other questionnaires.[28,83,118]

Some suggest that psychologic profiles may not accurately predict who is at risk for LBP.[29,90] Obviously, psychologic factors are associated with LBP and with its prognosis. Several studies have demonstrated that the MMPI of patients with poor treatment outcomes changes during the course of their illnesses.[5,32,47,68,117] Which comes first, though—the back disorder or psychologic problems? Other theories suggest that the individual prone to back pain for psychologic reasons is a passive individual who is afraid of interpersonal conflict. Therefore, the social and occupational withdrawal of the back patient is motivated by a desire to escape emotional stress in these situations. Recent Swedish studies have shown that those with the least desirable working environment are less likely to return to work.

SOCIAL FACTORS

A high incidence of social problems has been found in back patients. Their general social situation and economy is on the average less good in back patients, and many back patients suffer from drug and alcohol abuse.[63,112] Divorces and family problems are also more frequent. The educational level has been found to be low in some studies. Whether some social factors are the cause or the result of LBP is difficult to assess.

OTHER FACTORS

Smoking was identified as significantly associated with LBP episodes in Vermont,[31] Connecticut,[49] Denmark,[10] Finland,[36] and Sweden.[102] In a study of Swedish industrial workers, Svensson and Andersson[102] speculated that coughing led to increased intradiscal pressure and thus to increased spine loading and LBP. This conclusion is supported by a Danish study,[10] which identified coughing but not smoking as important in the etiology of low back complaints. The Vermont study,[31] however, indicated that coughing alone was insufficient to account for the observed differences in LBP complaints. It might be speculated that smokers have emotional, recreational, or occupational differences from nonsmokers, although multivariate analysis did not confirm that speculation.

SUMMARY

Many individual factors are associated with the incidence and prevalence of low back complaints. For convenience, these factors are summarized in Table 7.4. LBP is first experienced early in life, and the incidence increases with age. There is no increase after age 40 in males, and in females there is no increase after age 55. The highest incidence of operation for disc herniations is at age 40 for both sexes. LBP is equally common in both sexes, but women in physically heavy jobs had increased prevalence of LBP compared to males. There is little evidence that anthropometric factors such as height, weight, body build, limb length or body indices have any relationship to LBP. Postural deformities other than severe scoliosis do not predispose to LBP. Decreased mobility, particularly flexion, and decreased strength is found in those with LBP. It is not known whether these attributes are primary or secondary to LBP. The role of improved physical fitness in preventing LBP is not completely clear, although there is some evidence in favor of improved fitness. The risk of a back injury increases if the strength requirements of the job exceed the worker's strength. Disc degeneration is greater in those involved in heavy work. Osteoporosis and spondylolisthesis are both associated with increased LBP. Severe mental health problems are no more common in LBP patients, but changes in the MMPI are observed. Those with elevated MMPI scores have a poorer prognosis than those with average MMPI scores. Social problems are greater in LBP patients. LBP patients have increased exposure to smoking, but the etiology is unclear.

BIBLIOGRAPHY

1. Ad Hoc Committee on Low Back X-Rays: Low-back x-rays. Criteria for their use in placement examinations in industry. *J Occup Med* 1964; 6:373.
2. Addison R, Schultz A: Trunk strengths in patients seeking hospitalization for chronic low back disorders. *Spine* 1980; 5:539.
3. Alston W, Carlson KE, Feldman DJ, et al: A quantitative study of muscle factors in the chronic low back syndrome. *J Amer Geriatr Soc* 1966; 14:1041.
4. Battié MC: *The Reliability of Physical Factors as Predictors of the Occurrence of Back Pain Reports*. Goteborg, Sweden, Acad Avhandling, 1989.
5. Beals RK, Hickman NW: Industrial injuries of the back and extremities. *J Bone Joint Surg* 1972; 54:1593.
6. Bergquist-Ullman M. Larsson U: Acute low back pain in industry. A controlled prospective study with special reference to therapy and confounding factors. *Acta Orthop Scan [Suppl]* 1977; 170:1.
7. Berkson M, Schultz A, Nachemson A, et al: Voluntary strengths of male adults with acute low back syndromes. *Clin Orthop* 1977; 129:84.
8. Biering-Sorensen F: Low back trouble in a general population of 30-, 40-, 50-, and 60-year old men and women. Study design, representativeness and basic results. *Dan Med Bull* 1982; 29:289.

9. Biering-Sorensen F. *The Prognostic Value of the Low Back History and Physical Measurements* (thesis). University of Copenhagen, 1983.

10. Biering-Sorensen F. Thomsen C: Medical, social and occupational history as risk indicator for low-back trouble in a general population. *Spine* 1986; 11:720–725.

11. Bistrom O: Congenital anomalies of the lumbar spine of persons with painless backs. *Ann Chir Gynaecol Fenn* 1954; 43:102.

12. Björness T: Low back pain in persons with congenital club foot. *Scan J Rehab Med* 1975; 7:163.

13. Blumetti AE, Modesti LM: Psychological predictors of success or failure of surgical intervention for intractable back pain, in Bonica JJ, Albe-Fessard DG (eds): *Advances in Pain Research and Therapy,* vol. 1. New York, Raven Press, 1976. pp 323–25.

14. Bradford DS, Moe JH, Winter RB: Scoliosis and kyphosis. Operative management of idiopathic scoliosis, Rothman RH, Simeone FA (eds): *The Spine* vol 1, ed 2. Philadelphia, Saunders, 1975 pp 347–348.

15. Brown JR: Lifting as an industrial hazard. *Amer Industr Hyg Assoc J* 1973; 34:292.

16. Burwell RG, Fraser MA: An anthropometric study of patients with low back pain syndromes. Presented at the International Study of Lumbar Spine meeting, Paris, France, May 1981.

17. Cady LD, Bischoff DP, O'Connel ER, et al: Strength and fitness and subsequent back injuries in fire-fighting. *J Occup Med* 1979; 21:269.

18. Caplan PS. Freedman LMJ, Connelly TP: Degenerative joint disease of the lumbar spine in coal miners—a clinical and x-ray study. *Arthritis Rheum* 1966; 9:693.

19. Carr JE, Brownsberger CN, Rutherford RD: Characteristics of symptom-matched psychogenic and "real" pain patients on the MMPI. *Proc 74th Ann Convention Amer Psychol Assoc* 1966; 1:215.

20. Chaffin DB, Park KS: A longitudinal study of low back pain as associated with occupational weight lifting factors. *AIHAJ* 1973; 34:513.

21. Chaffin DB, Herrin GD, Keyerling WM: Preemployment strength testing. An updated position. *J Occup Med* 1978; 20:403.

22. Collis DK, Ponseti IV: Long term follow-up of patients with idiopathic scoliosis not treated surgically. *J Bone Joint Surg* 1969; 51:425.

23. Cox GB, Chapman CR, Black RF: The MMPI and chronic pain: The diagnosis of psychogenic pain. *J Behav Med* 1978; 1:437.

24. Dehlin O, Berg S, Andersson GBJ, et al: Effect of physical training and ergonomic counseling on the psychological perception of work and on the subjective assessment of low-back insufficiency. *Scan J Rehab Med* 1981: 13:1–9.

25. Evans W, Jobe W, Siebert F: A cross-sectional prevalence study of lumbar disc degeneration in a working population. *Spine* 1989; 14:60–64.

26. Fairbank JCT, Pynsent BP, Van Poortvliet JA, et al: Influence of anthropometric factors and joint laxity in the incidence of adolescent back pain. *Spine* 1984; 9:461.

27. Fisher FJ, Friedman MM, Demark RE Van: Roentgenographic abnormalities in soldiers with low back pain: A comparative study. *Amer J Roentgen* 1958; 79:673.

28. Forrest AJ, Wolkind SN: Masked depression in man with low back pain. *Rheumatol and Rehabil* 1974; 13:148.

29. Freeman C, Calyson D, Louks J: The use of the MMPI with chronic low back pain patients with a mixed diagnosis. *J Clin Psychol* 1976; 32:532.

30. Frymoyer JW, Pope MH, Kristiansen T: Skiing and spinal trauma. *Clin Sports Med* 1982; 1:304.

31. Frymoyer JW, Pope MH, Clements JH, et al: Risk factors in low back pain. An epidemiological survey. *J Bone Joint Surg* 1983; 65:213.

32. Gentry WD, Newman MC, Goldner JL, et al: Relation between graduated spinal block technique and MMPI for diagnosis and prognosis of chronic low back pain. *Spine* 1973; 2:210.

33. Giles LGF, Taylor JR: Low-back pain associated with leg length inequality. *Spine* 1981; 6:510.
34. Gyntelberg F: One year incidence of low back pain among male residents of Copenhagen aged 40−59. *Dan Med Bull* 1974; 21:30.
35. Hasue M, Fujiwara M, Kikuchi S: A new method of quantitative measurement of abdominal and back muscle strength. *Spine* 1980; 5:143.
36. Heliovaara M: *Epidemiology of sciatica and Herniated Lumbar Intervertebral Disc.* Helsinki, Finland, Research Institute for Social Security, 1988; pp 1–147.
37. Hirsch C. Jonsson B, Lewin T: Low back symptoms in a Swedish female population. *Clin Orthop* 1969; 63:171.
38. Hodgson S. Shannon HS, Troup JDG: *The Prevention of spinal Disorders in Dock Workers.* Report to National Dock Labour Board, London, 1974.
39. Horal J: The clinical appearance of low back disorders in the city of Gothenburg, Sweden. *Acta Orthop Scand [suppl]* 1969; 118:1.
40. Hossenlopp CM, Leiber L, Mo B: Psychological factors in the effectiveness of acupuncture for chronic pain, in Albe-Fessard DG, Bonica JJ (eds): *Advances in Pain Research and Therapy,* vol. 1. New York, Raven Press, 1976, pp 803–809.
41. Hrubec Z, Nashold BS Jr.: Epidemiology of lumbar disc lesions in the military in World War II. *Am J Epidem* 1975; 102:366.
42. Hult L: The Munkfors Investigation. *Acta Orthop Scand (suppl)* 1954a; 16:1.
43. Hult L: Cervical, dorsal, and lumbar spinal syndromes. *Acta Orthop Scan [suppl]* 1954b; 17:1.
44. Hussar AE, Guller EJ: Correlation of pain and the roentgenographic findings of spondylosis of the cervical and lumbar spine. *Am J Med Sci* 1956; 232:518.
45. Ikata T: Statistical and dynamic studies of lesions due to overloading on the spine. *Shikoku Acta Med* 1965; 40:262.
46. Imrie D. Personal communication, 1983.
47. Jamison K, Ferrer-Biechner MT, Brechner VL, et al: Correlation of personality profile with pain syndrome, in Bonica JJ, Albe-Fessard DG (eds): *Advances in Pain Research and Therapy,* vol. 1. New York, Raven Press, 1976, pp 317–321.
48. Kellgren JH, Lawrence JS: Osteoarthrosis and disk degeneration in an urban population. *Ann Rheum Dis* 1958; 17:388.
49. Kelsey JL: An epidemiological study of the relationship between occupations and acute herniated lumbar intervertebral discs. *Int J Epidemiol* 1975; 4:197.
50. Kelsey JL: Epidemiology of radiculopathies. *Adv Neurol* 1978; 19:385.
51. Kelsey JL, Hardy RJ: Driving of motor vehicles as a risk factor for acute herniated lumbar intervertebral disc. *Am J Epidemiol* 1975a; 102:63.
52. Kelsey JL, Ostfeld AM: Demographic characteristics of persons with acute herniated lumbar intervertebral disc. *J Chron Dis* 1975b; 28:37.
53. Kettelkamp DB, Wright DG: Spondylolysis in the Alaskan Eskimo. *J Bone Joint Surg* 1971; 53:563.
54. Keyserling WM, Herrin GD, Chaffin DB: Isometric strength testing as a means of controlling medical incidents on strenuous jobs. *J Occup Med* 1980; 22:332.
55. Kostuik JP, Israel J, Hall JE: Scoliosis surgery in adults. *Clin Orthop* 1973; 93:225.
56. Kostuik JP, Bentivoglio J: The incidence of low back pain in adult scoliosis. Submitted for publication, 1982.
57. LaRocca H, Macnab I: Value of pre-employment radiographic assessment of the lumbar spine. *Canad Med Ass J* 1969; 101:383.
58. Lawrence JS: Rheumatism in coal miners, Part III. Occupational factors. *Br J Indus Med* 1955; 12:249.
59. Lawrence JS: Rheumatism in cotton operatives. *Br J Indus Med* 1961; 18:270.
60. Lawrence JS, Molyreux MK, Dingwall-Fordyce I: Rheumatism in foundry workers. *Br J Industr Med* 1966; 23:42.

61. Lawrence JS: Disc degeneration: Its frequency and relationship to symptoms. *Ann Rheum Dis* 1969; 28:121.
62. Magora A: Investigation of the relation between low back pain and occupation. 2. Work History. *Indus Med Surg* 1970; 39:504.
63. Magora A: Investigation of the relation between low back pain and occupation. 5. Psychological aspects. *Scan J Rehabil Med* 1973; 5:191.
64. Magora, A: Investigation of the relation between low back pain and occupation. 7. Neurologic and orthopedic conditions. *Scand J Rehabil Med* 1975; 7:146.
65. Magora A, Schwartz A: Relation between the low back pain syndrome and x-ray findings. 1. Degenerative osteoarthritis. *Scand J Rehabil Med* 1976; 8:115.
66. Magora A, Schwartz A: Relation between low back pain syndrome and x-ray findings. 3. Transitional vertebra (mainly sacralization) *Scand J Rehabil Med* 1978; 10:135.
67. Magora A, and Schwartz A: Relation between the low back syndrome and x-ray findings. 4. Lysis and olisthesis. *Scand J Rehabil Med* 1980; 12:47.
68. McCreary C, Turner J, Dawson E: The MMPI as a predictor of response to conservative treatment for low back pain. *J Clin Psychol* 1979; 35:278.
69. McNeill T, Warwick D, Andersson G, et al: Trunk strengths in attempted flexion, extension, and lateral bending in healthy subjects and patients with low back disorders. *Spine* 1980; 5:529.
70. Merriam WF, Burwell RG, Mulholland FC, et al: A study revealing a tall pelvis in subjects with low back pain. *J Bone Joint Surg* 1983; 65:153.
71. Mooney V, Cairns D, Robertson J: The psychological evaluation and treatment of the chronic back pain patient. A new approach (part 2). *Orthopaedic Nurses' Assoc J* 1975; 2:187.
72. Moreton RD: So-called normal backs. *Indus Med Surg* 1969; 38:216.
73. Nachemson AL: Back problems in childhood and adolescence (in Swedish). *Lakartidningen* 1968; 65:2831.
74. Nachemson AL, Lindh M: Measurement of abdominal and back muscle strength with and without low back pain. *Scand J Rehabil Med* 1969; 1:60.
75. Nilsonne U, Lundgren KD: Long-term prognosis in idiopathic scoliosis. *Acta Orthop Scand* 1968; 39:456.
76. Nordgren B, Schek R, Linroth K: Evaluation and prediction of back pain during military field service. *Scand J Rehabil Med* 1980; 12:1.
77. Nummi J, Jarvinen T, Stambej U, et al: Diminished dynamic performance capacity of back and abdominal muscles in concrete reinforcement workers. *Scand J Work Environ Health [suppl]* 1978; 4:39.
78. Onishi N, Nomara H: Low back pain in relation to physical work capacity and local tenderness. *J Human Ergol* 1973; 2:119.
79. Paillas JE, Winninger J, Louis R: Role des malformations lombo-sacrees dans les sciatiques et les lombalgies: Etude de 1.500 dossiers radio-cliniques dont 500 hernies discales verifiees. *La Presse Med* 1969; 77:853.
80. Pedersen OF, Petersen R, Staffeldt ES: Back pain and isometric back muscle strength of workers in a Danish factory. *Scand J Rehabil Med* 1975; 7:125.
81. Pheasant HC, Gilbert D, Goldfarb J, et al: The MMPI as a predictor of outcome in low back surgery. *Spine* 1979; 4:78.
82. Phillips EL: Some psychological characteristics associated with orthopaedic complaints. *Curr Pract Orthop Surg* 1964; 2:165.
83. Pilowski I, Spence ND: Pattern of illness behaviour in patients with intractable pain. *J Psychosom Res* 1975; 19:279.
84. Pope MH: Risk indicators in low back pain. Published in special edition on "Current trends in low back pain research." *Ann Med* (Helsinki, Finland). 1989; 2195:387.
85. Pope MH, Bevins T, Wilder DG, et al: The relationship between anthropometric, postural, muscular, and mobility characteristics of males, ages 18–55. *Spine* 1985; 10:644.

86. Pope MH, Rosen JD, Wilder DG, et al: The relation between biomechanical and psychological factors in patients with low back pain. *Spine* 1980; 5:173.
87. Redfield JT: The low back x-rays as a pre-employment screening tool in the forest products industry. *J Occup Med* 1971; 13:219.
88. Riihimäki H: Back disorders in relation to heavy physical work (thesis). Helsinki, Finland, Institute of Occupational Health, 1989, pp 1–72.
89. Riihimäki H, Wickstrom G, Hanninen K, et al: Predictors of sciatic pain among concrete reinforcement workers and house painters—a five year follow-up. *Scand J Work Environ Health* 1989; 15:415.
90. Rosen JC, Frymoyer JW, Clements JH: A further look at validity of the MMPI with low back patients. *J Clin Psychol* 1980; 36:994.
91. Rowe ML: Preliminary statistical study of low back pain. *J Occup Med* 1963; 5:336.
92. Rowe ML: Disc surgery and chronic low back pain. *J Occup Med* 1965; 7:196.
93. Rowe ML: Low back pain in industry. A position paper. *J Occup Med* 1969; 11:161.
94. Rush WA, Steiner HA: A study of lower extremity length inequality. *Am J Roentgen* 1946; 56:616–623.
95. Schultz A, Andersson G, Ortengren R, et al: Loads on the lumbar spine, validation and biomechanical analysis by measurements of intradiscal pressures and myoelectric signals. *J Bone Joint Surg* 1982; 64:713.
96. Shaffer JW, Nussbaum K, Little JM: MMPI profiles of disability insurance claimants. *Amer J Psychiatry* 1972; 129:403.
97. Sorensen KH: *Scheuermann's Juvenile Kyphosis* (thesis) Copenhagen, Munksgaard, 1964.
98. Spangfort EV: The lumbar disc herniation. *Acta Orthop Scand [suppl]* 1972; 142:1.
99. Splithoff CA: Lumbosacral junction. Roentgenographic comparison of patients with and without backaches. *JAMA* 1953; 152:1610.
100. Sternbach RA, et al: Chronic low-back pain. The "low-back loser." *Postgrad Med* 1973; 53:135.
101. Svensson H-O, Andersson GBJ: Low back pain in forty to forty-seven year old men. I. Frequency of occurrence and impact on medical services. *Scand J Rehabil Med* 1982; 14:47.
102. Svensson H-O, Andersson GBJ: Low back pain in 40–47 year old men: Work history and work environment factors. *Spine* 1983; 8:272.
103. Svensson HO, Vedin A, Wilhelmsson C, et al: Low back pain in relation to other diseases and cardiovascular risk factors. *Spine* 1983; 8:277.
104. Svensson H-O, Andersson GBJ, Johansson S, et al: A retrospective cross-sectional study of low back pain in 38–64 year old women. Frequency of occurrence and impact on medical services. *Spine* 1988; 13:548–552.
105. Tauber J: An unorthodox look at backaches. *J. Occup Med* 1970; 12:128.
106. Tilley P: Is sacralization a significant factor in lumbar pain? *J Am Osteopath Assoc* 1970; 70:238.
107. Torgerson BR, Dotter WE: Comparative roentgenographic study of the asymptomatic and symptomatic lumbar spine. *J Bone Joint Surg* 1976; 58:850.
108. Valkenburg HA, Haanen HCM: The epidemiology of low back pain, in White AA III, Gordon SL (eds): *Symposium on Idiopathic Low Back Pain*. St. Louis, Mosby, 1982, pp 9–22.
109. Videman T, Numminen M. Troup JDG: Lumbar spinal pathology in cadaveric material in relation to history of back pain, occupation and physical loading. Submitted for publication, 1990.
110. Waring EM, Weisz GM, Bailey SI: Predictive factors in the treatment of low back pain by surgical intervention, in Bonica JJ, Albe-Fessard DG, (eds): *Advances in Pain Research and Therapy,* vol 1. New York, Raven Press, 1976, pp 939–42.
111. Weber H: Lumbar disc herniation. A controlled, prospective study with ten years of observation. *Spine* 1983; 8:131.

112. Westrin C-G: Low back sick-listing. A nosological and medical insurance investigation. *Acta Soc Med Scand* 1970; 2–3:127.

113. Westrin C-G: Low back sick-listing. A nosological and medical insurance investigation. *Scand J Soc Med [suppl]* 1973; 7:1.

114. Wiikeri M, Nummi J, Riihimaki H, et al: Radiologically detectable lumbar disc degeneration in concrete reinforcement workers. *Scand J Work Environ Health* [suppl 1] 1978; 4:47.

115. Wilfling FJ, Klonoff H, Kokan P: Psychological, demographic and orthopaedic factors associated with prediction of outcome of spinal fusion. *Clin Orthop* 1973; 90:153.

116. Wiltse LL: The effect of the common anomalies of the lumbar spine upon disc degeneration and low back pain. *Orthop Clin N Am* 1971; 2:569.

117. Wiltse LL, Rocchio PD: Preoperative tests as predictors of success of chemonucleolysis in the treatment of the low-back syndrome. *J Bone Joint Surg* 1975; 57:478.

118. Woodforde JM, Merskey H: Personality traits of patients with chronic pain. *J Psychosomatic Res* 1972; 16:167.

PART III

Patient Care

8

Evaluation of the Worker with Low Back Pain

John W. Frymoyer, M.D.
Scott Haldeman, M.D., D.C., Ph.D.

The evaluation of a worker with low back pain always starts with a history and a physical examination. Most workers with acute symptoms recover spontaneously in a short period of time and do not require further tests. Others with recurrent or chronic symptoms or with neurologic deficits may require imaging, electrodiagnostic, or laboratory studies. Throughout this chapter we emphasize selected use of tests based on specific indications derived from the history and physical examination, as well as the need to correlate the test results, history, and physical examination to develop a rational basis for treatment.

STANDARD MEDICAL EVALUATIONS

Medical History

A complete history should contain the following information.

Description of Symptoms.—The events surrounding the onset of symptoms should be detailed. For example, did the symptoms occur following a lifting episode? If so, what was the size and weight of the object being lifted? What was the lifting posture? Or, was there a fall? If the onset has been gradual, changes in overall health, work requirements, recreational activities, and possible contributing psychosocial factors such as job stress should be elicited.

The pain pattern should be clarified, including intensity, localization, the radiation of pain or numbness in the leg or groin, factors that accentuate the pain, such as body posture, coughing, or sneezing, and factors that relieve pain such as rest or movement and response to medications. The time of day when pain is most prominent is important information. For example, does the pain worsen through the day? This suggests mechanical low back pain. Is the pain worse when the patient first arises in the morning and then improves during the day? This suggests a spondyloarthropathy. Is the pain most severe at night? Does it awaken the worker? These are signs of a possible tumor or infections.[7]

Neurologic symptoms associated with the low back episode should be identified, including sensory changes (numbness, tingling), subjective sense of lower-extremity muscular weakness in coordination of the lower extremities, and changes in bladder and bowel control or sexual function.

History of Prior Episodes.—If the worker has had previous low back pain episodes, information should be elicited regarding these episodes to determine such things as causative factors, pain patterns, and factors that relieve or accentuate the pain. The success or failure of a particular treatment, including surgery, as well as the frequency and duration of disability are important predictors of response to current treatment[21] and risk for future disability.

Associated Symptoms and Diseases.—A general inquiry should be made into the patient's overall health. This includes significant medical diseases such as diabetes or vascular disease, prior surgery, and the relationship, if any, of low back symptoms to bodily function, such as bladder and bowel habits and menstrual periods in the female.

Drug Use and Abuse.—The current use of drugs of any type should be understood because of the possible adverse reactions of certain drugs when used in combination. Because the abuse of narcotics is a prevalent problem, this information should be sought but may be difficult to elicit. Intravenous use of illegal drugs is an important source of infection and attempts should be made to determine any such habits.

Functional Assessment.—Functional assessment should include a determination of the activities of daily living. Has the pain affected not only work but recreational activities? Does the worker have any knowledge about his spine, for example, has he attended a low back school?

At the completion of the history, the clinician should have created a plausible differential diagnosis and identified areas that will be of major concern during the physical examination, determined the probable need for further diagnostic studies, and have obtained some information about the possible risk for disability. A variety of forms exist to collect the information, one of which is shown in Table 8.1.

The Reporting of the History in an Injured Worker

Besides the history obtained in all back pain patients, an additional history must be obtained in the injured worker. Unlike the majority of patients who seek care for low back pain, injured workers are involved to some extent in a situation with legal implications. Injured workers who recover completely may never be questioned and may receive all benefits without difficulties. It is the responsibility of the physician, however, to present the facts surrounding an injury so that they can be interpreted by an employer, insurance agent, or attorney. The following five pieces of information must be clearly differentiated in the history. We place them here to reemphasize their importance.

Preinjury Activities and Occupational Requirements.—There should be a description of the normal daily activities the injured worker was capable of performing, including sports and recreational activities but, more important, job requirements for sitting, standing, bending, lifting, carrying, pushing, reaching, or pulling. Without this information, the clinician cannot estimate when an injured worker could return to work.

Preinjury Status.—This is primarily a discussion of prior injuries to the same areas, with a discussion of prior treatment and periods of disability. It is also necessary to know whether the worker was already having a degree of back pain and had some preexisting impairment of functional capacity. Some understanding of unrelated preexisting impairments helps a physician answer questions as to apportionment of an impairment and how the injury affected a worker's ability to return to normal employment.

TABLE 8.1
Data Collection Form for LBP.

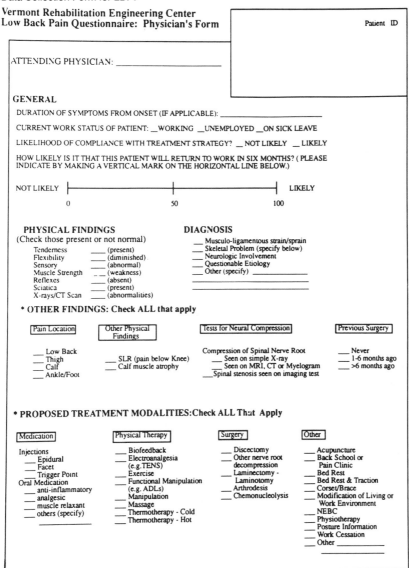

Vermont Rehabilitation Engineering Center
Low Back Pain Questionnaire: Physician's Form

Patient ID

ATTENDING PHYSICIAN: _____

GENERAL

DURATION OF SYMPTOMS FROM ONSET (IF APPLICABLE): _____

CURRENT WORK STATUS OF PATIENT: __WORKING __UNEMPLOYED __ON SICK LEAVE

LIKELIHOOD OF COMPLIANCE WITH TREATMENT STRATEGY? __ NOT LIKELY __ LIKELY

HOW LIKELY IS IT THAT THIS PATIENT WILL RETURN TO WORK IN SIX MONTHS? (PLEASE INDICATE BY MAKING A VERTICAL MARK ON THE HORIZONTAL LINE BELOW.)

NOT LIKELY |————————————|————————————| LIKELY

0   50   100

PHYSICAL FINDINGS
(Check those present or not normal)

Tenderness	____ (present)
Flexibility	____ (diminished)
Sensory	____ (abnormal)
Muscle Strength	____ (weakness)
Reflexes	____ (absent)
Sciatica	____ (present)
X-rays/CT Scan	____ (abnormalities)

DIAGNOSIS

____ Musculo-ligamentous strain/sprain
____ Skeletal Problem (specify below)
____ Neurologic Involvement
____ Questionable Etiology
____ Other (specify) _____
_____

* OTHER FINDINGS: Check ALL that apply

Pain Location	Other Physical Findings	Tests for Neural Compression	Previous Surgery
___ Low Back		Compression of Spinal Nerve Root	___ Never
___ Thigh	___ SLR (pain below Knee)	___ Seen on simple X-ray	___ 1-6 months ago
___ Calf	___ Calf muscle atrophy	___ Seen on MRI, CT or Myelogram	___ >6 months ago
___ Ankle/Foot		___Spinal stenosis seen on imaging test	

* PROPOSED TREATMENT MODALITIES:Check ALL That Apply

Medication	Physical Therapy	Surgery	Other
Injections	___ Biofeedback	___ Discectomy	___ Acupuncture
___ Epidural	___ Electroanalgesia	___ Other nerve root	___ Back School or
___ Facet	(e.g.TENS)	decompression	Pain Clinic
___ Trigger Point	___ Exercise	___ Laminectomy -	___ Bed Rest
Oral Medication	___ Functional Manipulation	Laminotomy	___ Bed Rest & Traction
___ anti-inflammatory	(e.g. ADLs)	___ Arthrodesis	___ Corset/Brace
___ analgesic	___ Manipulation	___ Chemonucleolysis	___ Modification of Living or
___ muscle relaxant	___ Massage		Work Environment
___ others (specify)	___ Thermotherapy - Cold		___ NEBC
_____	___ Thermotherapy - Hot		___ Physiotherapy
			___ Posture Information
			___ Work Cessation
			___ Other _____
			_____

Description of Injury.—Apart from the standard information as to whether it was a twist, lift, or fall type of injury, many workers' compensation forms require information as to the location and time of injury and whether it was perceived to be due to defective equipment or negligence by another worker. Such information allows an employer to look into and correct any dangerous area in the workplace.

Postinjury Treatment.—Where possible, a list of each physician consulted, each test performed, and the exact nature of any therapy, medication, or other treatment should be obtained. This may reduce unnecessary duplication of diagnostic and treatment procedures. Often, records may then be obtained that provide further information on the injured worker's diagnosis and response to care. Attempts to return to work and the tolerance of the patient to such attempts are useful in determining whether the worker will be able to return to the normal occupation.

Current Status.—The exact status of the injured worker at the time of consultation is important. Is the worker still under treatment or anticipating treatment? Are the symptoms stable, improving, or getting worse? Is the injured worker working in the normal occupation or some other occupation?

Physical Examination

The physical examination consists of inspection, measurements, palpation, percussion, and specialized tests. It is useful to develop a system for the examination because it reduces the time involved, is least likely to aggravate the symptoms, and ensures a complete evaluation. A flowchart is suggested in Table 8.2. Modifications of this format may be required as a function of the worker's ability to stand, move, and sit.

Standing Posture.—Body movements, gait, and standing posture indicate the immediate severity of symptoms and give an estimate of functional limitations. A normal, unguarded gait and posture implies symptoms of minimal severity, whereas a guarded gait accompanied by postural disturbances, such as scoliosis, usually indicates that the symptoms are severe. The ability of a patient to hop, squat, walk in tandem, and stand in place (the Romberg test) measures balance and coordination.

Range of Motion.—The pelvis should be controlled by the examiner (Fig. 8.1), while the range of flexion-extension, lateral bend, and axial rotation are observed. The pattern of motion is important as well as its magnitude. Sometimes a break in the progression of a smooth arc of motion occurs, often accompanied by flattening of the lumbar spine. This phenomenon typically occurs during flexion or extension and is sometimes called the instability catch. The motions in the various planes can be quantified by measuring devices, presented in Chapter 16.

Chest expansion may also be measured. Reductions below 1.5 cm suggest spondyloarthropathies.[7]

Gross Muscle Strength.—The worker is instructed to walk on heels and toes. Ability to perform these tasks suggest intact function of the L5 and S1 nerve roots. Quadriceps function (L2, L3, and L4 roots) may be assessed by asking the individual to either squat and rise or to climb up and down from a chair, leading first with the right and then with the left leg.

Supine Examination.—A systematic examination should include abdominal palpation for tenderness or masses. Evaluation of the peripheral pulses (groin, back of the knee, dorsum of the foot) may also be done at this time if a vascular lesion is suspected. Patients who are not responding to treatment for acute low back pain or who have chronic complaints should have a breast and pelvic examination (female) or a rectal examination (male). Examination of the lower extremities is used to determine the presence or absence of any significant joint deformities and to assess neurologic function. Measurement of leg length and atrophy

TABLE 8.2
Flowchart for the Examination of the LB Injured Worker.

Patient Standing	Posture	Scoliosis
		Lordosis—kyphosis
		Muscle spasm
	Gait	
	Range of motion	Flexion
		Extension
		Lateral bend
		Axial rotation
	Screening muscle strength test	Heel-toe walk
		Quads test (stairs)
Patient Recumbent (supine)	Measurements	Circumferences
		Leg length
	Neurologic exam	Reflex Ankle jerk
		Knee jerk
		Posterior tibial
		Sensation
		Muscle strength
	Nerve tension signs	Hip ROM
		Straight leg raising
		Confirmatory tests
		Abdominal exam
		Peripheral pulses
Recumbent (prone)	Neurologic	Complete sensation including perineum
		Femoral stretch test
	Palpation	Muscle spasm
		Spinous processes
		Interspinous spaces
		Sacroiliac joints
Seated	Observation	Seated posture
	Neurologic	"Flip test"
		Confusional SLR
Ancillary		Rectal
		Pelvic exam (female)

Source: The authors of this chapter.

should be included. As illustrated in Figure 8.2, we use a simple method for determining the level of circumferential measurement of the thigh and calf. Small differences in circumference (less than 1 cm) have little meaning because of measurement error. Hip motion should also be evaluated.

Neurologic Examination.—A neurologic examination may be done throughout the examination and in all positions. Coordination of the extremities, the evaluation of gait for weakness, and the manner in which the patient moves on the examination table give

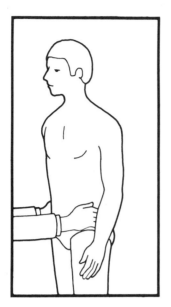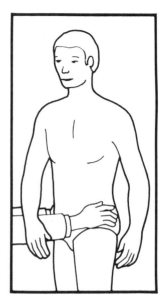

FIG 8.1.
Motion may be measured in flexion, extension, lateral bend, and axial rotation. The examiner should place hands on the pelvic girdle to control these motions, particularly axial rotation and lateral bend.

important neurological information. Knee (quadriceps) and ankle (Achilles) reflexes may be obtained in either the sitting or supine positions. In some patients, the posterior tibial or adductor reflex may be elicited. The posterior tibial reflex is present bilaterally in approximately 40 to 50% of normal subjects.[11] Thus, the bilateral absence of the reflex has no meaning. Sensation is determined by means of a sterile, sharp object (pinprick), light touch, a vibrating tuning fork, and the ability of the patient to feel position. Nonspecific loss of sensation must be differentiated from well-defined dermatomal loss which, in turn, must be differentiated from loss in the distribution of a peripheral nerve. The testing of muscle strength should include dorsiflexors and invertors (L4, L5 roots); plantar flexors and evertors (S1, S2 roots); muscles, knee extensors, and hip adductors (L2, L3, L4); and hip

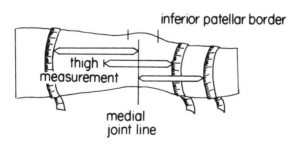

FIG 8.2.
For measurement of thigh and calf circumference, a reference landmark is selected, using either the medial knee joint line or the inferior border of the patella. A standard pen is used to determine the distance above and below that landmark, at which circumferential measurments will be made. Hence the name the BIK pen measurement.

flexors (T12, L1, L2, L3). The Babinski sign and the presence of clonus are measures of upper-motor neuron (spinal cord, brain) involvement and should also be elicited. Figures 8.3, 8.4, and 8.5 illustrate these neurologic tests.

Nerve Root Tension Signs.—The evaluation of nerve root tension signs is an important part of the examination. The authors prefer to logroll the limb initially to measure hip flexibility and then carry out a gentle range of motion of the hips prior to testing the straight leg raising. The straight leg raising maneuver has been described in many ways and under many names.[9,68] The simplest approach is to elevate the leg with the knee extended, with the examining hand placed on the pelvis to guard against pelvic motions (Fig. 8.6). The test is recorded as a positive nerve root tension sign when sciatica (posterior leg pain) is reproduced. The degree of elevation necessary to produce the symptoms is recorded and may be more precisely quantified by use of a spondylometer (see Chapter 16). Often, the individual complains of low back pain rather than sciatica. In this circumstance, the degree of elevation should be recorded, but the test is not positive for nerve root tension. Straight leg raising may also be restricted by tightness of the hamstrings, or the worker may report an aching discomfort behind the knee. Again, this should be recorded but is not a positive straight leg raising test. Sometimes sciatic pain occurs in the opposite leg as the test is being performed. This finding is referred to as contralateral or crossed-positive straight leg raising

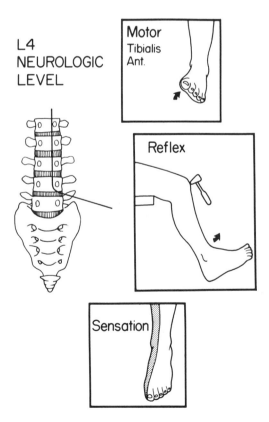

FIG 8.3.
Tests for neurologic function of the L4 root include the knee jerk, quadriceps strength, and sensory areas.

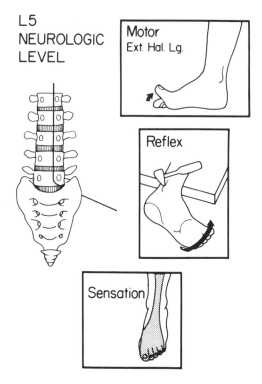

FIG 8.4.
Tests for neurologic function at the L5 root include decreased strength and sensation. The posterior tibial reflex when present is a useful confirmatory test, but it is bilaterally absent in 50% of all patients.

test[77] and is a highly specific finding for lumbar disc herniation. A variety of confirmatory tests have been described for straight leg raising.[68,69] Only two are discussed here, since they are used quite commonly.

Lasegue's Sign.—The hip and knee joints are flexed 90 degrees and then the knee extended to the point where sciatica is produced. The test may be further refined by dorsiflexing the foot.

Internal Rotation Test.—This is a straight leg raising test that is performed until sciatica is reproduced. The leg is then lowered to a level where the sciatica is relieved. Internal rotation of the hip is then performed and the test recorded as positive if sciatica is again produced. An alternative is to apply pressure behind the knee (bowstring test) after the leg has been lowered.

Examination in the Prone Position.—The worker is placed in the prone position. Gentle palpation of the spine processes, interspinous spaces, paraspinal muscles, sacroiliac joint, and sciatic nerve is then carried out. The examination should not be limited to the lumbar spine but should also include the thoracic spine because diseases in that location sometimes cause low back pain. Tenderness of the sciatic nerve implies inflammation, which often accompanies a lumbar disc herniation. This is most easily done in the sciatic notch.

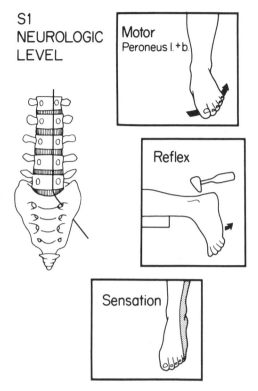

FIG 8.5.
Tests for neurologic function of the S1 root.

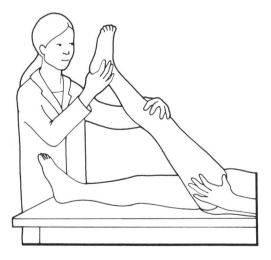

FIG 8.6.
The classic straight leg raising test done with the patient recumbent.

The neurologic examination should also be completed. Loss of pinprick sensation may be established for the back of the leg, particularly in the gluteal cleft and perianal region. Loss of sensation in this area is highly suggestive of cauda equina dysfunction.[1] The hamstring muscle strength (L4–L5) may also be assessed. In this position, a determination often may be made of the nerve root tension on the L2, L3, and L4 nerve roots, which form the femoral nerve. The femoral stretch test is performed with the examiner's hand placed on the buttocks. The hip remains in the extended position while the knee is flexed. A positive test is reproduction of anterior thigh pain. The test's validity decreases as soon as the examiner feels the pelvis rocking into extension.

Sitting Posture.—The neurologic examination may be performed equally well in the sitting as in the supine position. Some specialized tests (the Waddell signs) to be described later may also be done sitting. A variant of the SLR is shown in Figures 8.7a and 8.7b. It is also helpful to observe the worker's sitting posture. Often patients with acute sciatica support the body weight on the arms or actually shift the weight off the side with pain.

Principles of Palpation.—Palpation is performed in each of the examining positions. It is virtually impossible to determine the nature and location of the pain that a patient is complaining of or the biomechanic activities that influence the pain without actively palpating the area of complaint. Initial palpation includes laying the examiner's hands on the area of pain. Often it is necessary to palpate multiple structures such as the spinous processes, paraspinal muscles, sacroiliac joints, and iliac crests and the psoas, piriformis, quadratus lumborum, and gluteal muscles. As already noted, palpation of the abdomen, testicles, kidneys, inguinal area, or pelvic structures gives information on possible visceral or referred origin of the back pain.

When palpating the musculoskeletal structures, so-called layer palpation may be useful. This is performed by (1) palpating superficially over the skin for cutaneous hyperalgesia, (2) palpating the subcutaneous fascia for mobility of the skin over deeper structures (such mobility can be inhibited by scar tissue), (3) palpating the muscles and tendons for spasm and tenderness, which may be associated with inflammation or so-called nodules or trigger points (the latter phenomenon is widely described but its exact significance beyond localization of common areas of tenderness is not clear), (4) palpating bone, including spinous processes, ligaments, and bursa. This requires a knowledge of the anatomy of these structures, and often any localized tenderness or masses must be compared to palpation of similar structures on the asymptomatic side or in an asymptomatic area.

The palpation of structures during motion of the spine has been given pathologic connotation by certain enthusiasts, but this has yet to be proved. Nonetheless, the principle of palpating a joint as it goes through its range of motion and at the limits of range of motion is no different in the spine than it is in peripheral joints such as the knee, shoulder, or finger. This is performed by putting the hand and fingers on one area of the spine while the spine is moved through its range. This is followed by stressing the spine at its limit of motion. Catches, crepitation, painful arcs, restriction of motion, and pain on stressing the spine may be assessed in this way.

Tests for Nonorganic Signs.—A variety of specialized tests have evolved to test the reproducibility and consistency of patient responses. The best described and researched of these tests are those described by Waddell and associates.[72] These tests should alert the

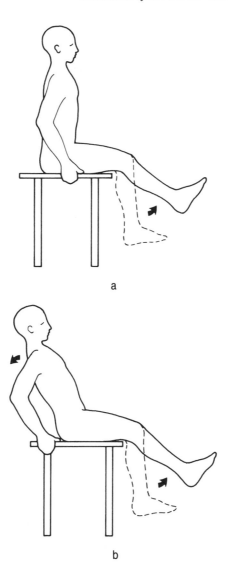

a

b

FIG 8.7. Seated SLR

The patient is sitting, and a straight leg raising maneuver is performed, usually by extending the leg from the knee bent to the fully extended knee position (a). In this exam, the patient is often told that the knee is being examined. If the patient has complained of sciatic pain on the recumbent straight leg raising, but the sitting straight leg raising (SLR) test is negative, it may be suggestive of malingering behavior. When an SLR maneuver is performed with a seated patient (b), the patient may experience exacerbation of the sciatica and attempt to shift into the extended spinal position, thus minimizing the degree of SLR elevation. The so-called flip test is one confirmatory test of nerve root entrapment.

examiner to the possibility of psychologic distress or malingering or both. These tests are of greater importance in evaluating the worker who is failing to respond to simple conservative measures within the expected time interval than they are in evaluation of patients with acute symptoms. Five types of physical signs are described; within each group specific tests are carried out.

Nonspecific Tenderness.—*Superficial*: The skin overlying the entire lumbar area is lighly pinched. Generalized tenderness is considered a positive sign.

Nonanatomic: The patient describes deep tenderness when one palpates over a wide area of anatomic structures. For example, a positive test would be a patient who describes local tenderness in the thoracic spine, paraspinal muscles, pelvis, and sacrum that does not follow any known syndrome or anatomic pattern.

Simulation Tests.—The object of these tests is to give the patient the impression that a specific test is being performed when in fact the test is not being performed.

Axial Loading: Compressive load is applied to the head. Persons complain of neck pain, but this maneuver rarely reproduces back pain. Reproduction of back pain is therefore a positive test.

Rotation: The shoulders and pelvis are passively rotated together so that no actual spine motion occurs, yet the patient believes rotation is being tested. Reproduction of back pain is a positive test.

Distraction Tests.—The object of this group of tests is to distract the person in such a fashion that a test that has been experienced as positive under one set of circumstances now becomes negative in the distracted patient. An example is the distraction straight leg raising test: The usual method is to have the worker sit and perform the straight leg raising test maneuver under the assumption that the knee, foot, or ankle are being examined (Fig. 8.7b). If the patient complains of pain reproduction with the straight leg raising test being performed in the supine position and not in the sitting position, the test is considered positive.

Regional Disturbances.—In general, pain distributions are a function of known anatomic pathways and structures. Interpretation of the examination therefore depends upon the patient giving non-anatomic, or non-physiologic responses to testing.

Weakness.—In a positive test, voluntary muscle contraction is accompanied by recurrent giving way, producing motions similar to a cogwheel. Alternately, a patient may show weakness on testing yet use good strength spontaneously.

Sensory.—Alterations in sensibility to touch and pinprick occur in a nonanatomic pattern, of which the most common varieties are the "stocking-glove" distribution, or diminished sensation over the entire half of the body or over one quadrant of the body.

Overreaction.—During the entire examination the person demonstrates overreactive behavior characterized by excessive verbalization of pain, facial expression signifying pain, collapsing episodes, and sweating. Waddell and associates have demonstrated that when three of five categories of tests are positive, there is a high probability of nonorganic pathology. In specific, they have used these tests to identify the individual who needs further psychologic assessment.

Formulation of the History and Physical Examination.—At the completion of the history and physical examination, a general formulation may be made of the worker's low back problem, including (1) decisions regarding the immediate need for further diagnostic tests, (2) an initial therapeutic plan, (3) a preliminary determination of the immediate disability, and (4) an outline of reasonable expectations for return to work. The following questions are helpful in making this formulation.

1. Has the worker had a major traumatic event (for example, a fall) that is sufficient to produce structural injury? A history of major injury combined with a physical examination that shows local tenderness, swelling, and skin discoloration should alert the examiner to this possibility. Obviously, the presence of such an injury, particularly when accompanied by any sign of neurologic impairment, should lead to careful transport of the patient to the nearest hospital or trauma center. Radiographic examination is required in this group.

2. Does the worker have an underlying disease process that might weaken structures to produce acute structural injury, despite the magnitude of the force being less than usually anticipated to produce such an injury? Persons who have taken cortisone or its derivatives, those with chronic debilitating diseases (for example, rheumatoid arthritis), and those with known neoplasms are examples of workers at risk. Osteoporosis may also contribute to lower resistance of tissues to trauma. In this group, spinal radiographs are warranted.[38]

3. Does the worker have some other, nonmusculoskeletal causation of low back pain that requires immediate attention? Although this is unlikely to occur in an industrial setting, identification of an abdominal mass that is pulsatile would be cause for immediate action (aneurysm of the aorta).

4. Does the worker have significant neurologic dysfunction? For example, a person with acute low back and leg pain, diminished muscle strength in lower extremities, and diminished sensation in the perianal area would warrant immediate attention because of suspected cauda equina lesion.

The probability that any of these events might occur in industry is low, but the four decisions are important because of the potential preventable loss of function or the need for early intervention. In most instances, the individual undergoing evaluation either does so in the setting of recurrent or chronic low back pain with an acute exacerbation or at the first episode of low back pain with trauma insufficient to produce bony injury.

DIAGNOSTIC STUDIES

For the majority of workers, further diagnostic studies are not required. The major determinations to be made include whether the individual can continue work at that time or requires some form of therapeutic intervention, most commonly bedrest or reduced activity.

Under the following circumstances, further diagnostic studies are indicated in addition to the four indications listed previously.

1. The worker is experiencing chronic and increasing low back pain with or without associated neurologic symptoms.
2. The worker is experiencing recurrent episodes that are increasing in frequency or intensity.
3. The worker is not responding within the anticipated time period to treatment of the acute symptoms (usually two to three weeks).

The further evaluation of the worker depends on pain patterns and severity of symptoms.

Laboratory Studies

Blood Tests.—A variety of blood tests may be used in the evaluation of the worker with low back pain. Table 8.3 lists these tests, the meaning of the measurement, and the low back conditions in which abnormalities might be detected.[7,22,24,38,55,71]

It is apparent from reviewing Table 8.3 that abnormalities in laboratory studies are not commonly found with low back pain. Obtaining these tests therefore depends upon clinical suspicion of infection, tumor, or a spondyloarthropathy. They are not indicated as a general screening test in low back disease.

Spinal Radiography

Liang and Komaroff[45] and Deyo and Diehl[10] have outlined the reasons for taking spinal radiographs at the time of an acute low back pain episode. These include the indications given in Table 8.4. Liang and Komaroff estimated the risk of missing serious pathology and cost savings by using this strategy. The risks were extremely low, and the cost savings were high. If radiographs have been done within the past two years and the worker does not fulfill the indications listed in Table 8.4, there is minimal probability that interval changes will either change the diagnosis or influence treatment.[67]

The preferred method for spinal radiography is a standing anteroposterior and lateral radiograph centered at the L4–L5 level.[59] The radiographic findings that are considered insignificant have already been presented in Chapter 3. Some radiologists also add a lumbosacral spot lateral film, which they feel gives important information about the lumbosacral joint. In general, we do not agree with that approach unless the lateral film does not adequately visualize that area.

Additional Plane Radiographic Studies

Oblique Radiography.—Oblique radiographs usually are not warranted and add unnecessarily high x-ray exposure for the information to be gained in routine use.[67] In a patient with spondylolisthesis, the technique is useful in determining the integrity of the pars interarticularis. The test may also be useful in the small subset of patients with a bony tumor. The routine use of the oblique film to obtain information about the facet joints is of limited value.[67]

Flexion/Extension Radiography.—In Chapter 3 information was presented about "segmental instability" and some of the controversy that surrounds that diagnosis in patients with degenerative spinal conditions. To demonstrate instability, the person must be mobile; an attempt to obtain films during acute symptoms is unlikely to be useful. The films may be obtained in either the seated or standing postures; the worker is instructed to flex the spine maximally, and a radiograph is taken. Maximal extension is then requested, and a second radiograph taken. An alternative is to place a backpack to produce compression loading, followed by traction to obtain compression unloading.[17] A variety of criteria have been presented to determine a positive test and the intra- and interobserver errors calculated.[13,29,39,46,54,60,78] Figure 8.8 presents the currently favored method.[13] Woody and associates[78] have calculated that a positive test is only valid when there is a minimum of 4-mm forward translation at the L4–L5 and L3–L4 levels and a 6-mm backward translation at the L5–S1 level. This type of information may also be used to assess the integrity of a previously performed spinal fusion.[18]

Tomograms.—Tomography is a historic method used to give multiplanar radiographic cuts in either the anteroposterior or lateral views. This method has been largely replaced by other imaging techniques, although it may occasionally be useful in assessing a spinal fusion's integrity, spinal tumors, and some fractures.

TABLE 8.3
Usefulness of Clinical Laboratory Studies in Diagnosing Low Back Pain

Test	What Test Measures	Low Back Conditions Where Altered
Complete Blood Count Hematocrit hemaglobin	A measure of volume of circulating red blood cells.	May be diminished in systemic diseases, i.e. neoplasm, & in chronic spinal infections.
White blood count & differential	Amount & type of circulating white blood cells.	Total white blood cell and shifts in differential may be present in spinal infections or occasionally in spondyloarthropathies.
Sedimentation Rate	Non-specific test of inflammation.	Increased in spinal infections, may be increased in neoplasms & spondyloarthropathies.
Chemistry Calcium Phosphorus	A measure of circulating calcium & phosphorus.	Calcium is elevated in hyperparathyroidism, may be elevated with primary & secondary osseous tumors, alterations in the distribution of calcium & phosphorus accompany many metabolic disorders but are normal in osteoporosis.
Alkaline Phosphatase	Enzyme associated with bone formation. Therefore elevation implies increased bone formation.	May be elevated in primary or secondary osseous neoplasms.
Acid Phosphatase	An enzyme associated with tumors metastatic to bone.	Increased in prostatic tumors.
Serum Proteins (albumin globulin protein electrophoresis) protein.	Measurement of amount & type of circulating.	Elevations of one fraction of globulin is associated with multiplemyeloma.
HLA 27-B Antigen	A circulating antigen	Usually individuals with spondyloarthropathies are HLA 27-B positive. Note 6–8% of males have this antigen and therefore its presence is not confirmatory of a spondyloarthropathy.

TABLE 8.4
Indications for Spinal Radiographs in Acute Low Back Pain*

INDICATION	SIGNIFICANCE
Age greater than 50 years	Risk of tumor, severe degeneration
History of severe trauma	Fracture likely
History of osteoporosis	Compression fracture
Known primary cancer	Suggest spinal cancer or possible infection
Unrelenting pain at rest	
Unexplained weight loss	
History of corticosteroids	Risk factors for spinal infection
Organ recipient	
AIDS	
Diabetes mellitus	
Drug abuse	
Alcohol abuse	Greater risk for fractures
Findings suggestive of spondylitis	
Neurologic defect	R/O bony, tumor or infectious cause

*Adapted from Liang/Komoroff[45] and Deyo/Diehl[10]

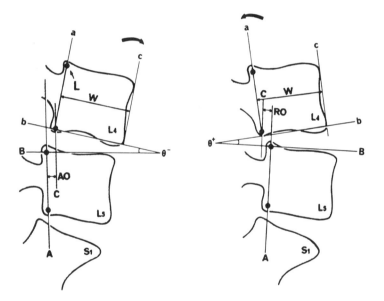

FIG 8.8.
To determine the amount of horizontal displacement on the flexion-extension views, first find and mark on each vertebra of the motion segment the remnants of Luschka's joints (*L*). Join the landmarks of the upper vertebra by a line (*line a*), and repeat the procedure for the lower vertebra (*line A*). From the lower landmark of the upper vertebra a line drawn parallel to line A and C (*AO* for anterior olisthesis and *RO* for retrolisthesis) is the amount of horizontal displacement of the vertebra above, not taking magnification into account. To obviate inaccuracies due to the x-ray magnification factor, the horizontal displacement is measured in percentage of displacement. Draw a line (*line c*) from the anterior border of the upper end plate on the proximal vertebra. Measure the horizontal midbody width (*W*) of the upper body between lines *a* and *c*. The percentage of horizontal displacement is $HD\% = (AO$ or $RO/W) \times 100$. To measure angular displacement, draw line *b* perpendicular to line *a* from the inferior landmark on the vertebra above, and line *B* perpendicular to line *A* from the upper landmark of the vertebra below. The angle between the two lines is the angular displacement in degrees. (From Dupuis PR, Yong-Hing K, Cassidy JD, et al: Radiologic diagnosis of degenerative lumbar spinal instability. *Spine* 1985; 10:262. Used by permission.)

A variety of other imaging techniques are now available to assess patients who fulfill criteria for their use. We emphasize here that these tests are not routinely used in acute low back pain, and their indications are based on the patient's history and physical examination. In other words these tests are used to confirm a clinical suspicion and should not be used as a "fishing expedition." The important principle is that radiographic images are only as valid as their correlation with the clinical signs and symptoms. The reasons we emphasize this important principle follow.

1. Imaging abnormalities are common in individuals who have never had low back symptoms or sciatica. Hitselberger and Witten[31] found myelographic evidence of lumbar disc herniations in 30% of their study population; Wiesel and associates[75] identified CT scan evidence of lumbar disc herniation or spinal stenosis in an equivalent percentage of an asymptomatic survey population; Boden et al.[4] similarly identified disc herniations and spinal stenosis in volunteers by magnetic resonance imaging (MRI); and Holt[32] found abnormal discograms in 40% of a prison population. All of this information emphasizes the issues of sensitivity, specificity, and predictive value of any imaging study. As a reference point, these values are given in Table 8.5 for lumbar disc herniation. At present no carefully controlled studies have determined the sensitivity or specificity of these tests for spinal stenosis and other diseases of the lumbar spine.

2. In addition to the significant imaging abnormalities, such as lumbar disc herniation, a number of other findings are commonly observed, the clinical significance of which are either questionable or as yet unknown. The most common of these follow: (1) disc space bulging observed in CT scans and MRI (this finding is nonspecific); (2) abnormal MRI images on the T2 weighted scan indicative of "disc degeneration" (the significance of this finding is not fully established, but in general it is thought to be nonspecific); (3) facet arthropathy.

3. Labeling a patient with a diagnosis such as disc degeneration on the basis of imaging studies alone may lead to unnecessary restrictions being placed on the individual, or worse, the worker self-restricting activities or assuming the existence of a serious and progressive disease.

4. Misinterpretation of the significance of an imaging study may lead to misguided

TABLE 8.5
Sensitivity and Specificity of Diagnostic Tests for Herniated Lumbar Disc*.

Diagnostic Test	Sensitivity	Specificity
CT scanning	0.92	0.88
Metrizamide myelography	0.90	0.87
Iophendylate myelography	0.80	0.90
Diskography	0.83	0.78
Epidural venography	0.87	0.70
Electromyography	0.92	0.38

* From Hudgins WR: The predictive value of myelography in the diagnosis of ruptured lumbar discs. *J Neurosurg* 1970;32:152. Used by permission.

therapeutic decisions. A review of the causes of failure in lumbar disc excision frequently shows that the imaging studies were poorly correlated with the clinical findings, and poor judgment was exercised in the selection of the patient for operation based on these findings.

Following is a review of the imaging techniques currently available.

Lumbar CT Scan

The CT scan is a powerful tool in the diagnosis of low back disease.[8,64] The disadvantages are that it involves significant radiographic exposure, many of the observed "abnormalities" exist in asymptomatic subjects, and the method is not necessary to determine the causation of pain in most low back pain sufferers. Much of the role for CT scan is being supplanted by MRI. In general, CT scan gives greater information about the bony structures, while MRI gives greater information about soft tissue structures. Furthermore, MRI is a more costly test and is not universally available. The indications, therefore, vary according to the availability of the test and the judgment of the doctor ordering the test. With this caveat, the indications are presented:

1. *Suspected Herniated Nucleus Pulposus.* The patient presents clinical symptoms and physical findings of lumbar disc herniation and has failed to respond to conservative management. Consideration is being given to surgical intervention (Fig. 8.9).
2. *Spinal Stenosis.* The patient has the clinical symptoms or plane radiographic findings that strongly suggest spinal stenosis (Fig. 8.10).
3. *Spinal Trauma.* CT scan is invaluable in assessing spinal fractures because of the detail of bony architecture it reveals. The test is rarely required in patients with simple compression fractures.

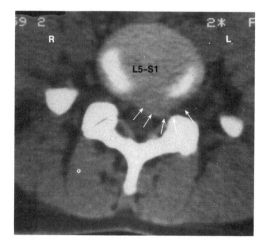

FIG 8.9.
A lumbar CT scan at the L5–S1 level is shown. This patient had low back pain, followed by sciatica in the S1 root distribution. His ankle reflex was absent, sensation was decreased on the lateral aspect of the foot, and the straight leg raising was positive at 25 degrees. These physical findings correspond with the large, well-lateralized lumbar disc protrusion at L5–S1, (*arrows*).

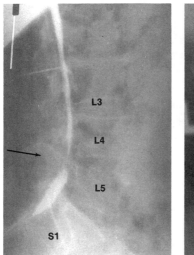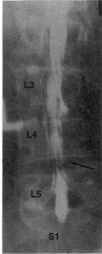

FIG 8.10.
This lateral myelogram shows narrowing of the dye column at multiple levels, indicative of spinal stenosis. The most dramatic change is at the L4–L5 level, where there is complete block to the dye flow, best seen on the lateral and to a lesser degree on the AP film (*arrows*).

4. *Spinal Tumors*. CT scan plays a major role in the localization and staging of primary and metastatic bone tumors. It adds to information obtained from the MRI.

5. *Postsurgical*. CT scan remains a powerful tool for the assessment of the integrity of a spinal fusion. Multiplanar reformatting of the images and three-dimensional reconstructions (reference) reveal information not readily available from any other source.

In addition to these general indications, CT scan may be useful in a few patients with suspected spondyloarthropathies and in whom other simpler tests have not confirmed the diagnosis. It may also be useful in combination with either myelography (myelographically enhanced CT) or discography (disco CT). These topics are discussed later in this chapter.

Magnetic Resonance Imaging

MRI is the most exciting imaging technique currently available for evaluation of low back disorders. The technique involves no ionizing radiation and produces a detailed picture of soft tissues previously unavailable. It is a costly test, however, and should not be used for general screening or for nonspecific reasons.[8,49]

1. *Lumbar Disc Herniation*. Many authorities now believe MRI is the imaging technique of choice. Masaryk[48] has calculated the sensitivity and specificity of the test; these are, respectively, 89% and 82%. The test can distinquish a sequestered from a bulged disc and is therefore critical when percutaneous discectomy is being considered.[48] The "myelogram" effect produced by the T1 weighted image also gives information not available from CT scan. If paramagnetic contrast media are used to enhance the image, differentiation of scar from disc material is possible with a high level of sensitivity[36] (Fig. 8.11).

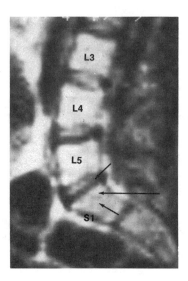

FIG 8.11.
A lateral of a magnetic resonance image (MRI) study. The vertebrae appear white, while the disc protrusion, which is avascular, is shown at the L5–S1 level (*arrow*).

2. *Spinal Stenosis.* MRI appears to be the imaging technique of choice for these conditions in the majority of patients.[49] Again, the myelogram effect of the T1 weighted image is a critical feature (Fig. 8.11).

3. *Spinal Tumors and Infections.* Because MRI is responsive to the actual physiology of tissues, it more accurately identifies the extent of many tumors and infections, particularly the soft tissue involvement. It also is extremely sensitive to tumors of neurologic origin. Unlike CT scan, extending the study into the thoracolumbar spine does not involve additional exposure to x-ray and, thus, information about this area can be obtained without added risk or cost.

4. *Spinal Trauma.* This is an area of controversy. Usually simple radiographs suffice (Fig. 8.12). The MRI gives more information than does CT scan about the integrity of neurologic structures but less information about bony structures. We believe and continue to use CT scan in these patients, but we more often utilize MRI in addition and do not perform myelograms in these patients.

5. *Failed Low Back Surgery.* MRI is invaluable for these patients; it is the first method that allows the differentiation of scar from recurrent disc.[36] This important feature is possible because of paramagnetic contrast media such as gadolinium, which produces images 98% sensitive to scar versus disc.

Discography

This test has been highly controversial, primarily because of the nonspecificity of the test, based on the data of Holt.[32] The details of this controversy have been presented in detail.[14,70,73] This controversy is also central to the issue of disc disruption. Our approach is as follows:

1. *Lumbar Disc Herniation.* We do not use discography in patients with lumbar disc herniation, relying instead on CT or MRI. A very small subset of patients with the clinical

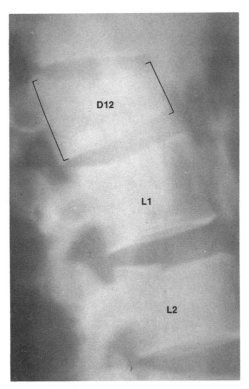

FIG 8.12.
This worker fell off a scaffolding 6 feet high, landing in the seated position. He had immediate pain but was neurologically intact. The lateral radiograph shows a typical wedge compression fracture with greater loss of vertebral body height anteriorly (*arrow*).

signs and symptoms of disc herniation, such as a radiculopathy, do not have the causation of their symptoms clarified by those tests. If we believe there is no significant psychologic or other factor accounting for their complaint, discography is combined with CT scan to provide a "disco-CT." The usefulness of this test has been promoted by Sachs, Vanharanta, et al.[66,70] (Fig. 8.13).

2. *Spinal Stenosis.* There is no role for discography in the diagnosis of spinal stenosis.

3. *Low Back Pain.* It is here that the controversy regarding discography is most apparent. If a patient is assessed as having continuing and disabling low back pain that is clearly mechanical, phychological factors are minimal or absent, and the patient has not responded to rehabilitative efforts, we believe there is a defined role for discography. The critical features of a positive test are that the injection faithfully reproduces the patient's symptoms and that the subsequent "disco CT" demonstrates disruption of the disc and tracting of the dye toward the side of symptoms if the patient has unilateral leg complaints.

4. *Surgical Planning.* Again, there is major controversy. Some authorities believe the extent of a proposed fusion should be determined by discography. For example, if the major pathology is at L4–L5 and an L4 to the sacrum fusion is planned, proponents would advocate discography at L3–L4. If this test is positive, they would extend the fusion to that level. In our view, this decision must be balanced against the reduced rate of fusion that accompanies each additional level fused, versus the risk of later symptoms if the fusion is

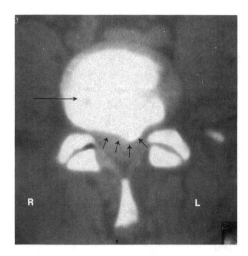

FIG 8.13.
This worker had low back pain with later development of left leg pain. A CT scan and MRI were interpreted as equivocal. A discogram was then performed with radiographic contrast media injected into the L5–S1 disc. The dye is shown as white in the subsequent CT scan (*arrows*), and the focal disc protrusion at L5–S1 on the left is confirmed (*arrows*).

not extended to incorporate the diskographically abnormal level. We believe the information available does not support sufficient risk or later failure to warrant the additional risk and reduced fusion rate.[18]

5. *Failed Surgery.* The major role of discography is in the patient with a failed spinal fusion, in which case the issue is whether or not pain is coming from the disc under a pseudoarthrosis. Again, this issue is controversial, but we have found the technique useful when no other source of continued pain was identifiable (Fig. 8.14).

Myelography

Myelography is the historic benchmark for the diagnosis of many lumbar spine disorders such as disc herniation, spinal stenosis, and neurologic tumors. The contrast media injected intrathecally may either be fat soluble (Pantopaque) or water soluble.[34,63] Fat-soluble contrast media have been virtually abandoned because of their association with arachnoiditis and the fact that water-soluble dyes give far better resolution of nerves and cauda equina. Myelography is not a benign procedure, and complications occur in 10 to 20% of patients undergoing this examination, including headache and seizures. These complications are mose common when the examination is negative and when the condition being evaluated is compensable.[30] Today, the indications for myelography are rapidly diminishing and being supplanted by MRI, although some favor its use in spinal stenosis and some spinal fractures with neurologic involvement. When the myelogram is followed by the CT scan, very accurate measurements of the thecal sac are possible. The calculation of the cross-sectional dimensions of the sac remain the single most well-established method for the diagnosis of spinal stenosis.[3] (Refer to Fig. 8.15.) Its use in the failed low back surgery patient has also been largely replaced by MRI. The ability of myelography to identify pathology in these patients, however, was shown in a report where 13% of patients with failed low back surgery were found to have unsuspected pathology.[61]

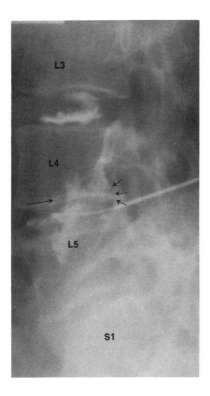

FIG 8.14.
This worker had a seated fall and subsequently developed disabling low back pain. He underwent an intensive rehabilitation program, during which time psychologic studies were normal. He was highly motivated to return to work, but soon after doing modest lifting his severe symptoms recurred. An MRI showed disc degeneration at L3–L4 and L4–L5. A discogram was performed that totally reproduced his back symptoms at L4–L5. The lateral radiograph shows the dye in place and significant disruption of the L4–L5 disc (*arrows*). He was treated by fusion and has returned to work.

Perhaps the most important lesson is that indications for CT scan and MRI should be based on the historic indications for myelography, which include an understanding of the important complications that accompany this examination.

Venography

This technique is mentioned only for its historic interest. It is rarely employed today.

Radionucleotide Scanning

A radionucleotide scan involves the injection of a radioactive isotope, which is selectively taken up by bone or other tissues.[25] Following the injection, the entire body or a focal area such as the spine is evaluated. If the radionucleotide is selectively taken up by bone (technetium), increased uptake is associated with increased bone formation or destruction. If the radionucleotide is taken up by soft tissues (gallium, indium-labeled neutrophils), the test is a measure of the blood flow and inflammatory response in these tissues.

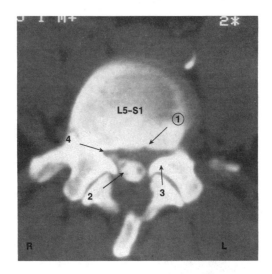

FIG 8.15.
This CT scan was obtained after a myelogram (myelographically enhanced CT scan) was performed. The caudal sac (*2*) and right S1 nerve root (*4*) are clearly outlined. A disc (*1*) is obliterating the S1 root on the left, consistent with his symptoms. Notice that the facets are overgrown, producing narrowing of the lateral recesses (*3*), adding to the nerve compression. His left leg pain was relieved by bony decompression of the left root canal, and removal of the focally bulging disc.

A bone scan is indicated primarily in patients whose clincial histories or pain suggests a neoplasm or infection. The test is used under the following circumstances:

- The individual has a history of known primary tumor or radiographic evidence suggestive but not confirmatory of neoplasm or infection.
- The individual has a pain pattern suggestive of tumor, and radiographs are normal but serologic abnormalities such as elevations of serum acid or alkaline phosphatase are present.
- The individual has severe pain after disc excision or elevations of fever accompanying low back pain. In these circumstances, the gallium scan is more sensitive than the technetium scan. Indium scanning, however, which is useful in peripheral joints, has been found to be very insensitive to spinal infections and is not useful.[16]
- An adolescent has low back pain associated with sports—which is known to increase the risk of spondylolysis—and plain radiographs do not show this condition or demonstrate only sclerosis in the region of the pars interarticularis.[76]

Other studies: A number of other techniques are useful in the evaluation of selected workers with low back pain. These include electrodiagnostic evaluation, possibly thermography, pain-provocative or local anesthetic injections. and psychologic assessment.

ELECTRODIAGNOSTIC STUDIES

The documentation of the presence or absence and the location of neurologic deficits is one of the most important diagnostic decisions to be made. In patients with acute pain of a few days duration, even if there is some intermittent paresthesia or pain in the legs, electrodiagnostic studies are not necessary. In addition, in patients with well-defined unequivocal neurologic deficits on clinical examination that correlate with pathology electrodiagnostic studies are seldom needed unless legal or some other reason for documentation is required. In patients who have chronic back pain with leg pain, however, weakness or sensory changes that cannot be adequately explained or do not fit any obvious pathology, electrodiagnostic testing is the most useful method of documenting the presence or absence of neurologic deficits.[28] These tests also have the capacity to localize the deficits and to determine crudely the chronicity and degree of deficit.

Modern computer technology has added considerably to the acumen of the electrodiagnostician, who can now utilize a wide variety of tests to study lower-extremity nerves. The temptation to indiscriminately perform every study possible must be avoided, as these tests may be uncomfortable and expensive. The determination of which tests should be performed must be made by considering the questions that arise from the clinical examination. These tests should be considered an extension of the clinincal examination of the nervous system.[26]

Electromyography

This test remains the mainstay of most electrodiagnosticians. Electromyography (EMG) is quite specific and may give some estimate as to the chronicity of denervation. This is due to the fact that muscular denervation follows a well-defined course. In the first two to four weeks the EMG is inevitably normal, because denervation sensitivity of the muscle membrane has not set in. This is one reason that most clinicians do not order an EMG until at least four to six weeks after an injury. From one month to 9 to 12 months after a nerve injury acute denervation may be documented due to irritability of the muscle membrane, which spontaneously produces fibrillation and positive sharp waves. After 9 to 12 months the nerve begins to reinnervate muscles, resulting in polyphasic potentials that may be recorded on muscle contraction. EMG also has the capacity to determine the level of radiculopathy or peripheral neuropathy. It must be kept in mind, however, that some variation in the innervation of muscles between patients does exist.

Reflex Studies

The studies included under this heading are the F-responses, H-reflexes, and bulbocavernosus reflex.

The F-response allows for the determination of motor conduction along the length of the nerve, including the nerve root. It measures conduction only in motor fibers, however. The sensitivity of this test is diminished by the fact that the major nerves in the lower extremities contain fibers from more than one root level. The test has one advantage over EMG in that it becomes positive immediately after an injury.

The H-reflex is probably the most widely used test after EMG for the evaluation of lumbar radiculopathy. This reflex is of value only at the S1 root level, but it is reported to have a 90% correlation with S1 radiculopathies.[5]

The bulbocavernosus reflex is a method for evaluating the S2–S4 nerve roots and cauda equina. It is of value when a large central disc herniation is felt to be causing bowel or bladder disturbance.[27]

Peripheral Nerve Conduction Studies

The major differential diagnoses for foot and leg numbness or weakness include radiculopathy, generalized peripheral neuropathy, and nerve entrapment or focal injury.

Saal et al.[65] reported a number of cases where peripheral neuropathies had been picked up in the routine electrodiagnostic consultation for radiculopathy. The testing of both motor and sensory nerve conduction measurement should be considered under the following circumstances:

1. *Tarsal tunnel syndrome*: Numbness in the foot can be caused by entrapment of the plantar branches of the posterior tibial nerve. The measurement of motor conduction in these tests is relatively easy. Sensory nerve conduction in these nerves is more difficult and not always obtainable.

2. *Peroneal neuropathy*: This most commonly occurs at the fibular head but may occur by direct trauma at other sites. Because peroneal lesions cause weakness in dorsiflexion of the foot and numbness over the big toe area (usually in the web), it is easily confused with an L5 radiculopathy.

3. *Peripheral neuropathies*: Generalized peripheral neuropathies may cause numbness, burning, and weakness in the legs. Such symptoms are usually bilateral and are easily distinguished from radiculopathy by careful clinical examination. Nonetheless, individuals with diabetes, a history of heavy alcohol use, or a family history of peripheral neuropathy should be investigated and the degree of deficits documented.

4. *Femoral neuropathies*: These neuropathies are very uncommon but may be confused with L3 or L4 radiculopathy and, where indicated, femoral nerve conduction may be measured as it passes out of the pelvis.

Somatosensory Evoked Responses (SERs)

The development of inexpensive computer equipment that can average multiple responses has allowed for the recording of potentials over the peripheral nerves, plexuses, spinal cord, and brain on stimulation of peripheral sensory nerves. The tests fall into the following categories, depending on the type of nerve stimulated.

1. *Mixed-nerve SERs*. The nerves most commonly tested in the lower extremities are the posterior tibial and peroneal nerves. This method is excellent for testing of spinal cord and central sensory pathways but is very insensitive to radiculopathies due to the multiple nerve roots represented in these nerves. The test is widely used for the diagnosis of spinal cord lesions, including thoracic and cervical stenosis, hematomas, tumors and multiple sclerosis. They are also used for the monitoring of spinal cord function during spinal surgery for scoliosis or major deformity where trauma or traction on the spinal cord is a consideration. The effects of general anesthesia on these tests, however, must be understood in order to avoid misinterpretation.[44]

2. *Pudendal evoked potentials*. This somatosensory evoked response is obtained by stimulating branches of the pudendal nerve. Along with the bulbocavernosus reflex response, it is used to evaluate neurologic disturbance of bowel, bladder, and sexual dysfunction.[27]

3. *Small sensory nerve SERs*. These potentials are obtained on stimulation of the sural, superficial peroneal, and saphenous nerves, which are felt to fairly accurately reflect the S1, L5, and L4 nerve roots. There remains controversy as to whether these tests are more or less sensitive than dermatomal SERs or EMG in diagnosing radiculopathies.

4. *Dermatomal SERs*. These potentials are only measured over the brain, but they may be obtained on stimulation of an area of the skin. They are useful in investigating symptoms of anesthesia over an area, but they appear not to be as sensitive as the EMG and reflex studies in documenting radiculopathy. When clearly abnormal, however, these responses

may be the only way of documenting a purely sensory radiculopathy. DSERs have also been used for the intraoperative monitoring of surgical decompression of specific nerve roots, although this should still be considered experimental.

Motor Evoked Responses

The ability to stimulate the cerebral cortex or spinal cord using a magnetic stimulator and to record responses in various muscle groups is now being investigated. This test has the capacity to measure motor pathways in the spinal cord and is currently being investigated for the diagnosis of radiculopathy.

Thermography

Disturbances in nerve root function are sometimes accompanied by alterations in local blood flow, producing secondary localized abnormalities in tissue temperature. These temperature changes may be measured by thermography. The proponents of this method cite its advantages: it is noninvasive, it measures physiologic dysfunction, and it is highly sensitive.[23,33,58] However, many believe the test is nonspecific and adds no useful information in most spinal diseases.[20,47] The most important disadvantage is that the use of thermography to objectify a physiologic disturbance in patients with compensable low back pain is unproven and is considered inadmissible evidence in some state jurisdictions. The only potentially useful effect appears to be in the documentation of reflex sympathetic dystrophy.

Pain Provocation and Relief

In Chapter 4, it was stressed that for a structure to be considered pain-productive, it must be possible to produce symptoms when the structure is noxiously stimulated and to relieve symptoms when its nerve supply is blocked by local anesthesia. This principle has been applied to the facet joints, nerve roots, painful nodules associated with fibromyalgia, and, less selectively, through the use of intra- and extradural injections of local anesthetics.

Facet Joint Block

No uniform criteria exist for the use of facet joint blocks.[2,15,52,53,57] This procedure appears indicated mainly in patients with chronic or recurrent low back pain that is failing to respond to conservative management, particularly when CT scan has demonstrated local facet abnormalities or when the plane radiographic picture or flexion/extension films are suggestive of segmental instability.[19] Another relative indication is to provide temporary pain relief for patients with low back pain so that more complete flexion and extension radiographs may be obtained. Because definition of facet syndrome and segmental instability are variable and the criteria imprecise, the selection of the patient and joints to be injected are uncertain. In fact, studies of these patient populations indicate that the usefulness of this technique may be far less than previously thought.[37] The ability of these techniques to provide lasting relief are minimal; less than 20% of patients treated have sustained reduction of symptoms six months after the injection.

There is, however, a specific use of facet injection applicable to patients who have degenerative cysts of the facets. These cysts may be identified by CT scan or MRI and are a rare but important cause of sciatica. Traditional treatment has been surgical.[56] An alternative is to perform a facet block, inject a radiopaque contrast media to outline the cyst and confirm its communication with the facet joint, and then inject a cortisone derivative. Ninety percent of patients treated by this technique had continuing relief after one year.[42]

Nerve Root Block

Selective injection of a nerve root can be a useful test in a patient with a monoradiculopathy. Simultaneous injection of a radiopaque contrast media outlines the nerve root far beyond the foramina and thus has the potential to identify unusual causes of extraforaminal compression. These tests are generally reserved for a few patients with complex pain problems and are not routinely used.[40,41]

Differential Spinal Block

Intra- or extrathecal injections of local anesthetic, accompanied by careful positioning of the individual to allow the anesthetic to rise slowly in the spinal canal, has been used as a diagnostic test in patients with chronic pain problems. The technique and its interpretation are both controversial and beyond the scope of this book.[6,51]

Other Local Injections

Some clinicians inject several other structures such as ligaments, myofascial nodules, and the sacroiliac joint. The use of these injections for either the diagnostic evaluation or treatment of patients has yet to be proved. Injecting steroids into an inflamed trochanteric bursa may relieve pain in that area. Injection into fibromyalgic nodules may cause temporary relief of the tenderness in that area, but it rarely has long-term effects.

Psychologic Tests

Some workers present with psychologic maladjustments or maladaptive coping mechanisms, which either directly relate to the causation of low back pain or affect their ability to cope successfully with their symptoms. This topic is considered in detail in Chapter 4, and we have included Waddell's tests earlier in this chapter to help the examiner identify the patient at risk. A variety of other tests have also been considered, including structured psychiatric interviews and various psychologic profiles such as the MMPI.[43] The simplest, clinically useful alternative is the pain drawing[62] (Fig. 8.16). This test may be easily applied in an office or industrial setting.

SUMMARY

Previous chapters have emphasized that most episodes of low back pain are self-limiting. In this chapter we emphasize that an organized history and physical examination determine the cause of symptoms, guide treatment, and estimate the risk of disability. Thus, further studies are not necessary in the majority of workers with low back pain. If the episode is recurrent or chronic, or if specific symptoms (night pain) or signs (neurologic involvement) indicate the potential for a significant pathologic condition, then further tests may be necessary. Plain radiographs are the most common starting point, and specific indications are presented for their use. Laboratory studies are warranted in only a very small group of patients, most of whom are not an issue in occupationally related low back pain.

A variety of sophisticated imaging techniques are available, but the most useful are CT scan, magnetic resonance imaging, and electrodiagnostic testing. These tests should be obtained for specific reasons and not simply because the individual has low back pain. The interpretation of these tests should be done with a knowledge of the significant findings as

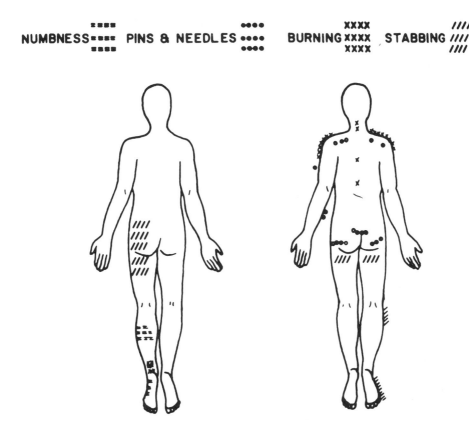

NUMBNESS ∎∎∎∎ **PINS & NEEDLES** ●●●● **BURNING** XXXX **STABBING** ////

FIG 8.16.
A variety of pain drawings are used. Typically the patient is told to draw the location of pain using some code for pain (XX), numbness (OO), tingling, or other sensory changes. In usual instances, the drawings include both front and back views. Depicted here are two drawings of the posterior view of a patient, one from a patient with clear-cut sciatica, the other from a patient with numerous psychologic problems. Notice, in the second case, that pain is depicted as being external to the body and located in multiple areas. (From Ransford AO, Cairns D, Mooney V: The pain drawing as an aid to the psychologic evaluation of patients with low back pain. *Spine* 1976; 1:127. Used by permission.)

opposed to findings such as disc bulging, which is nonspecific. Their ultimate importance, in most cases, is the confirmation of a condition that is suspected or apparent by history and physical examination. Other tests, such as laboratory investigations, bone scans, and pain-provocative studies, are useful for a small subset of workers and are not generally employed. The recognition of psychologic disturbances is of importance, however, such disturbances may be suspected from the pain drawing and confirmed by more sophisticated test techniques.

The ultimate goal of all of these tests is to provide a basis for further rational therapy. Thus, it is critically important to make decisions that correlate the history, the physical examination, and the confirmatory test when deciding on therapy. Conversely, decisions based on imaging and other studies where the clinical symptoms and signs are not closely correlated is associated with a high potential for less than optimal therapeutic response and continued disability.

BIBLIOGRAPHY

1. Aho AJ, Auranen A, Pesonen K: Analysis of cauda equina symptoms in patients with lumbar disc prolapse. Preoperative and follow-up clinical and cystometric studies. *Acta Chir Scand* 1969; 135:413.
2. Badgley CE: The articular facets in relation to low back pain and sciatic radiation. *J Bone Joint Surg* 1941; 23:481.
3. Bell GR, Rothman RH, Booth RE, et al: A study of computer-assisted tomography: II. Comparison of metrizamide myelography and computed tomography in the diagnosis of herniated lumbar disc and spinal stenosis. *Spine* 1984; 9:552–556.
4. Boden SD, Davis DO, Dina TS, et al: The incidence of abnormal lumbar spine MRI scans in asymptomatic patients: A prospective and blinded investigation. Presented at the meeting of the International Society for Study of the Lumbar Spine, Kyoto, Japan, 1989.
5. Braddon RC, Johnson EW: Standardization of H-reflex and diagnostic use in S1 radiculopathy. *Arch Phys Med Rehabil* 1974; 55:161–166.
6. Brown MD: Diagnosis of pain syndromes of the spine. *Orthop Clin N Am* 1975; 6:233.
7. Calin A: Ankylosing spondylitis, in Kelley WN, Harris ED, Ruddy S, et al. (eds): *Textbook of Rheumatology*. Philadelphia, Saunders, 1981.
8. Chafetz N, Genant HK: Computed tomography of the lumbar spine. *Orthop Clin N Am* 1983; 14:147.
9. Cram RH: A sign of sciatic nerve root pressure. *J Bone Joint Surg* 1953; 35:192.
10. Deyo RA, Diehl AK: Lumbar spine films in primary care: Current use and effects of selective ordering criteria. *J Gen Intern Med* 1986; 1:20.
11. Donaghy RMP: The posterior tibial reflex. A reflex of some value in the localization of the protruded intervertebral disc in the lumber region. *J Neurosurg* 1946; 3:457.
12. Dupuis H: Belastung durch mechanische Schwingungen und moegliche Gesundheitsschaedigungen im Bereich der Wirbelsaeule. *Fortschritte der Medizin* 1974; 92:618.
13. Dupuis PR, Yong-Hing K, Cassidy JD, et al: Radiologic diagnosis of degenerative lumbar spinal instability. *Spine* 1985; 10:262.
14. Executive Committee of the North American Spine Society: Position statement on discography. *Spine* 1988; 13:1343.
15. Fairbank JCT, Park WM, McCall IW, et al: Apophyseal injection of local anesthetic as a diagnostic aid in primary low back pain syndromes. *Spine* 1981; 6:598.
16. Fitzgerald R: Personal communication.
17. Friberg O: Lumbar instability: A dynamic approach by traction-compression radiography. *Spine* 1987; 12:119.
18. Frymoyer JW, Hanley EN Jr., Howe J, et al: A comparison of radiographic findings in fusion and nonfusion patients ten or more years following lumbar disc surgery. *Spine* 1979; 4:435.
19. Frymoyer JW, Selby, DK: Segmental instability: Rationale for treatment. *Spine* 1985; 10:280.
20. Frymoyer JW, Haugh LD: Thermography: A call for scientific studies to establish its diagnostic efficacy. *Orthopaedics* 1986; 9:699.
21. Frymoyer JW, Cats-Baril WL: Predictors of low back pain disability. *Clin Orthop* 1987; 221:89.
22. Galen RS: The predictive value of laboratory testing. *Orthop Clinics N Am* 1979; 10:287.
23. Getty CJ: "Bony sciatica"—The value of thermography, electromyography, and water-soluble myelography. *Clin Sports Med* 1986; 5:327.
24. Goldsmith RS: Calcium, phosphate, and vitamin D. *Orthop Clin N Am* 1979; 10:319.
25. Goldstein HA: Bone scintigraphy. *Orthop Clin N Am* 1983; 14:243.
26. Haldeman S: The electrodiagnostic evaluation of nerve root function. *Spine* 1984; 9:42–48.
27. Haldeman S: Pudendal nerve evoked spinal, cortical and bulbocavernosus reflex responses. Methods and application, in Cracco RQ, Bodis-Wollner I (eds): *Evoked Potentials. Frontiers of Clinical Neurosciences*, vol 3. New York, Alan R Liss, 1986.

28. Haldeman S, Shouka M, Robboy S: Computed tomography, electrodiagnostic and clinical findings in chronic Workers' Compensation patients with back and leg pain. *Spine* 1988; 13:345–350.

29. Hanley EN Jr, Matteri RE, and Frymoyer JW: Accurate roentgenographic determination of lumbar flexion-extension. *Clin Orthop* 1976; 155:145.

30. Herkowitz HN, Romeyn RL, Rothman, RH: The indications for metrizamide myelography. *J Bone Joint Surg* 1983; 65:1144–1149.

31. Hitselberger WE, Witten RM: Abnormal myelograms in asymptomatic patients. *J Neurosurg* 1968; 28:204.

32. Holt EP Jr: The question of lumbar discography. *J Bone Joint Surg* 1968; 50:720.

33. Hubbard J, Maultsby J, Wexler CE: Lumbar and cervical thermography for nerve fiber impingement: A critical review. *Clin J Pain* 1986; 2:131.

34. Hudgins WR: The predictive value of myelography in the diagnosis of ruptured lumbar discs. *J Neurosurg* 1970; 32:152.

35. Hudgins WR: Computer-aided diagnosis of lumbar disc herniation. *Spine* 1983; 8:604.

36. Hueftle MG, Modic MT, Ross JS, et al: Lumbar spine: Postoperative MR imaging with Gd-DTPA. *Radiology* 1988; 167:817.

37. Jackson RP, Jacobs RR, Montesano PX: Facet joint injection in low-back pain. A prospective statistical study. *Spine* 1988; 13:966.

38. Johnston CC JR, Epstein S: Clinical, biochemical, radiogaphic, epidemiologic, and economic features of osteoporosis. *Orthop Clin N Am* 1981; 12:559.

39. Knutsson R: The instability associated with disk degeneration in the lumbar spine. *Acta Radiol* 1944; 25:593.

40. Krempen JF, Smith BS: Nerve-root injection. A method for evaluating the etiology of sciatica. *J Bone Joint Surg* 1974; 56:1435.

41. Krempen JF, Smith BS, DeFreest LJ: Selective nerve root infiltration for the evaluation of sciatica. *Orthop Clin N Am* 1975; 6:311.

42. Kurz LT, Garfin SR, Bjorkengren AG, et al: Intraspinal synovial cysts: Radiologic documentation of their facet communication (abstract). *Orthop Trans* 1986; 10:510.

43. Lawlis GF, McCoy CE: Psychological evaluation: Patients with chronic pain. *Orthop Clin N Am* 1983; 14:527.

44. Leuders H, Gurd A, Hahn J, et al: A new technique for intraoperative monitoring of spinal cord function: Multichannel recording of spinal cord and subcortical evoked potentials. *Spine* 1982; 7:110–115.

45. Liang M, Komaroff M: Roentgenograms in primary care patients with acute low back pain. A cost effectiveness analysis. *Arch Int Med* 1982; 142:1108.

46. Macnab I: The traction spur. An indicator of segmental instability. *J Bone Joint Surg* 1971; 53:663.

47. Mahoney L. McCulloch J, Csima A: Thermography in back pain. 1. Thermography as a diagnostic aid in sciatica. *Thermology* 1985; 1:43.

48. Masaryk TJ, Ross JS, Modic MT, et al: High resolution MR imaging of sequestered lumbar intervertebral discs. *AJNR* 1988; 9:351.

49. Modic MT: MRI of the spine. Chicago, Year Book Medical Publisher, 1988.

50. Modic MT, Masaryk T, Boumphrey F, et al: Lumbar herniated disk disease and canal stenosis: Prospective evaluation by surface coil MR, CT, and myelography. *AJNR* 1986; 7:709.

51. Mooney V: Alternative approaches to the patient beyond the help of surgery. *Orthop Clin N Am* 1975; 6:331.

52. Mooney V: The syndromes of low back disease. *Orthop Clin N Am* 1983; 14:505.

53. Mooney V, Robertson J: The facet syndrome. *Clin Orthop* 1976; 115:149.

54. Moran FP, King T: Primary instability of lumbar vertebrae as a common cause of low back pain. *J Bone Joint Surg* 1957; 39:6.

55. Nawab RA, Azar HA: The laboratory diagnosis of plasma cell myeloma and related disorders. *Orthop Clin N Am* 1979; 10:391.

56. Onofrio BM, Mih AD: Synovial cysts of the spine. *Neurosurg* 1988; 22:642.
57. Paris SV: Anatomy as related to function and pain. *Orthop Clin N Am* 1983; 14:475.
58. Pochaczevsky R: The value of liquid crystal thermography in the diagnosis of spinal root compression syndromes. *Orthop Clin N Am* 1983; 14:271.
59. Pope MH, Hanley EN, Matteri RE, et al: Measurement of intervertebral disc space height. *Spine* 1977; 2:282.
60. Posner I, White AA III, Edwards WT, et al: A biomechanical analysis of the clinical stability of the lumbar and lumbosacral spine. *Spine* 1982; 7:374.
61. Pyhtinen J, Lahde S, Tanska E-L, Laitinen J: Computed tomography after lumbar myelography in lower back and extremity pain syndromes. *Diagn Imag* 1983; 52:19.
62. Ransford AO, Cairns D, Mooney V: The pain drawing as an aid to the psychologic evaluation of patients with low back pain. *Spine* 1976; 1:127.
63. Rothman RH: Patterns in lumbar disk degeneration. *Clin Orthop* 1974; 99:18.
64. Rothman SLG, Glenn WV Jr: *Multiplanar CT of the Spine.* Baltimore, University Park Press, 1985.
65. Saal JA, Dillingham MF, Gambard RG, et al: The pseudoradicular syndrome: Lower extremity peripheral entrapment masquerading as lumbar radiculopathy. A report of thirty-one cases. Presented at the meeting of the North American Spine Society, Banff, Canada, June 25–28, 1987.
66. Sachs BL, Vanharanta H, Spivey MA, et al: Dallas discogram description: A new classification of CT/discography in low-back disorders. *Spine* 1987; 12:287.
67. Scavone JG, Latshaw RF, Rohrer G: Use of lumbar spine films. Statistical evaluation at a university teaching hospital. *JAMA* 1981; 246:1105.
68. Scham SM, Taylor TKF: Tension signs in lumbar disc prolapse. *Clin Orthop* 1971; 75:195.
69. Troup JDG: Straight-leg raising (SLR) and the qualifying tests for increased root tension: Their predictive value after back and sciatic pain. *Spine* 1981; 6:526.
70. Vanharanta H, Guyer RD, Ohnmeiss DD, et al: Disc deterioration in low-back syndromes. A prospective, multi-center CT/discography study. *Spine* 1988; 13:1349.
71. Van Lente F: Alkaline and acid phosphatase determinations in bone disease. *Orthop Clin N Am* 1979; 10:437.
72. Waddell G, McCulloch JA, Kummel E, et al: Nonorganic physical signs in low back pain. *Spine* 1979; 5:117.
73. Weinstein J, Claverie W, Gibson S: The pain of discography. *Spine* 1988; 13:1344.
74. Wiesel SW: Personal communication, 1989.
75. Wiesel SW, Tsourmas N, Feffer HI, et al: A study of computer-assisted tomography. I. The incidence of positive CAT scans in an asymptomatic group of patients. *Spine* 1984; 9:549.
76. Wiltse LL, Widell EH Jr, Jackson DW: Fatigue fracture: The basic lesion in isthmic spondylolisthesis. *J Bone Joint Surg* 1975; 57:17.
77. Woodhall B, Hayes GJ: The well-leg-raising test of Fajersztajn in the diagnosis of ruptured intervertebral disc. *J Bone Joint Surg* 1950; 32:786.
78. Woody J, Lehmann T, Weinstein J, et al: Excessive translation on flexion-extension radiographs in asymptomatic populations. Presented at the meeting of the International Society for the Study of the Lumbar Spine, Miami, Florida, April 13–17, 1988.

9

Treatment of the Acutely Injured Worker

Gunnar B.J. Andersson, M.D., Ph.D.
John W. Frymoyer, M.D.

INTRODUCTION

The title of this chapter could lead a reader to the erroneous assumption that workers with acute low back pain have developed their pain from an injury. In fact, the number of workers who suffer an obvious spinal injury from a fall, direct blow, or other trauma are in the minority. Most workers sustain their injury from some other, less obvious event, usually related to lifting or overexertion. The events leading up to the acute onset of symptoms are frequently vague and, as noted in previous chapters, the physical findings are nonspecific. Further confusing the problem is that, when there is the potential for compensation, workers are far more apt to identify a work-related event as the precipitant cause. Regardless of cause, the vast majority of workers with acute symptoms are no different from the individuals who develop low back pain during recreation or from no obvious cause. The treatment of these acutely injured workers is the topic of this chapter.

As discussed elsewhere in this book, the natural history of LBP episodes is quite favorable, with rapid recovery being the rule rather than the exception (Chapter 4). As a reminder, Figure 9.1 illustrates the expected recovery rate for all cases of LBP with or without leg pain.[1,4,21] More than 70% of those affected recover in two to three weeks, 90% in six weeks. When symptoms persist more than seven weeks, the condition is chronic and usually requires a totally different diagnostic and therapeutic approach.[21]

Such a favorable natural history should be reassuring to the patient, treating physician, and supervisor. It also has important implications for research, which attempts to determine which treatments are effective. A basic principle in the scientific research on low back disease is the use of the randomized, controlled prospective study. This means that patients are randomly allocated to either a treatment group using the method under study or a control group. In the ideal study, the control group receives no treatment and therefore should represent the natural history of the untreated problem, which is already very favorable for most acute low back pain.[6] The barriers to this type of research are formidable. As a result, only a small number of such studies have been performed, and our information about what treatments are truly effective is limited. This issue has been discussed by Deyo,[6] and similar conclusions were reached by the Quebec Task Force,[21] a panel of experts drawn from many disciplines. After analyzing over 600 published articles, the task force concluded that only a few treatments for low back pain and sciatica have established scientific validity.

In this chapter we review the available treatment options, emphasizing methods that

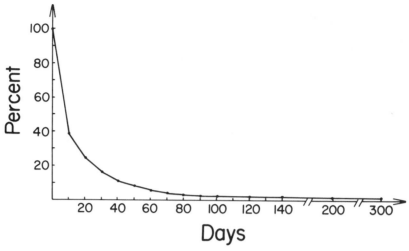

FIG 9.1.
Proportion of patients still sicklisted as a function of time. Refer to text for details about the study. (From Andersson GBJ, Svensson H-O, Oden A: The intensity of work recovery in low back pain. *Spine* 1983; 8:880–884. Used by permission.)

have been validated by scientific study, and then describe our preferred method. Before presenting this information, it is important to emphasize the goals for treatment of the acutely injured worker.

THE GOALS OF TREATMENT

Three main treatment goals should be set for the acutely injured worker: (1) reduction of pain and discomfort, (2) rapid return to function and work, and (3) avoidance of recurrent or persisting symptoms leading to chronicity. These goals are best accomplished by a structured approach.[4,25] The three goals require separate attention, and on occasion they may conflict with each other. Reduction of pain may be a deterrent to rapid return to work and function, and chronicity or recurrence may follow from inadequate attention to factors not directly related to the pain. Most important, the natural history for recovery should always be kept in mind. If an individual patient is not recovering at the expected rate, a careful analysis to determine the possible causes of pain should be performed and the treatment plan altered accordingly.

The attainment of these goals starts immediately on the initial encounter with the back-injured worker. In the acute phase pain may be highly variable, ranging from modest aching to intense symptoms. When pain is severe, there are often difficulties in undressing, and the patient is afraid to move, cough, sneeze, or laugh for fear of further pain. As the treating medical professional takes a history, attention must first be given to the patient's comfort. During the physical examination time and patience are required to allow the patient's fear of increasing pain and spasm to subside and to let the patient gain confidence in the physician and treatment. When the history and physical examination are complete, the patient should be informed of the benign nature of the illness and given the assurance that recovery in a relatively short time is likely. The choice of treatment is then based on the severity of the acute symptoms.

AMBULATORY TREATMENT

Many workers with modest symptoms are actually not in need of any treatment and can in fact remain at work. If the worker is normally involved in heavy labor, short-term light duty may be necessary. It is the policy of many companies not to allow light duty and to require the worker to be "100% capable" before returning to work. Although the issue is certainly complex, industry should at least be aware that the cost may be higher to themselves and the worker if the 100% healthy policy is enforced, particularly when the symptoms are of modest severity. Several studies in a variety of industries have shown that keeping the worker at the job site reduces the duration of time lost from work and results in significant cost savings.[20,25] An important part of this strategy is to have on site a health professional who is knowledgeable about low back pain. Yet another dividend from this type of enlightened industrial policy has been a significant reduction in the number of workers requiring later surgery.

MEDICATIONS

The use of narcotic medications, muscle relaxants, and tranquilizers have all been advocated, and they are widely used in the treatment of low back pain. These drugs are rarely necessary and, in fact, many have unpleasant side effects. There is little question that the worker with severe symptoms may require the short-term judicious use of a narcotic such as codeine. Both the patient and the treating physician should have a clear plan for stopping the narcotic within two to three days. If a narcotic such as codeine does not give adequate pain relief, a more serious spinal disorder such as an infection or tumor should be suspected. Unfortunately, with the significant problem of drug abuse in our society, thought should also be given to the possibility that substance abuse might be a complicating factor when the acute symptoms require ongoing narcotics.

A wide variety of drugs are termed muscle relaxants, yet few have been shown to have a direct effect on muscle spasm, and most are central nervous system depressants, that is, tranquilizers. The side effects are varied and may include unexpected mood alterations, such as depression, and diminished mental and physical acuity. For this reason, these drugs should be used cautiously, particularly if it is a goal to keep the patient working. Again, short-term use for patients with more severe symptoms is acceptable mainly to relax the patient so that rest is easier.

The drugs of choice in low back pain are nonnarcotic analgesics, most of which have some antiinflammatory properties that may also add to their effectiveness. The most safely and commonly used drugs are aspirin compounds, acetaminophen, and ibuprofen. Most of these drugs have been subjected to scientific scrutiny and have been shown to relieve pain effectively but have only minimal effect on the rate of functional recovery.[6,24] NSAIDs (nonsteroidal antiinflammatory medication) is recommended, particularly if rhizopathy exists.

MANIPULATION

Manipulation has been the source of much controversy. Contrary to popular opinion, there is no single form of manipulation. The techniques range from rather gross and forceful rotations of the spine to a relatively gentle, low-amplitude thrust. Because there are so many forms and schools of manipulation and because of the benign natural history of back pain it has been difficult to establish the effectiveness of this treatment form. There is sufficient evidence, however, to reach the following conclusions[3,14,18]:

1. In acute low back pain one or two manipulations are effective in reducing pain severity and may slightly improve the rate of functional recovery.
2. The effectiveness of manipulation appears to be limited to the first one or two weeks, having little benefit thereafter. Therefore, its primary use is in acute low back pain and not in subacute and chronic conditions.
3. Repetitive or multiple manipulations have no demonstrated effectiveness, nor is there evidence that manipulation either corrects chronic low back conditions or prevents recurrences.
4. The mechanism by which manipulation causes its effects is unknown, although there are many theories. The least plausible one is that manipulation realigns a spine that is out of alignment or replaces a displaced tissue or structure.

BEDREST

The time-honored treatment for low back pain has been bedrest. Historically, this treatment was often extended for many days, or even weeks, frequently reinforced by the use of traction. Until recently, the effectiveness of such treatment was uncertain. Wiesel et al.[24] have reported prospective studies in young male military recruits and found that seven days of bedrest was more effective than ambulatory treatment. Later, Deyo, Diehl, and Rosenthal[7] performed a study in which he and his associates demonstrated that two days of bedrest was as effective as seven days. Moreover, the short term of bedrest reduced the period of dysfunction. Three months later the test subjects were reevaluated, and no differences were found with respect to chronicity or recurrence of symptoms.

MODALITIES

Modalities is a commonly used term referring to a variety of applied treatments, usually given by physical therapists. Included in this category are heat, cold (ice), massage, diathermy, and ultrasound. Although there are strong proponents of each method, the scientific basis of these treatments is at best conjectural. Whether heat works better than cold is probably best discovered by experience with a given patient rather than by making a categorical statement applicable to all patients. Massage feels good to many patients. Diathermy and ultrasound, however, have no proven therapeutic effects in low back pain, and therefore consideration should be given to cost versus benefit. Other modalities that may have some effectiveness in chronic low back pain are not a consideration in patients with acute symptoms. The most important of these is transcutaneous electrical nerve stimulation (TENS). A key point in the use of modalities is not to persist. Passive therapy has negative effect if prolonged, as discussed later in this chapter.

TRACTION

Traction is one of the oldest treatment forms, yet it has been rigorously evaluated in only a few studies. Traction may be given by gravity reduction methods, such as hanging upside down (sometimes called inversion therapy), by autotraction devices, and by motorized tables. There is almost no data about traction in acute low back pain, but one study concluded that traction had no additional benefits to bedrest alone.[19] Two other studies limited their patient selection to those with low back pain and sciatica and suggested a modest but significant effect on pain relief.[12,17]

EXERCISE PROGRAMS

In the acute phase of low back pain there is little role for exercise programs. In fact, flexion exercises may increase the pressure within the intervertebral discs and accentuate symptoms, particularly if the patient has low back pain and sciatica. Kendall and Jenkins[15] compared exercise programs and concluded there was only modest effectiveness once symptoms had become reduced to a tolerable level. Isometric exercises appeared to be the most effective. In the past decade there has been increased enthusiasm for spinal extension exercises, a position promoted by MacKenzie, whose name is often attached to those programs. An independent study by Donaldson, Silva, and Murphy[9] of the "MacKenzie method" showed the technique to be effective in patients with low back pain, with or without sciatica, but no adequate control group was included. In subacute back pain, Vanharanta, Videman, and Mooney[22] found that extension therapy was more effective than traction or back school.

More important than muscle-strengthening exercises has been the use of aerobic exercise. By *aerobic exercise* is meant any physical activity that increases the heart rate; it does not mean specific aerobic exercise classes. Chöler et al.[4] have shown that this effectively hastens the functional recovery. Alternative exercises applicable to acute symptoms are walking, swimming, and the use of stationary bikes. Underlying this treatment program is an increasing amount of basic biomechanical knowledge about spinal support structures and muscle that indicates the beneficial effect of physical activity on muscle, ligament, bone, and intervertebral disc.

BACK SCHOOL

The topic of education in the treatment and prevention of occupational low back disorders is presented in detail in Chapter 15. Suffice it to say that this form of treatment is effective in the acute and subacute phase of back pain, and it increases the rate of functional recovery.

AUTHORS' RECOMMENDED TREATMENT

The information given above demonstrates that effective treatment is limited to a relatively small group of simple, cost-effective measures that can improve the rate of pain relief and functional recovery. Unfortunately, none of these treatments have been proved to be effective in the prevention of recurrent low back pain.

Patients with less severe pain who can remain ambulatory are encouraged to do so, and medications are usually limited to aspirin or one of the nonsteroidal antiinflammatory medications (NSAIDs).

For patients with more severe pain, treatment for the first two days is modified bedrest and medication. The patient may arise for meals and to use the toilet. When in bed, the patient is encouraged to lie on the side or back with the hips or knees flexed. The bed should be arranged for maximum comfort, with a bolster or pillows placed behind the knees to achieve hip and knee flexed position. The patient should be taught to rise from bed without imposing additional strain on the back. This is accomplished by first logrolling and then using the legs over the edge of the bed as a counterbalance while pushing off with the arm. Medications used over the first few days are limited to aspirin or acetaminophen. Propoxyphene, codeine, and oxycodone may occasionally be given if pain is very severe. Careful instructions are given to use these medications sparingly. A mild laxative may be necessary because of the constipating effect of narcotics. NSAIDs have analgesic as well as antiinflammatory effect. The choice is empiric, since most of the newer NSAIDs have similar effects, although some agents are more effective than others in an individual patient. The side effects vary also, but all can cause gastric irritation. The cost also varies considerably, and this is an additional consideration. Muscle relaxants are rarely indicated. Hot packs and cold treatment may be used at the patient's discretion.

On the third day, patients are encouraged to begin a program of gradually increasing their activity, which should include walking for short distances. Several walks a day of 500 to 1,000 meters (half a mile) are encouraged. Gentle movements in flexion, extension, and lateral bending over the initial one-fourth of the normal range of motion should also be started at this time. Each day the number of movements is increased and the range is increased. Additional walking is encouraged. Sitting is discouraged and kept to a maximum of a half hour at a time. Driving is also discouraged, except for short distances. The patient is told to report any significant deterioration, including the development of sciatica, urinary retention, or loss of bowel or bladder control.

The first follow-up visit is usually one week after the onset of symptoms. Radiographs are now obtained if there has been no significant improvement and are definitely indicated if there is worsening or if sciatica is present. Usually, radiographs are not necessary because recovery is ongoing and often nearly complete. The patient is then encouraged to return to work if the job requirements are sedentary or light. If the job is manual labor, a light-duty return is encouraged, although many companies do not have this option open. Increasing physical activity is advantageous, particularly for those who do heavy work because they have an increased risk of becoming chronic low back sufferers. As shown by Chöler et al.,[4] active and well-managed treatment hastens recovery (Fig. 9.2). Wiesel, Feffer, and Rothman[25] found that instituting a treatment algorithm allowed earlier return to work and significant savings in cost.

All workers should be advised to continue conditioning exercises to promote cardiovascular fitness, and they should also be advised in proper material handling techniques and back care.

If the worker is not improving, and the physical examination and radiographs do not

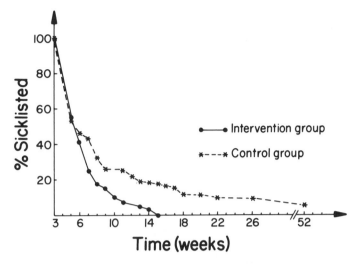

FIG 9.2.
Proportion of treated patients still sicklisted after 3 to 52 weeks: intervention group vs. control group. (From Chöler U, Larsson R, Nachemson A, et al: *Back pain—attempt at a structural treatment program for patients with low back pain.* SPRI Report 188, Social Planerings-och Rationaliseringsintstitut Rapport, Stockholm, 1985.)

reveal any significant pathology, ongoing bedrest is not recommended. Continued use of a NSAID is acceptable for pain management but not the use of a narcotic medication. We encourage continued walking, and we often enroll the worker in a physical therapy program designed to promote mobility but not heavily focused on muscle strengthening or on the use of "modalities." Reevaluation takes place weekly. If improvement has not occurred in one month, then radiographs are obtained in all patients, unless done previously. Based on the physical findings, additional studies may be contemplated during the interval between four weeks and six weeks. A definite decision may also be made as to whether the patient has a problem that might require surgery (rare) or whether an aggressive rehabilitation or work-hardening program will suffice. This approach is particularly important if no significant disease is discovered.

TREATMENT OF ACUTE BACK AND LEG PAIN

Workers who complain of pain radiating down one or both legs in a nerve root distribution represent a more severe subset of acutely injured workers. In these patients possible nerve root pressure, tension, and inflammation should be tested. The details of the physical examination of these individuals are outlined in Chapter 8. The straight leg raising (SLR) test is the most important clinical test in a suspected disc herniation, being almost always positive. If the test is positive on the affected side when the opposite leg is raised (crossed Lasègue or well leg raising test), the patient almost certainly has a herniated disc.[13] As discussed in Chapter 2, this type of sciatic pain must be differentiated from the nonspecific pain that most patients experience and that can sometimes affect the buttocks and thighs.

The acute care of these patients is similar to that of the "uncomplicated" low back pain patient. Although the recovery is slower, a significant number of patients recover without surgery. Hakelius[13] found that 50% of patients with sciatica were improved at four weeks and 90% in 90 days, a finding confirmed by Andersson, Svensson, and Oden.[1] This finding should strongly support a conservative attitude, particularly since Weber[23] found that patients with confirmed disc herniations treated conservatively were indistinguishable from operated patients 5, 10, and 15 years later.

Again, we present the scientific evidence for effective treatment, followed by our recommended approach.

Bedrest

There is almost no information about how effective bedrest is in the treatment of sciatica. In his study, Deyo[6] suggested but did not prove that two days might be as effective as seven days. What does seem evident is that treatment for more than a week is probably not effective. More important, continued and prolonged inactivity has harmful effects on joints, muscles, discs, and ligaments.[11]

Traction

As noted previously, two studies suggest that sciatica is improved by the addition of traction, but the benefit is at best marginal.[12,17]

Nonsteroidal Antiinflammatory Medications

Similar to the case of low back pain alone, nonsteroidal antiinflammatory medications appear to be effective in reducing the pain of sciatica. This issue has been studied specifically for phenylbutazone (Butazolidin) and indomethacin,[9] two drugs that are rarely used today.

Cortisone

Some physicians and surgeons use oral cortisone in an initially high dose (40–50 mg of prednisone), which is rapidly tapered over the next five to seven days. There is little evidence to show that this is uniformly successful. Historically, it was popular to inject cortisone or one of its derivatives into the intradural space, similar to the route used for a spinal anesthetic. This treatment has been implicated in the later development of nerve scarring. An alternative that does not have this complication is the epidural injection, in which the cortisone derivatives are injected into the epidural space, usually with some form of local anesthetic. The results of this treatment are controversial. In one prospective, randomized study this method was shown to be effective in patients with sciatica,[8] while in another it was ineffective.[5] The latter study has been criticized (and we agree), because the treatment effectiveness was determined 24 hours after the injection. It is our clinical experience, confirmed by others,[26] that the effects of the injection may become more apparent over the course of a few days to a week or more.

Other Treatments

There is no information to suggest that manipulation, "modalities," or corsets and braces have any beneficial effects on either pain reduction or functional restoration of acutely injured workers with sciatica.

Authors' Preferred Method

Initial bedrest is recommended for injured workers with sciatica. The patient must be clearly told to notify the physician if increasing weakness occurs, and particularly to report urgently any change in bladder or bowel control. As is discussed in Chapter 4, the loss of bladder or bowel control may indicate a massive disc herniation, which occurs in 1 to 2% of patients with a known acute disc hernia.[16]

The duration of the initial bedrest is typically two days, although patients with severe pain and a strongly positive SLR may be counseled to have bedrest for up to seven days. Again, we do not reinforce the need to stay absolutely at rest, permitting the patient to be up for toilet and meals. The use of analgesics and antiinflammatory medications is encouraged, but the antiinflammatory drugs should be taken on a regular dosage, rather than sporadically, to achieve their full beneficial effects. If symptoms improve (confirmed by an increasing tolerance to straight leg raising), the patient is encouraged to begin walking, swimming, or stationary bicycling quite early. Return to work may be encouraged as soon as the worker is adequately comfortable, but definite restrictions should be made on lifting, prolonged sitting, long-distance driving, and awkward body postures for a minimum of six weeks. If the worker is improving at four weeks, it is worthwhile to consider more vigorous exercise, although sit-ups should probably be avoided for three months because they increase intradiscal pressure. By three months, the individual should be fully able to engage in all activities but should definitely have instruction in proper lifting techniques.

The exceptions to this approach comprise four groups of patients:

1. The injured worker who develops loss of control of bladder or bowel function. These individuals require urgent imaging studies and emergency surgery if a massive disc herniation is confirmed. No more than 1 to 2% of individuals with a disc herniation fall into this category.

2. The injured worker who develops progressive significant muscle weakness, such as foot drop. Although a delay in surgery of up to 12 weeks has been shown to have no effect on the recovery,[13] we see little merit in this period of delay. This group comprises no more than 5 to 10% of patients with documented disc herniation.

3. The injured worker who is having unrelenting pain, no change in or worsening of the straight leg raising test, and who has had adequate conservative treatment. In Weber's study,[23] this group involved 15% of all patients. Delay is appropriate only if there are signs of improvement.

4. The injured worker who has had a documented previous attack of sciatica within the past two years, has received adequate therapy, and now has a recurrence. Repeating conservative treatment in this group of patients is unrealistic, unless the individual wishes to choose this alternative again.

The diagnostic approach and surgical treatment for these patients is discussed in Chapter 8.

SUMMARY

The treatment of the acutely injured worker should begin as soon after the injury as possible. If symptoms permit, the worker should remain at the job site and be given light-duty work, with an anticipation of rapid return to full capacity. If symptoms are more severe, a short period of rest, analgesics, and antiinflammatory medications is followed by early functional restoration as the principal methods of treatment. Return to work should be possible for the majority after a few days or weeks. When symptoms persist for four to six weeks a more thorough investigation is advisable, because the worker should have recovered at this time. When sciatica is present, the same general principles are followed, although the recovery may be slower than for the worker with low back pain alone. Worsening of sciatica, muscle weakness, or recurrent sciatica are relative indications to consider imaging studies at four to six weeks and possible surgical intervention. In a small minority of patients, loss of bladder or bowel control constitutes an acute emergency and an urgent need for imaging studies and surgical intervention. Most patients with sciatica do not require surgery, however, and should be functional within three months.

BIBLIOGRAPHY

1. Andersson GBJ, Svensson H-O, Oden A: The intensity of work recovery in low back pain. *Spine* 1983; 8:880–884.
2. Bell GR, Rothman RH: The conservative treatment of sciatica. *Spine* 1984; 9:54–56.
3. Brumarski DJ: Clinical trials of spinal manipulation: A critical appraisal and review of the literature. *J Manipulative Physiol Ther* 1984; 7:243–249.
4. Chöler U, Larsson R, Nachemson A, et al: *Back pain—attempt at a structured treatment program for patients with low back pain* (in Swedish). SPRI Report 188, Social Planerings-och Rational Isesingsinstitut Rapport, Stockholm, 1985.
5. Cuckler JM, Bernini PA, Wiesel SW, et al: The use of epidural steroids in the treatment of lumbar radicular pain: A prospective randomized, double-blind study. *J Bone Joint Surg* 1985; 67:63–66.
6. Deyo RA: Conservative treatment for low back pain: Distinguishing useful from useless therapy. *JAMA* 1983; 250:1057–1062.
7. Deyo RA, Diehl AK, Rosenthal M: How much bed rest for acute low back pain? *N Engl J Med* 1986; 315:1064–1070.
8. Dilke TFW, Burry HC, Grahame R: Extradural corticosteroid injection in management of lumbar nerve root compression. *Br Med J* 1973; 2:635–637.
9. Donaldson R, Silva J, Murphy K: The centralization phenomenon, its usefulness in evaluating and treating radiating pain. *Spine* 1990; in press.
10. Frymoyer JW: Back pain and sciatica. *N Engl J Med* 1988; 318:291–300.
11. Frymoyer JW, Gordon SL (eds): *New Perspectives on Low Back Pain*. Park Ridge, Illinois, American Academy of Orthopedic Surgeons, 1988.
12. Gillström P, Ehrnberg A: Long-term results of autotraction in the treatment of lumbago and sciatica: An attempt to correlate clinical results with objective parameters. *Arch Orthop Trauma Surg* 1985; 104:294–298.
13. Hakelius A: Prognosis in sciatica: A clinical follow-up of surgical and nonsurgical treatment. *Acta Orthop Scand [suppl]* 1970; 129:1–76.
14. Haldeman S: Spinal manipulative therapy: A status report. *Clin Orthop* 1983; 179:62–70.
15. Kendall PH, Jenkins JM: Exercise for backache: A double-blind controlled trial. *Physiotherapy* 1968; 54:154–157.
16. Kostuik JP, Harrington I, Alexander D, et al: Cauda equina syndrome and lumbar disc herniation. *J Bone Joint Surg* 1986; 68:386–391.

17. Larsson U, Chöler U, Lidström A, et al: Auto-traction for treatment of lumbago-sciatica: A multicentre controlled investigation. *Acta Orthop Scand* 1980; 51:791–798.

18. Ottenbacher K, DiFabio RP: Efficacy of spinal manipulation/mobilization therapy: A meta-analysis. *Spine* 1985; 10:833–837.

19. Pal B, Magnion P, Hossain MA, et al: A controlled trial of continuous lumbar traction in the treatment of back pain and sciatica. *Br J Rheumatol* 1986; 25:181–183.

20. Spengler DM. Personal communication. 1989.

21. Spitzer WO, Le Blanc FE, Dupuis M, et al: Scientific approach to the assessment and management of activity-related spinal disorders: A monograph for clinicians. *Spine* [suppl 1] 1987; 12:1–59.

22. Vanharanta H, Videman T, Mooney V: McKenzie exercises backtrack and back school in lumbar syndrome. *Ort Trans* 1986; 10:533.

23. Weber H: Lumbar disc herniation: A controlled prospective study with ten years of observation. *Spine* 1983; 8:131–140.

24. Wiesel SW, Cuckler JM, DeLuca C, et al: Acute low back pain: An objective analysis of conservative therapy. *Spine* 1980; 5:324–330.

25. Wiesel SW, Feffer HL, Rothman RH: Industrial low back pain: A prospective evaluation of a standardized diagnostic and treatment protocol. *Spine* 1984; 9:100.

26. White AH, Denby R, Wynne G: Epidural injections for the diagnosis and treatment of low back pain. *Spine* 1980; 5:78–86.

10

Rehabilitation of the Patient with Chronic Low Back Pain

Rowland G. Hazard, M.D.
Leonard N. Matheson, Ph.D.
Thomas R. Lehmann, M.D.
John W. Frymoyer, M.D.

INTRODUCTION

Since low back pain (LBP) strikes 80% of all adults at some point in their lives, it must be considered part of normal life. Fortunately, about 90% of those afflicted recover comfort and function within two to three months.[3,27] The 10% who do not recover within a few months, however, have such a dismal prognosis that many do not ever recover sufficiently to return to work. It is this group of patients that poses the greatest problems in medical management and accounts for most of the costs. A recent study of back injuries at the Boeing Company[24] Spengler reported that 79% of the total cost for low back-injured patients were devoted to 10% of the cases with chronic disability. These epidemiologic features of the natural history of low back injury underscore the urgency with which the health, insurance, and industrial disciplines currently approach the apparent epidemic of chronic occupational back pain and disability.

When does acute pain become chronic? At a National Institute of Disability and Rehabilitation Research workshop in 1987,[4] there was general agreement that the chronic phase of low back pain begins about three months after onset. In comparison, a recent report from Quebec[25] suggests that chronic pain begins at seven weeks. While the time of the exact transition from acute to chronic phases of low back pain may be disputed, its significance is not. Entry into the chronic phase is marked by a sudden decline in symptomatic recovery despite assumed completion of tissue healing following initial trauma. This is at least in part due to the compounding of the original nociceptive event by a host of psychosocial issues and disability behaviors. As Waddell[26] has concluded, chronic back pain and disability are best understood as a complex biopsychosocial problem (see Chapter 2). Treatment is no longer a matter of straightening out a few "nuts and bolts" that have gone awry in the patient's back. In fact, a specific, curable cause for symptoms is rarely evident in these patients. For the vast majority of patients with chronic pain the traditional medical model of pathophysiologic diagnosis, specific treatment, and subsequent relief of pain proves ineffective.[6]

The worker disabled by chronic back pain faces problems on several fronts. Without a diagnosis, cure, or clear prognosis, the patient may pass from one practitioner to another in search of "the answer." In the meantime, the individual's role within the family, community, and work group may be profoundly altered. Often encouraged by physician and family alike, the patient may avoid activities that might cause reinjury. A progressive pattern of self-limitation from previous work and recreational activities often results in a general deconditioning syndrome,[20] which becomes a significant feature of disability in its own right. Self-image and personal confidence may dwindle because of curtailed capacities and social involvement. Compensation for lost wages often is insufficient to meet the family's financial demands, and the difference may erode accumulated savings. Dismissal shortly after returning to work is anticipated because of the potential for back injury liability in the employer's mind. In this setting, worker's compensation benefits appear to be the only financial salvation. Life changes of such magnitude are often associated with depression, anger, guilt, and anxiety. These conditions contribute to the experience of chronic pain in what becomes a vicious cycle of pain and situational distress. Drug and alcohol abuse may provide further complications. Most of the chronically disabled workers are beset by a wide variety of such problems. Rehabilitation amounts to an undoing of this disability process.

Fordyce[7] has pointed out the poor correlation between self-assessments of pain and observed functional capacity in patients with chronic low back pain. This discrepancy, labeled "symptom magnification" by Matheson[15] and "disability exaggeration" by Hazard et al.[10] makes assessment of work readiness extremely difficult in the usual medical office visit scenario. Nevertheless, clinicians traditionally rely on their patients' self-reports of pain and disability when recommending return-to-work dates, assessing work capacities, and rating impairment levels. Such estimations may come as the "final blows" in patient-physician relationships originally based on mutual expectations of biologic diagnoses and cures.

In the past 30 years, the failure of the traditional medical model in reducing occupational back pain and disability has spawned a variety of alternative approaches. For the most part, pain centers, work-hardening programs, and functional restoration centers share an appreciation for the complexity and interrelationships of the biologic and psychosocial issues involved in chronic low back disability. Therefore, treatment is frequently multidisciplinary. Programmatic therapy of chronic back pain is evolutionary, in that questions regarding the relative importance of the various therapeutic components, accountability, and even accreditation remain unanswered. The central problem lies in the nature of chronic pain itself, because it is virtually impossible to quantify objectively. Related outcomes such as physical capacity, psychologic well-being, coping skills, family adjustment, occupational fitness, and return to work are also difficult to quantify. The relative importance of these outcomes varies when considered by patients, health care providers, insurance carriers, and employers.[11] Recognizing these problems in quantification of therapeutic outcome, the remainder of this chapter addresses the basic elements of rehabilitation as well as the contents and outcomes of pain centers, work-hardening programs, and functional restoration centers.

STEPS IN REHABILITATION

Table 10.1 shows five steps taken in the rehabilitation process. Since each step takes time, it's not necessary to wait for mastery or achievement of each step before proceeding to the next. These steps include accepting the impairment, establishing goals, understanding barriers, reinforcing goals, and managing pain.

TABLE 10.1
Steps in Rehabilitation

- Accepting the impairment
- Establishing goals
- Understanding barriers
- Reinforcing goals
- Managing pain

Accepting the Impairment

The first step for the patient is accepting a realistic level of impairment. After the loss of any bodily function there is a period of mourning and anger and an unwillingness to accept the impairment as is. Some patients never get past this stage. The successful process is twofold: (1) accepting the reality of the loss and (2) accepting self-responsibility for adaptation. The patient with low back impairment faces particular difficulty, because the impairment is neither as visible nor as definitive as an impairment such as the loss of a limb. The lack of a clear pathophysiologic explanation for the pain frequently causes further frustration.

Others around the patient (family, physicians, employers, neighbors) may also have a difficult time seeing, understanding, and accepting that the LBP patient is disabled. The patient's failure to function is seen as weak, contrary to the work ethic, and questionably motivated. All of the patient's energies may be consumed in the search for an explanation that will restore credibility to his complaints. This often includes visits to many health professionals in an attempt to legitimize the problem, even to the point of seeking surgery.

Another typical reaction is anger. It is one order of anger to hurt in the first place, but a much higher order of anger to hurt and be suspected of malingering. This angle also misdirects the patient's energy. Getting even rather than getting well becomes the goal.

The patient's caretakers must understand and even anticipate these feelings. They must also explain the nature of the impairment and, if possible, the nature of the anatomic cause. Words that may frighten the patient, such as "degeneration" or "disintegration," should be carefully avoided. If the cause is unknown, the patient must be taught the possible sources of pain. The permanent nature of the impairment must be explained so that the patient's energy is no longer devoted to finding the cure but rather to restoring maximal function. The patient must not view the rehabilitation process as a treatment trial, nor should surgery be held out as a contingency if it is not already indicated. The rehabilitation process has to be viewed as the achievement of a clearly stated goal: function despite the impairment.

The patient is educated about the inherent conflict between disability and rehabilitation. With disability comes a dependency on others: doctors, family, insurance company, employer, and welfare. In contrast, the goal of rehabilitation is to become independent. The patient must become his or her own 24-hour-a-day therapist, who is knowledgeable and dependable in self-treatment. Once the problem is accepted as real and as one requiring self-responsibility, the next step is the establishment of goals.

Establishing Goals

The therapist must help the patient distinguish impairment from disability. The impairment is the patient's loss of bodily function. The disability is the patient's loss of capacity to cope with the physical and socioeconomic environment. The patient is taught that the presence of the impairment does not necessarily have to cause disability. Total disability and total rehabilitation are viewed as two ends of a yardstick. The major goal for the patient is to achieve maximal rehabilitation. Short- and long-term goals should be identified. The long-term goal of total independence and financial and emotional security may appear unattainable, and therefore short-term, attainable goals must be reached. Each short-term goal is considered a step toward more challenging objectives. Examples of short-term goals are achieving a certain level of repetitions in an exercise, acquiring certification of high-school equivalence, solving a family problem, working as a volunteer, or taking a lower-paying job and accepting lower socioeconomic status until return to a better position becomes possible. Achievement of each short-term goal reinforces positive behavior and helps restore confidence.

Understanding Barriers

The next step is learning more about the barriers that low back pain patients must overcome; these barriers may be invisible or hidden. Therapists teach patients about the barriers and alternate ways of dealing with them.

The barriers for the disabled low back pain patient may include fear, anger, work disincentives, misunderstanding, limited education, stressful life situations, the physical impairment itself, vocational limitations, and emotional instability. As described later in this chapter, several therapeutic disciplines may be required for crossing these barriers, including counseling, teaching, behavior modification, physical training, and vocational advice.

Reinforcing

Reinforcement involves the affective component of the learning experience. This affective learning is enhanced through the team or multidisciplinary approach, by peer pressure or patient group interaction, and by involving family members. Regular team conferences enhance communications within the team and with the patient. Regular team conferences allow all members to coordinate their approach and reinforce the learning experience.

Therapists must be compassionate and understanding but firm in demanding achievement of reasonable goals. For example, at the commencement of the Iowa rehabilitation program, patients were told to set and achieve their own goals.[12] Of the first 26 patients treated, however, none returned to work. A policy was developed of giving patients a termination date for their healing period and a release to return to work within a few weeks of discharge. In the subsequent 51 patients treated by this policy 17 returned to work and were still working six months later, 5 returned to work but lost their jobs because of the poor economy, 4 returned but were unable to function because of their backs, 3 went into vocational training, and 22 never attempted to return to work or retraining. Thus, a simple change in strategy (but not in program content) increased the reemployment rate from 0 to 45%.

Most patients improve while in the rehabilitation environment, but some regress after discharge. By teaching the family the concept of behavior modification, the home environment can become a rehabilitation environment. The family often controls the success or failure of the rehabilitation effort. Patients with severe disability have returned to work because the spouse played a strong affective role. The opposite may occur in other families.

Utilization of Pain Management Modalities

The fifth step in the rehabilitation process is the utilization of pain management techniques. Psychoactive modalities such as relaxation therapy, biofeedback, operant conditioning, and cognitive behavioral therapy may be useful. These are discussed later in this chapter.

Several authors have studied the role of transcutaneous electrical nerve stimulation (TENS) for pain control in LBP patients. In a controlled trial of subthreshold TENS, TENS unit with dual battery, and electroacupuncture applied to patients participating in a low back rehabilitation program, the electrical stimulation produced no noticeable effect on the overall rehabilitation results.[13]

Given the diversity of biologic, social, and psychologic barriers facing patients with chronic low back pain and disability, comprehensive rehabilitation must be multidisciplinary. Pain management, work hardening, and functional restoration with behavioral support have emerged as the foremost rehabilitation strategies. While these approaches overlap somewhat in content, each offers a particular focus, as outlined in Table 10.2. The treatment of choice may not be clear for a given patient, as there are no rigorous studies comparing the effectiveness of these approaches for various patient types. In general, functional restoration with behavioral support has had the best documented success in enabling people with chronic occupational low back disability to return to work.

PAIN CENTERS

In the past 20 years, more than 1,000 pain clinics have been developed in the United States for the treatment of patients with chronic pain. These programs include a wide variety of passive therapies, such as ultrasound, manipulation, massage, acupuncture, electrical stimulation, and facet and epidural injections. Some programs utilize these passive modalities and serve as little more than a triage for referral to other specialists, such as orthopedic surgeons, neurosurgeons, rheumatologists, anesthesiologists, psychologists, and psychiatrists. Other programs share a reliance on behavioral modification. Such programs are based on Fordyce et al.'s observation that the severity of chronic pain complaints often does not correlate with measured functional performance.[7] Acting on the fact that it is not possible to measure directly and change the subjective experience of pain,

TABLE 10.2
Relative Focus of Three Rehabilitation Approaches

Pain Center
- Passive modalities: heat, cold, acupuncture, ultrasound, electrical stimulation, nerve blocks
- Behavioral modification

Work-Hardening Program
- Graded work simulation
- Work feasibility evaluation and enhancement

Functional Restoration Program
- Physical retraining (sports medicine) guided by repeated measurements of functional capacities
- Occupational case management

---

pain center programs focus on modifying the behaviors generated by that experience. These behaviors may produce reinforcing consequences for the patient, such as attention from family members, compensation benefits, and so on. Without these consequences, the behaviors are "unrewarded" and therefore less likely to persist. A key feature of behavioral methods is the interruption of this self-perpetuating cycle of pain, behavior, and environmental consequences. The fundamental goal of most behavioral approaches is the reduction of disability through behavioral change rather than the direct diminution of pain. With or without the above-mentioned passive modalities, pain centers use such behavior-related techniques as group and individual counseling, hypnosis, stress-management, biofeedback, educational classes, and family sessions. The intensity of these programs ranges from occasional outpatient treatment to intensive inpatient programs. As the content of these programs varies, so does the disciplinary representation by medical subspecialists, counselors, physical and occupational therapists, and so on.

The efficacy of the pain center approach to chronic back pain rehabilitation is controversial.[2,8] Differences in program content and pretreatment patient characteristics defy generalizations of therapeutic effectiveness. The disparate criteria of pain reduction and decreased pain behaviors further obscure comparisons between programs and the relationships of specific program contents and outcome.

To date, there does not appear to be conclusive evidence that isolated aspects of pain center programs reduce subjective reports of pain, though improvements in activity level, medication use, and other pain-related behaviors have been reported.[8] Detoxification, particularly from narcotic analgesics, is usually more appropriate in the pain center setting than in less medically oriented programs.

WORK HARDENING

Work hardening is a comparatively recent rehabilitation approach for patients with chronic occupational low back pain. Work hardening was developed in the mid-1970s at Rancho Los Amigos Hospital in Downey, California. Graded work-simulation tasks, which mimicked tasks the injured worker would be required to perform when returning to work, were designed to promote physical and emotional conditioning. Work hardening has become popular throughout the United States, Canada, and Australia as a means of rehabilitating individuals who are occupationally disabled. In late 1988, more than 500 programs in the United States identified themselves as providing work-hardening services.[18]

As with many new therapeutic developments, content and quality vary among work-hardening centers. In 1988, the Work Hardening National Advisory Board of the Commission on Accreditation of Rehabilitation Facilities developed Guidelines for Accreditation of Work Hardening Programs.[5] In addition to developing the basic standards that must be met for a work-hardening program to become accredited, the National Advisory Board developed a comprehensive definition of work hardening:

> Work hardening programs, which are interdisciplinary in nature, use conditioning tasks that are graded to progressively improve the biomechanical, neuromuscular, cardiovascular/ metabolic and psychosocial functions of the individual in conjunction with real or simulated work activities. Work hardening provides a transition between acute care and return to work while addressing the issues of productivity, safety, physical tolerances, and worker behaviors. Work hardening is a highly structured, goal oriented, individualized treatment program designed to maximize the individual's ability to return to work.[5]

The work hardening program usually has as its core team a physical therapist, occupational therapist, vocational therapist, and psychologist. This team meets weekly or more often to coordinate the patient's care and coordinates its efforts with the patient's physician.

The characteristic that distinguishes work hardening from previous treatment approaches is its use of work simulation on a graded basis. In a work-hardening program, the patient usually receives treatment on a five-days-per-week basis with the degree of daily involvement increasing to a full eight-hour day as the patient is able to tolerate such involvement. The patient is involved on a daily basis in a combination of tasks that provide physical conditioning and other tasks that simulate critical demands of a target occupation. The combination of tasks is undertaken within the context of an employment setting. The patient must arrive early each morning, as required by the anticipated job, and, as the program progresses, eventually remain in the "workplace" for a full day, taking rest breaks and a lunch break that are consistent with the work demands found in competitive employment.

The elemental frame of reference within which work hardening takes place is the set of work demands that employers place on workers in the competitive labor market. These basic work demands have been termed vocational feasibility factors and have been gathered into the feasibility evaluation checklist displayed in Figure 10.1.[14]

The feasibility evaluation checklist includes 21 factors that a 1979 study conducted at Rancho Los Amigos Hospital identified as the basic factors considered by employers in the competitive labor market. These factors are more basic than the skills, aptitudes, and physical capacities that workers bring to the workplace. The truth of this assertion may be seen in the context of this situation: an injured worker with a 10-year history of skilled labor has, through physical therapy, developed strength and endurance that is adequate for employment in her previous position. She returns to work after a six-month absence, demonstrating problems with early-morning attendance and ability to accept criticism from a supervisor. Because these were not demands placed on her during her six-month convalescence and therapy regimen, they are unresolved treatment issues. These issues are separate from the level of skill or aptitude the worker presents. If the patient continues to be late for work and resists criticism from a supervisor, employment will not continue even if she is the most skilled person in the work force. In most of these cases, the injured worker resolves these issues, remains in the workplace, and maintains employment. A substantial minority of injured workers, however, do not successfully adapt, and, even though they possess the attributes necessary to perform previous employment, they will not maintain employment. This is one reason that most formal vocational rehabilitation programs include a 60-day follow-up period, with active involvement provided by a vocational rehabilitation specialist. Most of this involvement focuses on dealing with feasibility issues. The magnitude of this problem is staggering. Considering 462 consecutive patients, Matheson[16] found that 35% of injured workers who had not worked for one year or longer demonstrated significant feasibility problems, which precluded return to work. The educational components of a rehabilitation program try to change the worker's attitudes to correct these feasibility problems.

The structure and goal orientation of an individually developed treatment plan are reviewed daily by the interdisciplinary team. Although early in the work-hardening program the goal of return to work may be quite general, as the program progresses the goal becomes more specific so that, usually no later than the midway point, one particular occupation is selected as the focus of treatment. Several specific services have been identified in the CARF guidelines, as outlined in Table 10.3.

FEASIBILITY EVALUATION CHECKLIST

EMPLOYMENT AND
REHABILITATION
INSTITUTE OF
CALIFORNIA

EVALUEE: _____
RATER: _____ DATE: _____
PDC LEVELS TESTED: _____

	PRESENT FUNCTION					IMPROVEMENT POTENTIAL					PRESENT FUNCTION					IMPROVEMENT POTENTIAL			
	NOT EVALUATED	EMPLOYABLE COMPETITIVE	EMPLOYABLE SHELTERED	NOT EMPLOYABLE		HIGH	MODERATE	LOW	UNCERTAIN		NOT EVALUATED	EMPLOYABLE COMPETITIVE	EMPLOYABLE SHELTERED	NOT EMPLOYABLE		HIGH	MODERATE	LOW	UNCERTAIN

Section One — Productivity

A. QUANTITY
Evaluee's dependable demonstrated output

B. QUALITY
Evaluee's dependable demonstrated output of acceptable units.

C. ATTENDANCE
Evaluee's demonstrated consistency in reporting to place of work on assigned work days.

D. WORK-PLACE TOLERANCE
Evaluee's demonstrated capacity to remain in the work-place on a dependable basis.

E. TIMELINESS
Evaluee's demonstrated consistency in reporting to place of work on time, returning from breaks on time, and leaving place of work at appointed time.

F. INSTRUCTABILITY
Evaluee's demonstrated ability to perceive, understand, and follow work instructions.

G. MEMORY
Evaluee's demonstrated ability to remember task instructions, work structure, and safety rules.

H. CONCENTRATION
Evaluee's demonstrated ability to focus attention on the task to which he/she is assigned.

Section Two — SAFETY

A. ADHERENCE TO SAFETY RULES
Evaluee's demonstrated adherence to industry safety rules.

B. USE OF PROPER BODY MECHANICS
Evaluee's demonstrated consistency in the application of proper body mechanics to job tasks.

C. WORK PLACE SAFETY
1. Audition
2. Vision
3. Sensation
4. Balance

D. USE OF PROTECTIVE BEHAVIOR
Evaluee's demonstrated use of common sense in protecting himself/herself and other workers from danger.

Section Three — Interpersonal Behavior

A. RESPONSE TO SUPERVISION
Evaluee's demonstrated ability to appropriately:
1. Accept direction from a supervisor
2. Adjust to different supervisors or supervisory styles.
3. Follow through with accepted directions.

B. RESPONSE TO FELLOW WORKERS
Evaluee's demonstrated ability to work in concert with other workers addressing the same task.

C. RESPONSE TO CHANGE
Evaluee's demonstrated ability to adjust to changes in work routine, assignments, and conditions.

D. GENERAL WORKER ATTITUDE
Evaluee's demonstrated dedication to work and his/her role as a worker.

Comments: _____
_____
_____
_____

FIG 10.1.
Feasibility Evaluation Checklist.

Work hardening assists the patient to develop a perception of himself as a worker. The patient's "work-ability" is developed, including the physical tolerance, emotional resiliency, and other traits necessary to return to employment and maintain employment in the competitive labor market.

Matheson reported great diversity of program layout and staffing patterns in 58 programs

TABLE 10.3
Guidelines for Work-Hardening Program Services

1. Practice, modification, and instruction in component work tasks
2. Development of strength and endurance related to the performance of work tasks
3. Education to teach safe job performance and prevent reinjury
4. Assessment of specific job requirements through job analysis
5. Education of the employer and family as to the individual's present status
6. Provision of a mechanism to promote self-management and responsibility
7. Evaluation of productivity, safety in the workplace, and worker behavior
8. Identification of skills transferable to other occupations

surveyed.[17] A typical program occupied a 2,500-square-foot industrial facility and was staffed by either an occupational therapist or physical therapist, with assistance from a vocational evaluator or psychologist and two technicians.

The CARF guidelines[5] require that each accredited program evaluate outcome in terms of the following outcome measures: (1) returned to work, (2) met program goals, (3) declined further services, (4) did not comply with organizational policies, (5) demonstrated limited potential to benefit, and (6) required further health care intervention.

Unfortunately, to date little emphasis has been placed on the collection of outcome data. When data are collected and reported, not all of these outcome measures have been applied. Additionally, no study has provided a control group for comparison. Although it may be argued that many work-hardening program participants have been rehabilitation failures and that the work-hardening program is a last chance, so that any success is an improvement over no treatment at all, this does not allow us to estimate a treatment effect separate from the effect that any sort of expenditure might have.

Another problem often encountered with outcome measures is that they are difficult to evaluate unless the reference group is considered. For example, some programs report outcome in comparison to all individuals who were accepted for the program. Other programs consider outcome in terms of all of the individuals who were referred for services, and a third type consider outcome only in terms of the people who completed the program. The length of time of disability is also important. Some programs accept only workers who are rapidly recovering from an acute injury and already have an 80 to 90% expectation of returning to their previous jobs. Other programs focus on patients with chronic disability, often after they have undergone unsuccessful surgical procedures, who may have a low feasibility for any type of competitive employment. The expectations for outcome must differ from group to group. Although reports of program effectiveness should be presented in terms of initial patient characteristics, such data are not currently available. Variation in patient populations may account for the wide range of work-hardening program outcomes reported by Niemeyer and Jacobs.[22] Selected data are presented in Table 10.4.

FUNCTIONAL RESTORATION

Functional restoration is the most recent programmatic development in the rehabilitation of workers with chronic back pain and disability. This approach responds to the disparity between evident pathology, severity of pain, and limitation of physical capacity by quantifying the physical behaviors the injured worker must regain to allow reemployment. Injured workers who are cautioned by physicians and families to protect their backs and who

TABLE 10.4
Outcome Data from Selected Work-Hardening Programs*

Program	Outcome
ERIC Work Rehabilitation Center Anaheim, California	About 85% of those admitted to work-hardening were able to return to feasible competitive employment by discharge, but only 50% of those who completed the work-hardening program returned to work, based on a 60-day follow-up. Most of the loss of effectiveness is due to postprogram case management problems.
Irene Walter Johnson Institute of Rehabilitation St. Louis, Missouri	Approximately 70% who have completed work hardening have returned to work.
Loma Linda University Medical Center WERC Program Loma Linda, California	Some 55% who entered work hardening returned to employment. About 15% entered vocational rehabilitation, 26% obtained further medical treatment.
Massachusetts General Hospital Industrial Rehabilitation Boston, Massachusetts	About 48% returned to same job with same employer; 8% returned to different job with same employer; 4% entered training program; 20% awaiting further medical management; 8% awaiting case settlement.
Piedmont Hospital Work Recovery Center Atlanta, Georgia	About 74% of workers who entered the work-conditioning program have returned to work.
Professional Services for the Injured Tacoma, Washington	Some 86% who have participated have returned to work.

*From Carlton, 1989; Rhomberg, 1989; Anzai, 1989; Fortenbach, 1989; Brandon, 1989, Holmes, 1989.[1]

may be further motivated toward inactivity by fear of reinjury become relatively decondi-tioned through loss of trunk strength, flexibility, and general cardiovascular fitness. Although they integrate behavioral modification and work-hardening techniques, func-tional restoration programs are distinguished by repeated measurement of strength, flex-ibility, and general fitness as objective guidelines for therapy and occupational planning.

A formal program of functional restoration with behavioral support begins with approximately one and one-half days of physical, psychosocial, and occupational evalua-tion, as outlined in Table 10.5. Self-assessments of pain and disability are measured with visual analog scales, pain drawings, and questionnaires such as the Oswestry Pain Questionnaire. Psychologic measures include the Minnesota Multiphasic Personality Inventory, the Millon Behavioral Health Index, the Beck Depression Inventory, and psychologic interviews. Specific physical capacity measurements include trunk flexibility using the 2 inclinometer system described by Mayer et al.[19] Trunk strength is measured isokinetically, using the CYBEX trunk extension/flexion machine. Frequent lifting capac-ity is measured by a protocol of loads progressing by 5-lb increments to patient tolerance or target heart rate achievement. General endurance is measured by arm and leg bicycle ergometers. General speed and dexterity are measured by the time required to complete a

TABLE 10.5
Quantitative Evaluation Variables

Pain and Disability Self-Reports	*Psychologic Measures*
• Quantitative pain drawings	• Personality inventories
• Visual analog scales	• Coping style questionnaire
• Questionnaires	• Depression questionnaire
	• Interview
Physical Capacities	*Social Factors*
• Trunk flexibility	• Work status
• Trunk strength	• Health care utilization
• Lifting capacity	• Worker compensation or litigation status
• Cycling endurance	
• Activities of daily living	

standardized obstacle course. Socioeconomic assessments include inventories of income and expenses, clarification of worker compensation or litigation status, return-to-work goal setting, and review of work history and aptitudes. After completion of initial data collection, multidisciplinary staffing focuses on the patient's return-to-work goals and on strategies for removing physical, psychologic, and social barriers between the patient and the patient's goals.

The intensive portion of the treatment program runs for three weeks, five and one-half days per week. The program is roughly divided into physical, psychologic, and occupational components. Physical training involves two daily sessions of floor exercises, trunk and extremity flexibility exercises integrated with relaxation techniques, and specific strengthening exercises for trunk and extremity muscle groups, using weight training (Fig. 10.2). General endurance is developed through stationary cycling. Activities involving rapid, unguarded movements include volleyball (Fig. 10.3). Occupational therapy involves work simulation and more general training in frequent and sustained lifting, pushing/pulling, prolonged postural maintenance of stressful positions, carrying, and so on. Physical exercise lasts approximately five hours per day. Therapists conduct daily classes in

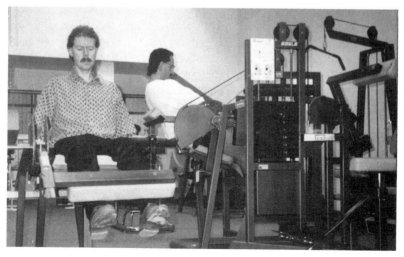

FIG 10.2.
Weight training in the gym is designed to strengthen trunk and extremity muscles.

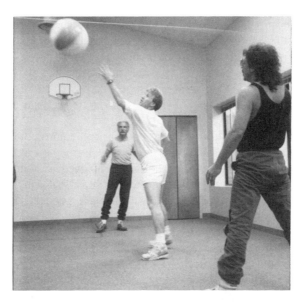

FIG 10.3.
Activities such as volleyball involve unguarded movements, challenging the patient's concepts of disability.

spinal anatomy, medications, diagnostic studies, compensation law, and acute pain management. Occupational counselors discuss job feasibility and facilitate the development of a specific return-to-work plan that fits the patient's needs and capacities. Psychologic intervention includes group and individual counseling on a daily or alternate-day schedule, and family counseling is done weekly. These sessions are designed to clarify the role of stress and emotions in pain behavior. Incapacitating emotional reactions to pain, including anger, depression, and frustration, are dealt with through open discussion and development of positive coping skills. Biofeedback and specific training in relaxation techniques are integrated with individualized physical strategies for dealing with acute pain episodes, and patients are encouraged to use relaxation techniques on a regular basis.

Following the three-week intensive program, multidisciplinary treatment continues for one and one-half to two days per week for up to six weeks, as the patient integrates improved physical capacity with a specific return-to-work plan.

In 1985, physician Tom Mayer and the staff of the Productive Rehabilitation Institute of Dallas for Ergonomics (PRIDE) reported on the content and outcome of their functional restoration program.[20] They initially evaluated 111 patients meeting the admission criteria of disability for at least four months and lack of evidence for a surgically correctable lesion. Thirty-eight of these patients formed a comparison treatment group when their insurance companies refused financial authorization for participation in the treatment program. The remaining 73 patients entered the program. Seven of these participants dropped out of the program, leaving 66 to graduate. Demographic characteristics, surgeries, duration of disability, worker's compensation status and medications were initially similar for the treatment and comparison groups. Following the three-week rehabilitation program, graduates were evaluated at three-month and one-year intervals. Nearly all patients in the study were evaluated for work status at year end, primarily by structured telephone interview. After one year, 86% of the program graduates were working or involved in occupational training programs. By comparison, only 20% of the dropout group and 45% of the comparison group were similarly employed. Additional surgery rates were lower in the treatment and comparison group than in the dropouts. Settlement of worker's compensation cases was significantly more common in the treatment group than in the comparison and dropout groups. Overall, program graduates enjoyed improved trunk strength, repetitive lifting capacity, and trunk flexibility. Self-assessments of pain and disability similarly improved.

In a later study a group of 116 treatment patients was compared to 72 nontreatment patients.[21] At the end of two years 87% of the treatment group contacted were working, whereas only 41% of the comparison group were employed. Additional surgery rates, health care visits, and reinjuries were approximately twice as great in the comparison group. Again, significant early improvements in physical parameters and self-assessments of pain and disability were found in the program graduates.

A similar program combining functional restoration with behavioral support was established at the New England Back Center in 1986. Using the PRIDE format of treatment, comparison, and dropout group distinctions, a prospective one-year study was conducted to test the efficacy of this program.[9] Initial patient characteristics of these groups were similar. All 90 patients meeting entry criteria of four months of continuous disability and absence of a surgically correctable lesion were evaluated with the tests listed in Table 10.5. These tests were repeated at the time of discharge from the three-week program, at 6 to 12 weeks thereafter, and at year end.

The final study groups involved 59 program graduates, 5 program dropouts, 17 comparison patients, and 6 crossover patients, who were denied insurance authorization for at least six months then treated and followed for six months. Of the original 90 patients, three refused participation.

One year after treatment, return-to-work rates were significantly higher for the program graduates, as illustrated in Figure 10.4. Program graduates who continued to be unemployed cited pain, pregnancy, retirement, schooling, cardiac disability, and lack of suitable work. Self-assessments of pain, disability, and depression as well as measured physical capacities improved significantly within the three weeks of treatment for program graduates. Although these initial improvements and self-assessments were well maintained through the year of follow-up, there was partial attrition of the physical capacity gains. Overall, program graduates' self-assessments of pain did not correlate well with work status, which might be expected in view of previously reported discrepancies between chronic pain complaints and physical capacities. Furthermore, isokinetic trunk strength and frequent lifting capacity were not significantly correlated with year-end work status.

The treatment group patients in the PRIDE and New England Back Center studies had been disabled for 12 to 19 months, on average, so the expectation of future work was very low. Therefore, the follow-up return-to-work rates are very encouraging. They demonstrate that even in workers with long-standing disability from work, with the psychosocial and physical deconditioning problems attending long-term disability, the combination of functional restoration guided by physical capacity measurements and behavioral support can be very effective in improving self-assessed pain, functional levels, and eventual work status.

Since most workers recover from acute occupational back injury without rehabilitation, and the cost of intensive functional restoration programs generally exceeds $5,000, it is clear that not everyone with an industrial back injury warrants such intensive care. Fredrickson investigated psychologic and physical predictors of success of rehabilitation for patients with chronic low back pain using the Minnesota Multiphasic Personality

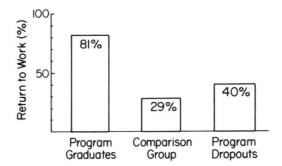

FIG 10.4.
Return-to-work status of patients with chronic low back disability one year after a functional restoration program (Hazard, 1989).

Inventory, personal interview, pain drawing, demographic data, and measurements of flexibility, strength, and endurance.[9] Demographic data were poor predictors, except in the case of patients more than 50 years old, who were far less likely to return to work following treatment than their younger counterparts. Worker's compensation and litigation were relatively strong predictors of poor outcome. Psychologic tests were poor predictors. The pretreatment prognostication of the interviewing psychologist and the estimation of the treatment staff when the patient was discharged from treatment were the best predictors of eventual return-to-work status. Politan evaluated 42 psychologic, physical, and medical variables, testing their correlation with the patients' eventual status as treated and reemployed, dropped out of treatment, or denied treatment.[23] Overall, the treatment success group was characterized by better pretreatment self-assessments of pain and disability, depression, Millon Behavioral Health Inventory scores, as well as more favorable surgical history and longer time-at-job and job-availability levels. It is hoped that this model and others will be refined and used to improve the prescription and cost effectiveness of intensive rehabilitation for workers with chronic back pain and disability.

BIBLIOGRAPHY

1. Anzai D, Wright M: Workers' evaluation and rehabilitation center. In Niemeyer LO, Jacobs K (eds). *Work Hardening: State of the Art*. Thorofare, NJ, Slack, Inc. 1989, pp 251–266; Brandon TL, Snyder L: Work Recovery Center Piedmont Hospital. In Niemeyer LO, Jacobs K (eds). *Work Hardening: State of the Art*. Thorofare, NJ, Slack, Inc., 1989, pp 209–221; Carlton RS, Niemeyer LO: Employment and Rehabilitation Institute of California. In Niemeyer LO, Jacobs K (eds). *Work Hardening: State of the Art*. Thorofare, NJ, Slack, Inc., 1989, pp 373–391; Fortenbach M: The Industrial Rehabilitation Program at Massachusetts General Hospital. In Niemeyer LO, Jacobs K (eds). *Work Hardening: State of the Art*. Thorofare, NJ, Slack, Inc., 1989, pp 184–190; Holmes MB, Mizoguchi JT: Professional services for the injured. In Niemeyer LO, Jacobs K (eds). *Work Hardening: State of the Art*. Thorofare, NJ, Slack, Inc., 1989, pp 336–356; Rhomberg S: Irene Walter Johnson Institute of Rehabilitation. In Niemeyer LO, Jacobs K (eds). *Work Hardening: State of the Art*. Thorofare, NJ, Slack, Inc., 1989, pp 231–249.
2. Aronoff GM, Evans WO, Enders PL: A review of follow-up studies of multidisciplinary pain units. *Pain* 1983; 16:1–11.
3. Berquist-Ullman M, Larsson U: Acute low back pain in industry. *Acta Orthop Scand Suppl*. 1977; 170:5–109.

4. Carron H: Chronic low back pain, in *Low Back Pain: Report of a Workshop,* Carron H (ed). Charlottesville, University of Virginia, 1987, pp 3–4.

5. Commission on Accreditation of Rehabilitation Facilities: *Standards Manual for Organizations Serving People with Disabilities.* Tucson, CARF, 1989, p 69.

6. Deyo RA: Conservative therapy for low back pain: Distinguishing useful from useless therapy. *JAMA* 1983; 250:1057–1062.

7. Fordyce WE, McMahon R, Rainwater G, et al: Pain complaint-exercise performance relationship in chronic pain. *Pain* 1981; 10:311–321.

8. Fordyce WE, Roberts AH, Sternback RA: The behavioral management of chronic pain: A response to critics. *Pain* 1985; 22:113–125.

9. Fredrickson BE, Trief PM, Van Beresen P, et al: Rehabilitation of the patient with chronic back pain: A search for outcome predictions. *Spine* 1988; 13:351–353.

10. Hazard R, Fenwick J, Kalisch S: Disability exaggeration in patients with chronic low-back pain: Correlations with psychological factors. Presented at the International Society for Study of the Lumbar Spine, Kyoto, 1989.

11. Hazard RG: Functional restoration and outcomes, in *Contemporary Care for Painful Spinal Disorders,* Mayer TG, Mooney V, Gatchel R (eds). Philadelphia, Lea & Febiger, 1990.

12. Lehmann TR: Personal communication, 1983.

13. Lehmann TR, Russell DW, Spratt KF, et al: Efficacy of electroacupuncture and TENS in the rehabilitation of chronic low back pain patients. *Pain* 1986; 26:277–290.

14. Matheson LN: Feasibility evaluation checklist. Rehabilitation Institute of Southern California.

15. Matheson LN: Symptom magnification, in *Work Capacity Evaluation.* Anaheim, ERIC, 1984, pp 39–49.

16. Matheson LN: Vocational feasibility and its assessment. Dallas, Industrial Musculoskeletal Health, University of Texas Health Science Center, 1988.

17. Matheson LN: National Program survey: Work hardening in the United States. *Industrial Rehabilitation Quarterly* 1988; Winter 1:1, 12–17.

18. Matheson LN: Work hardening accreditation. *Industrial Rehabilitation Quarterly* 1989; 2:1, 7–10, 14.

19. Mayer TG, Tencer AF, Kristoferson S, et al: Use of non-invasive techniques for quantification of spinal range-of-motion in normal subjects and chronic low-back dysfunction patients. *Spine* 1984; 9:588–595.

20. Mayer TG, Gatchel RJ, Kishino N, et al: Objective assessment of spine function following industrial injury: A prospective study with comparison group and one-year follow-up. *Spine* 1985; 10:482–493.

21. Mayer TG, Gatchel RJ, Mayer H, et al: A prospective randomized two-year study of functional restoration in industrial low back injury utilizing objective assessment. *JAMA* 1987; 258:1763–1767.

22. Niemeyer LO, Jacobs K (eds): *Work Hardening: State of the Art.* Thorofare, NJ, Slack, Inc., 1989.

23. Politan PF, Gatchel RJ, Barnes D, et al: A psychosociomedical prediction model of response to treatment by chronically disabled workers with low-back pain. *Spine* 1989; 14:956–961.

24. Spengler DM, Bigos SJ, Martin NA, et al: Back injuries in industry: A retrospective study. I. Overview and cost analysis. *Spine* 1986; 11:241–245.

25. Spitzer WO, LeBlanc FE, Dupuis M, et al: Scientific approach to the assessment and management of activity-related spinal disorders. *Spine* 1987; Suppl 12:S1—S59.

26. Waddell G: A new clinical model for the treatment of low-back pain. *Spine* 1987; 12:632–644.

27. White AWM: Low-back pain in men receiving workmen's compensation. *Can Med Assoc J* 1966; 95:50–56.

PART IV

Selection and Workplace Evaluation

11

Concepts in Prevention

Gunnar B.J. Andersson, M.D., Ph.D.

INTRODUCTION

There is widespread agreement that the problem of low back pain (LBP) is so great that it should be addressed with general preventive measures. While there are several alternative preventive models, none has been properly evaluated. The three main preventive approaches follow:

1. Designing the job to fit the worker
2. Selecting the appropriate worker for the job
3. Teaching the worker to use the correct work method

Each approach is discussed in separate chapters in the book. This chapter serves only as an introduction; the interested reader can find more substance in Chapters 12 through 14.

DEFINITIONS

Classic preventive medicine divides prevention into three categories:

1. *Primary prevention* efforts attempt to prevent the initiation of a disease. Primary prevention includes proper workplace design to reduce exposure and may also include preplacement screening to detect unusually susceptible workers and the teaching of proper work techniques.

2. *Secondary prevention* efforts attempt to modify the progression of a disease. In classic prevention theory, these include disease detection in a preclinical stage, where it can be addressed by treatment or exposure modification.

3. *Tertiary prevention* efforts attempt to minimize the consequences of a disease (or injury) once it has become clinically manifest. These include reducing disability from disease by optimal medical care and workplace modification. The prevention of treatment complications also falls into this category.

The three classes of prevention may be illustrated as in Figure 11.1. The process of prevention generally becomes more difficult and expensive once disease is established. All these prevention classes tend to overlap as they relate to LBP.

When discussing prevention, it is useful to differentiate between approaches applied to society in general (for example, fluoridation of drinking water) and more individual approaches (for example, advice against smoking). The first does not require the participation of the individual, that is, it is passive, whereas the second clearly does require

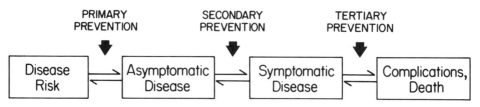

FIG 11.1.
The potential course of a disease and the opportunities for prevention.

participation, because it is active and therefore more difficult to accomplish. Changes at the workplace may be considered intermediate, requiring the good intentions of management and acceptance by workers.

PRIMARY PREVENTION

To institute true primary prevention of low back pain, the health care professional should know what constitutes the disease risk. Unfortunately, current knowledge lacks detail. LBP is a symptom, not a disease or an injury. The associations of LBP to workplace and individual factors are discussed in Chapters 6 and 7. Generally speaking, associations are weak. Occupational risk factors are more important for disability than for disease or injury, and few individual risk factors hold up to scientific scrutiny. This lack of knowledge could easily lead to a negative attitude toward prevention. In spite of superficial knowledge, however, considerable scientific evidence and commonsense knowledge permit specific suggestions for primary prevention programs. For example, it is known that low back pain may be caused by mechanical trauma, either isolated or repeated. Although the precise limits at which physical loads become harmful or the ways in which individual factors influence those limits are unknown, a great deal of useful information has been developed. That knowledge can be used to reduce the physical work load on the lower back. Dissatisfaction with work also increases the risk of injury and disability. That information may also be used in prevention.

The three main alternatives in primary prevention are each the subject of a chapter.

1. Preemployment screening programs are discussed in Chapter 13. Screening is clearly an area where primary and secondary prevention overlap and, indeed, some consider it entirely the latter.[1] Definitions important to screening procedures are given later in this chapter.

2. Improvements in work habits are discussed in Chapter 15. These improvements may be reached by both direct work-related instruction and general information (schooling) about the back and its optimal function. The importance of the external moments acting on the spine and how those are influenced by object weight, location, size, and density as well as by posture, dynamics and forces, asymmetries in loading, and various time factors (duration, frequency)—all these need to be understood and not simply memorized. It is well known that in spite of the fact that many workers learn how to handle objects at work and to avoid certain postures, using that knowledge in the stress of the working environment is difficult. Very few back schools today are aimed at primary prevention, and most have not been designed for that purpose. Rather, the concept of back school arose from a wish to

improve efficiency in patient care, prevent recurrences, and promote self-care (tertiary prevention). Back schools have not been evaluated from the perspective of whether the information is clearly understood or just temporarily memorized. Practical instruction at the workplace cannot be replaced by sound and slide programs and posters.

3. Changes at the workplace are outlined in Chapter 14. These changes include reduction of permissible loads (by recommendation or regulations), optimization of postures, and ergonomic design of the workplace, work tools, and work methods.

SECONDARY PREVENTION

This type of prevention shares some of the problems just mentioned, with the added problem of early disease (risk) detection. The medical profession's ability to identify asymptomatic "disease" that places the industrial low back at risk is poor. Periodic health evaluations therefore have limited value.

Secondary prevention and tertiary prevention tend to overlap, particularly with respect to recurrences. Previous low back pain, for example, increases the risk of a subsequent episode. Such knowledge is useful in both secondary and tertiary prevention.

TERTIARY PREVENTION

Selection of the appropriate therapy to reduce the disability and chronicity of LBP and to prevent recurrence may be the most immediate and practical prevention method, but it would be totally redundant if primary prevention could be made effective. Evaluation and therapy are discussed in Chapters 8 through 10, where we emphasize that early recognition of the problem and proper management are important methods of reducing chronicity and recurrence. Wiesel, Feffer, and Rothman[5] showed that early and careful management dramatically reduced the impact of low back pain on lost time at work, treatment cost, and direct cost to industry. These results have been confirmed by Chöler et al.[2]

The assessment of when a worker may be allowed to return to work safely after a back pain episode is based on incomplete scientific evidence. Room for improvement exists also in the issues of for whom and at which time modifications of the workplace and work method can aid in reducing LBP chronicity or recurrence. Even when chronic symptoms have developed, it is important to encourage work activities in some form to avoid chronic disability.

GENERAL CONSIDERATIONS IN SCREENING

Screening is the use of examinations or tests to detect previously unrecognized or unreported medical conditions or to detect risk factors. In the context of prevention of low back pain, risk factor detection is usually the goal. A worker at risk is one who, because of interaction between a personal risk factor of any kind and workplace exposure or demand, has an increased probability of developing low back pain or sustaining a back injury. Several options in worker selection and their advantages and limitations are discussed in Chapter 13. Definitions of some important terms—sensitivity, specificity, and predictive value—are given here. In calculating these screening parameters a cross-tabulation is used in which subjects are classified as to whether or not they are likely to develop a disease (injury) subsequent to screening (Fig. 11.2).

Sensitivity is a measure of a test's ability to identify correctly persons with a certain condition. It can be expressed as the fraction or percent of all persons with a condition who test positive (true positives):

$$\frac{\text{True Positive}}{\text{True Positive} + \text{False Negative}} \times 100\%$$

This means that if sensitivity is 95%, then 95 of a group of 100 people with a certain condition will have a positive test (true positive) and 5 will have a negative (false negative).

Specificity is a measure of a test's accuracy in correctly identifying persons who do not have the condition and who will test negative (true negatives).

$$\frac{\text{True Negatives}}{\text{True Negatives} + \text{False Positives}} \times 100\%$$

A test with a 95% specificity applied to a group of 100 persons who do *not* have a disease is negative in 95 (true negative) and positive in 5 (false positive).

The *predictive value* of a test may be either positive or negative. A positive predictive value is the ability to identify individuals at risk. It may be expressed as follows:

$$\frac{\text{True Positives}}{\text{True Positives} + \text{False Positives}} \times 100\%$$

A negative predictive value indicates the probability that a negative test will denote a person without a risk factor. It may be expressed as follows:

$$\frac{\text{True Negatives}}{\text{False Negatives} + \text{True Negatives}}$$

The predictive value depends on the actual frequency of a condition in the population. An example used by Rockey, Fantel, and Omenn[4] illustrates this: The exercise electrocardiogram (ECG) test is about 95% sensitive and about 95% specific for coronary artery disease (CAD). If this test is given to 1,000 patients with angina pectoris—a group in which

	Disease positive	Disease negative	
Positive test	a = true positives	b = false positives	(a+b)
Negative test	c = false negatives	d = true negatives	(c+d)
	(a+c)	(b+d)	

FIG 11.2.
Relationship of screening criterion and disease.

the frequency of CAD is 80%—of the 800 persons with CAD, 95% or 760 will have positive exercise ECGs. Of the 200 persons without CAD, 95% or 190 will have negative ECGs, but 10 will have positive tests. Therefore, the (positive) predictive value of the test is 760 divided by (760 + 10), or 98.7%.

What if the test were applied to healthy 18- to 30-year-old job applicants, a group in which the frequency of CAD is about 2%? If 1,000 applicants were screened, 19 of the 20 (95%) with CAD would have positive tests. Of the 980 applicants with CAD, 931 (95%) would have negative tests, but 49 would have positive tests. Therefore, the predictive value of the test is 19 divided by (19 + 49), or 28%. This means that only 28% of those with a positive test actually have CAD (true positive); the other 72% with a positive test are free of the disease (false positives). If such a test were used as a prerequisite for employment, 72% of those denied employment because of a positive test would have been misclassified.

Table 11.1 illustrates the dependence of the predictive value on disease prevalence. When the prevalence is 50% or higher, predictive value is marginally influenced by prevalence, but when it is below 10%, the ratio of true positives to false positives drops dramatically (Fig. 11.3).

Sensitivity, specificity, and predictive value require a standard to be calculated. These data are often unavailable, making it impossible to calculate predictive values correctly.

HOW TO DEVELOP A PREVENTION PROGRAM

When actually a program of prevention is being started, the first phase includes planning and education. Information is fundamentally important at this stage. The management, organized labor, and employees should be informed about methods, goals, risk factors, and the possibility of prevention. This may require brochures, posters, and presentations. Once the support of management and labor is secured, the second phase may be initiated. This stage involves actual screening—in the case of back injuries, screening of both worker and workplace. Specific subject and work-related risk factors are defined and analyzed before the third phase is started. The third phase includes implementation of the second-phase findings to alter the workplace, reassign workers, and institute education. A fourth phase should always include evaluations of the third-phase interventions and reinforcement of the principles of low back pain prevention.

TABLE 11.1
Predictive Value of a Positive Test as a Function of the Disease Prevalence. Laboratory Test with 95% Sensitivity and 95% Specificity.*

Prevalence of disease (%)	Predictive value of positive test
1	16.1
2	21.2
5	50.0
10	67.9
15	77.0
20	82.6
25	86.4
50	95.0

*From Galen RS: Selection of appropriate laboratory tests, in Young DS, et al (eds): *Clinician and Chemist: The Relationship of the Laboratory to the Physician.* Washington, DC, Assn for Clinical Chemistry, 1979. Used by permission.

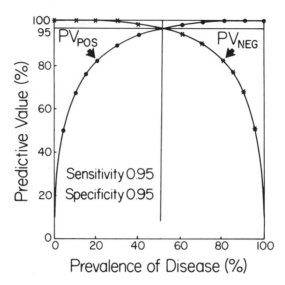

FIG 11.3.
Numerical values of PV$_{pos}$ and PV$_{neg}$ as a function of the prevalence when the sensitivity and specificity are 0.95.

SUMMARY

In spite of the less than concrete scientific evidence on the ultimate effectiveness of any of the proposed preventive routes and in light of the magnitude of the LBP problem, all avenues should be explored. Combined prevention programs have proved effective in reducing the frequency of low back complaints, at least in the shorter-term perspective. Prevention programs applied to society in general could benefit from the example of the successful caries-prevention program, which is introduced to people at all stages of life. Workers should be made aware that they themselves can influence their LBP, and they should be charged with that responsibility. The workplace should be improved as needed and work methods optimized. Workers should not have to exert themselves at or above their actual limits. A program of diagnosis, care, and rehabilitation should be put into immediate effect for the injured worker. Although these approaches will not eliminate low back pain, we hope they will reduce the extent of the problem.

BIBLIOGRAPHY

1. Anderson JAD: Occupational aspects of low back pain. *Clin Rheum Dis* 1980; 6:17–35.
2. Choler U, Larsson R, Nachemson A, et al: Back pain—Attempt at a structural treatment program for patients with low back pain (in Swedish). SPRI Report 188, SPRI, Stockholm, 1985.
3. Galen RS: Selection of appropriate laboratory tests, in Young DS, et al (eds): *Clinician and Chemist: The Relationship of the Laboratory to the Physician*. Washington, DC, Assn for Clinical Chemistry, 1979.
4. Rockey PH, Fantel J, Omenn GS: Discriminatory aspects of pre-employment screening: Low-back x-ray examinations in the railroad industry. *Amer J Law and Med* 1979; 5:197–214.
5. Wiesel SW, Feffer HL, Rothman RH: Industrial low back pain: A prospective evaluation of a standardized diagnostic and treatment protocol (unpublished manuscript). Washington, DC, The George Washington University Medical Center.

12

Workplace Evaluation

Don B. Chaffin, Ph.D.
Gunnar B.J. Andersson, M.D., Ph.D.
Malcolm H. Pope, Dir. Med. Sc., Ph.D.
Margareta Nordin, Ph.D.

RATIONALE FOR WORKPLACE EVALUATION

The need to describe manual work activities quantitatively was first recognized in the late nineteenth century. Since that time several systems have been developed to meet a variety of objectives for organizing workplaces and predicting the labor requirements to accomplish any job. Only recently, however, have any methods attempted to describe comprehensively the physically stressful aspects of work. This chapter describes several current workplace evaluation systems, particularly systems that concentrate on factors believed to contribute to the risk of low back pain (LBP).

One reason for the paucity of such systems is, as one might suspect, a general disagreement on precisely what should be measured. One survey of current research literature singled out the following physical workplace factors as important:[26]

1. Loads—measures of the vector forces and moments, lifting, pushing, pulling, and so on that act on the body during materials handling
2. Dimensions—measures of size, shape, and form of objects handled
3. Distribution of loads—measures of the location of the object's center of gravity with respect to the worker
4. Couplings—measures of the interface between the worker and the load (e.g., handle design parameters such as size, shape, location, coding, and texture)
5. Stability of load—measures of the consistency of the load's center of mass (e.g., liquids and bulky materials)
6. Workplace geometry—measures of the spatial properties of the task such as movement distances, directions, extent-of-motion paths, obstacles, and the nature of the destination (each of which affect worker posture)
7. Temporal factors—measures of the frequency, duration, and pace of work activities over the short and long term
8. Complexity—measures of manipulation requirements; objective of activity, tolerances for motion error
9. Environment—measures such as temperature, humidity, lighting, noise, vibration, foot traction, and toxic agents
10. Organization—measures of administrative factors such as use of teamwork,

machine pacing, work incentives, extended work shifts, job rotations, and personal protective devices
11. Psychologic factors—work satisfaction, autonomy, work overload, job security, expectations, inadequate resources, and so on

Although the list is far from complete, it does suggest that the etiology of LBP is quite complex and involves the interaction of many factors.

A practical difficulty with evaluation of workplaces for potential risks of physical trauma is that the literature is unclear about whether the process is attributable to acute or cumulative trauma. If the cause is normally a long-term overload process, then the workplace evaluation should include the temporal aspects of work, such as frequency and duration of exertions, fatigue, work-rest regimes, and so forth.

If, on the other hand, the etiology is predominantly acute trauma due to a peak stress or unexpected events (such as slipping and falling or being struck), then infrequent, unpredictable, atypical aspects of work such as emergency procedures, maintenance, machine setup, and perhaps leisure time activities should receive primary attention. A study by Herrin et al. attempted to develop some insight into this dilemma.[28] Their epidemiologic study rated the physical stresses of 55 different jobs in five plants. Almost 3,000 manual exertions were identified within these jobs. The jobs were ranked according to both peak exertion requirements (maximum strengths and L5–S1 compression forces) and average exertion levels (weighted by the frequency of performing each manual task in a job). Thus a job requiring a worker to load a heavy stock reel only once per shift and then simply monitor the machine's performance would be rated high for peak stress but low for average stress. Three years of medical data for the 6,912 workers populating the study jobs were then used to determine which analysis was better. The results seem slightly to favor maximum peak stresses as being better correlated with both the incident rate and severity rate of all types of musculoskeletal and overexertion injuries, but low back disorders were slightly better correlated with average job stress ratings than with peak stress ratings.

Given the present state of knowledge in this matter and the diversity of manual work in industry it appears that the risks of both acute and cumulative trauma to the low back must remain major concerns in industry. Hence it is necessary to apply multiple evaluation procedures.

HISTORIC PERSPECTIVE

Organizing the efforts of groups of workers has traditionally involved a sequence of three steps:[10]

Development of a Preferred Method

Assuming that a task or job can be performed using any number of different methods, it is important that a preferred method be defined. To develop a method, do the following:

- State the objective of the operation or activity.
- Identify methods that meet or exceed the objective.
- Implement feasible methods on a trial basis with assistance of experienced workers and supervisors.
- Select the best method that meets the objective.

Preparation of a Standard Practice

Preparing a standard practice requires that the preferred method be stated formally, which involves the following procedures:

- Sketch the workplace (including relevant dimensions and locations of all machines, objects to be handled, and tools used), and indicate where the operator normally sits or stands.
- List abnormal working conditions that could affect work performance (e.g., illumination, slippery flooring, heat).
- Document and publish the sequence of motions required of a worker to complete the operation.

Determination of a Time Standard

Time standards are determined either by having a skilled worker perform the operation while being timed or by consulting normative time data in the literature (e.g., synthetic time systems). Overall operation standard times can be predicted by accumulating the elemental standard times, which assume an experienced, well-trained worker.

Training of the Worker

Instruction sheets, verbal directions, and training aids must be developed and used to ensure that workers understand the job requirements and follow preferred work methods.

These three steps usually evolve from a management concern that labor may not be well utilized and that time may be wasted. As the cost of labor increases, more emphasis is invariably given to ensuring that each step is fully implemented by the industrial or production engineering functions of a well-managed plant. Within the last few decades, however, an additional concern has been imposed by top management, namely, that any operation must be accomplished safely. It is this relatively new awareness and concern for worker safety and health that makes job and workplace evaluation such an important function today. To understand better the role of conventional workplace evaluation in injury prevention and to give some perspective to the current practice of workplace evaluation, it is recommended that the reader consult the excellent textbooks available, for example, Barnes,[3] Niebel,[47] and Mundel.[45]

Perhaps the most influential of the early contributors to the field was Frederick W. Taylor. Taylor's *Principles of Scientific Management*[60] indicated the need for standardization of work methods, time studies, instruction of workers, selection of workers, and incentives for completing work correctly and on time. Taylor's study of shoveling rice, coal, and iron ore in 1898 was a rigorous and comprehensive investigation of the optimal design for a shovel in terms of size, shoveling frequency, and rest allocation necessary to maximize the total output of a group of workers.[11] Taylor showed that a shovel that would allow about 22 pounds (10.3 kg) of material to be lifted each time resulted in maximal total daily output for a group of physically strong workers. By a combination of careful selection and training of workers, provision of special shovels for materials of different weights, and bonuses for above-average output, he was able to demonstrate that 140 men could perform the work previously done by 400 to 600 workers.[11]

At about the same time, Frank and Lillian Gilbreth were advocating that manual activities in industry needed to be carefully categorized to minimize fatigue and monotony while maximizing productivity.[3] One of Frank Gilbreth's earliest and most often-quoted studies was of bricklaying.[22] By using photographs of the bricklayers in his construction business he was able to demonstrate that fatigue and wasted motion could be minimized and high output achieved if bricks were first sorted for good and bad bricks, oriented with the best side facing out, and delivered to the bricklayer at a comfortable working height by means of an adjustable scaffold. His methods resulted in a doubling of total output. His study also demonstrated the concept of division of labor. Since bricklaying tasks could be divided into skilled and unskilled portions, the necessary labor could also be divided among different workers (with different skills and presumably different wage rates).

Two specific methodologic contributions to the study of manual labor must be attributed to the Gilbreths. One is the use of micromotion study, which allows great attention to be given to categorizing individual body motions, referred to as "Therbligs" (an anagram derived from their name).[23] These basic motions were carefully timed; later they became the basis for one of the first predetermined time systems.

The Gilbreths' other methodologic contribution was the first cycleograph (or chronocycleograph), which was used to compare alternative motion sequences. A set of blinking lights (flashing at a known rate) was attached to the arm and hand of a worker, and a photograph was made with the camera shutter open for a prolonged period. The motion path was transcribed as a sequence of dots onto film. By measuring the numbers and displacements of the dots, the Gilbreths were able to measure and compare job motion requirements. Today this technique has been considerably enhanced by modern video and computer techniques to allow whole body motion studies, but the concept is virtually unchanged.

It should be clear that the general approach and investigative methods of work analysis developed by Taylor and the Gilbreths early in this century continue to be directly applicable to workplace evaluation today. Without the mechanisms and procedures of systematic work classification, time study, motion study, and motion analysis, it would be impossible to reduce job-induced musculoskeletal stress in industry.

The time necessary for Therbligs such as Move, Reach, Grasp, Position, Regrasp, Turn, Apply Pressure, Release, or Disengage is predictable. Additional allowances are necessary for Eye Focus and Travel Time (required to search for an object within the field of view) and for Motion of the Body, Legs, and Feet. Additional adjustments must be made for difficulty with simultaneous tasks (different usages of the hands may be incompatible). A standardized coding system for activities has been adopted. Table 12.1 gives examples of this coding system.

Benefits and Limitations of Traditional Performance Prediction Time Systems

In reviewing the preceding job evaluation technology, it may be noted that traditional time and motion study provides much essential information:

- The workplace documentation includes a sketch of the layout with major hand motions and distances noted. Such a sketch is essential for planning changes in the workplace layout.
- The analysis reveals the relative balance of work between the two hands. If the imbalance were great, it could contribute to asymmetric symptoms in workers (e.g., dominant hand disorders and syndromes).
- The analysis describes the extent of static holding activities required of each hand

TABLE 12.1
Coding Conventions for MTM Motion Analysis*

Code Example	Interpretation of Codes
R8C	Reach, 8 inches, Case C
R12Am	Reach, 12 inches, Case A, hand in motion at end
M6A	Move, 6 inches, Case A, object weighs less than 2.5 pounds
mM10C	Move, 10 inches, Case C, hand in motion at the beginning, object less than 2.5 pounds
M16B15	Move, 16 inches, Case B, object weighs 15 pounds
T30	Turn hand 30 degrees
T90L	Turn object weighing more than 10 pounds 90 degrees
AP1	Apply pressure, includes regrasp
G1A	Grasp, Case G1A
P1NSD	Position, Class 1 fit, nonsymmetrical part, difficult to handle
RL1	Release, Case 1
D2E	Disengage, Class 2 fit, easy to handle
EF	Eye focus
ET14/10	Eye travel between points 14 inches apart where line of travel is 10 inches from eyes
FM	Foot motion
SS16C1	Sidestep, 16 inches, Case 1
TBC1	Turn body, Case 1
W4P	Walk four paces

*Adapted from Barnes RM: *Motion and Time Study: Design and Measurement of Work*, ed. 6. New York, Wiley and Sons, 1968. Used by permission.

(such as those required in using the hand to hold an object in lieu of a jig). Such postural requirements may contribute to localized muscle fatigue.

Despite these benefits, however, several limitations are apparent in the traditional methods:

- Conventional systems rarely record the variability of loads handled, distances moved, and so on; therefore, extreme deviations about the atypical "average" are ignored. The fact that the total time required to complete a particular task is relatively insensitive (or robust) to this variability does not lessen the importance of this aspect in the etiology of LBP.
- Conventional systems virtually ignore posture as a predictor variable. Except for the grossest classifications (such as standing versus seated work) these systems ignore one of the Gilbreths' major contributions. Their early practice of filming motions was designed to identify systematically awkward postures and inefficient motions. The recent emphasis on developing simpler and quicker shortcut techniques and procedures for time prediction purposes may be self-defeating, especially in view of prevention of LBP.

- The systems require observations that may affect the way in which a task is conducted. Also, they are time consuming for the analysis.
- Perhaps the most important shortcoming of these methods is that they are designed to account for average job performance time. As such, no attention is given to infrequent or nonroutine work. Typically, tasks that require less than 5% of the total workday, such as occasional machine setups, maintenance, cleanup, or emergency procedures, are neither rigorously documented nor analyzed. Yet many follow-up accident or injury reports suggest that these undocumented, infrequent, yet required job tasks account for a large number of injuries and often involve manual exertions that produce peak musculoskeletal stresses.

Despite these limitations, however, traditional time and motion study forms a foundation for procedures aimed at enriching the evaluation of manual jobs. For routine, repetitive industrial work it is common to have analyses such as MTM available (Fig. 12.1). These should be sought out and used in evaluating manual jobs.

For unrepetitive, unstructured work it is more common to conduct work sampling studies to document job requirements. These, too, serve as a valuable starting place for improved job evaluation methods.

CONTEMPORARY JOB ANALYSIS SYSTEMS

The shortcomings of traditional time and motion analysis systems just discussed, coupled with a perceived need for more specific job data have led to several more contemporary approaches to improved evaluation of musculoskeletal stress on jobs. A few of these systems are described here. For a more detailed discussion see Chaffin and Andersson.[10]

Physical Stress Checklists and Surveys

A checklist of physical tasks sometimes can be used to document a job's general physical requirements. In such a procedure a job analyst observes the worker and checks off those

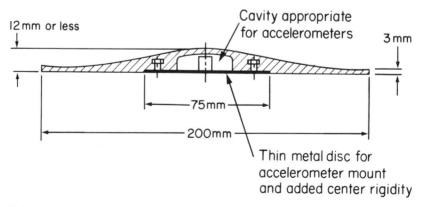

FIG 12.1.
Sample MTM analysis of lifting a tote box from a pallet to a workbench and removing a part from the tote box. (Adapted from Chaffin DB, Andersson GBJ: *Occupational Biomechanics.* New York, Wiley and Sons, 1984. Used by permission.)

activities performed on a list of 35 or more common manual tasks (e.g., bend trunk, pull with arm(s), lift with back). Such a list has been used in at least one study to improve job placement procedures for individuals with physical impairments.[52]

Another informative survey approach documents the average frequency of occurrence and weight handled during various standard manual tasks.[61] Koyl and Marsters-Hanson modified this procedure to include the recording of the hours during the day that each activity is performed.[37] By comparing these data with a clinical assessment of a person's mobility and strength, Koyl and Marsters-Hanson proposed that placement of individuals on specific jobs could be improved.[37] The Department of Labor has used such data to classify jobs subjectively, according to the general criteria given in Table 12.2.

Such physical stress survey data are important for identifying jobs that are potentially hazardous to a worker's musculoskeletal system. They are also applicable to jobs that are not highly repetitive, for which traditional methods are limited. In this sense the surveys indicate when special in-depth studies may be warranted. Such surveys are especially useful when combined with injury data analysis to motivate more intensive evaluations.

Lifting Limits in Manual Materials Handling

The *Work Practices Guide to Manual Lifting* offers specific recommendations for evaluating human lifting limitations in particular.[46] The *Guide* is intentionally simplistic in approach and application since it was intended for general industry use. The criteria include muscle strength and physical work capacities (aerobic) in addition to biomechanical aspects of disc compression.

The 1981 *Guide* specifically calls for the measurement of the following factors.

TABLE 12.2
Strength Requirement Classification Criteria Adopted by U.S. Department of Labor*

Degree of Strength	Amount of Lifting/Carrying	Posture; Other Activities
Sedentary Work	Occasional: 10 pounds maximum	Primarily sitting; walking and standing at most occasionally
Light work	20 pounds maximum 10 (or less) pounds frequently	Significant amount of walking or standing or Primarily sitting, but requiring pushing and pulling of arm and/or leg controls
Medium work	50 pounds maximum; 50 (or less) pounds frequently	Unspecified
Heavy work	100 pounds maximum; 50 (or less) pounds frequently	Unspecified
Very heavy work	Over 100 pounds allowed; 50 (or more) pounds frequently	Unspecified

*Adapted from Smith P, Armstrong TJ, Lizza GD: IE's can play crucial role in enabling handicapped employees to work safely, productively. *Indus Eng* 1982;14:98–105. Used by permission.

1. *Object weight* (L)—measured in pounds (or kilograms). If this varies from time to time, the average and maxima are necessary.
2. *Horizontal location of the hands* (H)—measured in inches (or centimeters) forward of the midpoint between the ankles. This distance is usually measured near the origin of lifting, wherein the low-back moment is judged to be greatest. A rule of thumb for this dimension is H = (W/2 + 6), where W is the horizontal width of the object (W/2 implies that the hands grip the object at its center, and 6 inches is assumed for foot and body clearance).
3. *Vertical location of the hands* (V)—measured in inches (or centimeters) above the midpoint between the ankles.
4. *Vertical travel distance* (D)—measured in inches (or centimeters) from the origin to the destination of the lift.
5. *Frequency of lifting* (F)—measured in lifts per minute, assuming continuous lifting for a period of one or eight hours.
6. *Duration of period* (P)—assumed to be either occasional (less than one hour) or continuous (for eight hours).

The *Guide* specifically ignores a number of important variables. In particular, the *Guide* is only applicable to these tasks:

1. *Smooth lifting.* The *Guide* assumes no accelerations of the load or human body. Obviously, with acceleration or jerking the stress to the low back can be substantially higher than that suggested by the *Guide*.

2. *Two-handed, symmetric* lifting in the sagittal plane. The *Guide* assumes that lifting is only two-dimensional, with both hands directly in front of the body, and does not involve twisting throughout the lift. It should be noted that as this book goes to press NIOSH is revising the 1981 *Guide*, and inclusion of asymmetric lifting evaluation should be expected.

3. *Moderate width object.* The hands are assumed to be separated no more than shoulder width. The handling of extremely wide objects (such as a standard sheet of plywood) is outside the scope of the *Guide*.

4. *Unrestricted standing posture.* The *Guide* assumes that there are no obstructions to interfere with the movement of the object, nor are there props or aids to facilitate the lifting. Lifting style is not considered beyond simple stoop versus squat techniques.

5. *Good handles* on the object. The *Guide* specifically ignores grip capability, which has been extensively studied outside the lifting context.

6. *Favorable environmental conditions.* It is assumed that heat and cold stress do not contribute to the burden on the individual and that a slippery floor is not important.

7. *No other work.* It is assumed that when not engaged in lifting the individual is essentially at rest, having no significant carrying, pushing, pulling, holding, or other such tasks.

The *Guide* presents two limits: the action limit and maximum permissible limit. The range between these limits is designed to reflect the variability between individuals in the U.S. working population. Full definitions follow.

1. *Maximum permissible limit* (MPL). This limit reflects a lift that produces 1,430 pounds (6,361 N) of compression on the L5–S1 disc, that creates a metabolic load for repeated lifting of 5.0 kcal per minute, or that is within the strength capabilities of only 25% of men and virtually no women.

2. *Action limit* (AL). This limit is algebraically equal to one-third of the MPL. An action limit creates 770 pounds (3,425 N) of compression on the L5–S1 disc, requires 3.5 kcal per minute for repeated lifting, or is within the strength capabilities of 75% of women and virtually all men.

MPL and AL are used to judge the physical stress associated with the lifting of an object of specific weight in a job. Depending on whether the weight is above or below each limit a different organizational response is required, as follows:

1. *Above MPL*—tasks that require engineering controls (e.g., fundamental job or task modifications in terms of H, V, D, F, P, or L, such as use of a hoist or modification of the workplace layout).
2. *Below the AL*—job tasks are of nominal stress and risk to most people.
3. *Between the AL and MPL*—job or lifting tasks require either engineering controls or administrative controls. Administrative controls include workforce selection (functional capacity testing) and training for fitness and awareness of job stresses and ways to limit them.

In algebraic form, the two NIOSH weight lifting limits are (in pounds of weight):

$$AL = 90 \ (6/H) \ (1 - 01 \ [V - 30]) \ (0.7 + 3/D) \ (1 - F/F_{max})$$

$$MPL = 3 \ (AL)$$

where

H ranges from 6 to 32 inches (15.2–81.3 cm)

V ranges from 0 to 70 inches (0–177.8 cm)

D ranges from 10 to (80 − V) inches (25.4–(203.2 − V) cm)

F ranges from 0.2 to F_{max}

and

F_{max} = 12 for continuous low lifting (P = 8 hr and V less than 30 in.)
= 18 for occasional high lifting (P = 1 hr and V less than 30 in.)
= 15 otherwise

To record job lifting data, a physical stress job analysis sheet such as that shown in Figure 12.2, should be used. This form shows the analysis for a single task of loading a reel of stock into a machine, as illustrated in Figure 12.3.

After the lifting evaluation is complete for *each* lifting task in a job, the resulting predicted action limits and maximum permissible limits are computed and added to the coding forms in the columns provided. These limits then can be compared line by line to determine the relative stressfulness of each lifting task.

Because the H distance is so critical in determining the amount of low back stress, it is prudent to measure H at both the origin and destination. The origin is usually associated with greater inertia resulting from accelerating the mass upward. If a great deal of control is

PHYSICAL STRESS JOB ANALYSIS SHEET

Department __Fabrication__   Date __2-18-90__

Job Title __Punch Press__   Analyst's Name __E.J.B.__

Task Description	Object Weight AVG MAX (NEWTONS)		Hand Location ORIGIN H cm	V cm	DESTINATION H cm	V cm	Task Freq	AL	MPL	Remarks
Load Stock	200	200	53	38	53	160	0			

FIG 12.2.
NIOSH job lifting analysis form filled in for the lifting task depicted in Figure 12.3. Note: The zero entry for task frequency denotes that the stock reel is loaded at a frequency of less than once every five minutes.

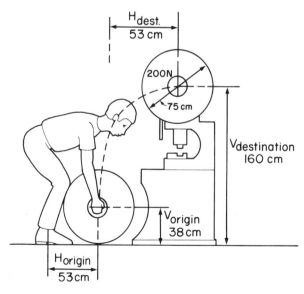

FIG 12.3.
Example of lifting stock into punch press. It is assumed that the worker steps forward with the load to place it atop press, that is, H remains constant, while V changes. (Adapted from Chaffin DB, Andersson GBJ: *Occupational Biomechanics.* New York, Wiley and Sons, 1984. Used by permission.)

also required in placing the load at the destination (i.e., in a precise location or with a fragile load), it may be more appropriate to use the destination H value.

The NIOSH *Guide* is a recent effort to control one type of manual materials handling, namely, the act of lifting in the sagittal plane. It attempts to be more comprehensive than previous efforts with respect to job evaluation methods, criteria used for limits, and control strategies. It is too early to discern the *Guide*'s long-term effects on controlling musculoskeletal injuries in industry, but anecdotal evidence is very supportive. Copies of the *Guide* are now available from the American Industrial Hygiene Association in Akron, Ohio. NIOSH is currently planning to enlarge the scope of the *Guide* to include evaluation of asymmetric lifting.

Static Strength Analysis

Because the NIOSH *Guide* applies only to symmetric lifting in the sagittal plane, a more generalized analysis scheme is often necessary to describe and evaluate manual work. One such scheme concentrates on static strength predictions.

One model compares the load moments produced at various body joints during any task to population capabilities.[21] The job analysis requirements are comparable to the NIOSH procedure, but they can be extended to pushing and pulling in directions other than orthogonal. Chaffin and Andersson give a complete description of the job analysis method and strength prediction model.[10]

In general, forces acting on the hands are viewed as vector quantities (in magnitude and direction) acting separately on each hand. The model combines the effects of these external loads with the effects of each body segment's weight for a given body posture (obtained from photographs or video images) in order to predict the moment load on each major body articulation. The resultant strength requirement for each major muscle group (to counteract this moment load) is then predicted for various strata of the population.

The model also predicts the compressive force acting on the L5–S1 disc for each posture and load condition being analyzed. For each task of interest, a general body posture of the legs and torso can either be assumed (via a computerized postural optimization scheme) or described by the job analyst (e.g., standing, stooping, squatting, leaning forward, sitting). Normally, a videotape of the job being performed is used to set the posture input values. Personal computer versions of the model, referred to as the Static Strength Prediction Programs™ are available through The University of Michigan's Software Office in Ann Arbor, Michigan.

Garg and Chaffin[21] and Chaffin and Andersson[10] include detailed discussions of the strength prediction and L5–S1 compression force model and computer algorithm. Stobbe[58] and Herrin[27] discuss the methods for assessing isometric strength in industry and predicting population norms. Battié[4] has recently challenged the concept of static strength testing and prediction for reported low back injury. In a large prospective study among aircraft industry employees the static strength test was not a significant predictor for reported low back injury. Hence, current knowledge of the applicability of generic strength testing needs further evaluation.

European Standards

For many years, some member states of the European community have had individual standards for lifting. It is only recently that the EEC has received a proposal for minimum health and safety requirements for handling heavy loads where there is a risk of back injury.[16] The draft regulations require that, if possible, heavy loads be moved with mechanical assistance, that the employee examine the physical effort and characteristics of the load, that management examine the individual characteristics of the worker and give the worker proper training and full information on the loads. Details such as those included in the NIOSH guide are not included in the directive. It is anticipated that the countries of the EEC will make laws to comply with this directive by 1991.

Psychophysical Strength Analysis

The psychophysical approach to assessment of strength does not assume an underlying mechanical model of a body, nor is it related to spinal loading per se. Rather, it focuses directly on the individual's perception of manual capability when doing a task.

Psychophysical scales have been developed in many practical problem areas. For example, the scales of effective temperature, loudness, and brightness were all developed with a psychophysical methodology.[30,56,57] Psychophysics has also been used by Borg in developing rating scales of perceived exertion (RPE);[6,7] by the Air Force in studies of lifting;[17,59] and by the Army in studies of treadmill walking[18,19] and in developing effort scales.[8,9]

Snook[53] summarized a series of seven studies conducted at Liberty Mutual Research Center that stand out for their comprehensiveness in the area of manual materials handling capacities, as did Ayoub et al.[1] The latter studies were restricted to lifting tasks only. Snook and his associates also provided the first analysis to relate psychophysical strength predictions to the increased risk of low back injury.

To evaluate the effectiveness of job design in the reduction of injuries (as well as the effectiveness of selection techniques and training procedures), 191 cases of low back injury from 32 states were investigated.[54] Questionnaire results revealed that about 25% of policy-holder jobs involve manual materials handling tasks that (on a psychophysical rating scale) are acceptable to less than 75% of the workers. Half of the low-back injuries were associated with these jobs, indicating that workers are three times more susceptible to low back injury when performing a manual handling task that is acceptable to less than 75% of the working population. This suggests that, at best, two out of every three low back injuries associated with heavy manual handling tasks can be prevented if the tasks are designed to fit at least 75% of the population. The third injury will apparently occur anyway, regardless of the job. The other low back injuries not associated with heavy manual handling tasks will also occur. It can be concluded that up to one-third of industrial back injuries can be obviated by the careful and proper design of manual handling tasks.

To evaluate the relevant percentages of the population, Snook[54] presented summary tables for industrial males and females, itemizing psychophysical limits on lifting, lowering, pushing, pulling, and carrying for each of the following task variables:[54]

1. Vertical region (knuckle height to floor level, or shoulder height to knuckle height, or arm reach to shoulder height)
2. Object width (horizontal dimensions)
3. Distance moved (vertical dimensions for lift, horizontal dimensions for pushing and carrying)
4. Frequency of exertion (in repetitions per minute)

One shortcoming of this analysis is the referencing of the vertical dimensions of the task to a particular individual's anthropometry rather than to absolute coordinates.

A similar study by Ayoub et al. provided prediction models for maximum psychophysical lifting capacity as a function of worker and task variables.[1] Six regression equations were generated for each lifting region: floor to knuckle; floor to shoulder; floor to reach; knuckle to shoulder; knuckle to reach; and shoulder to reach. Experiments were conducted at frequencies of 2, 4, 6, and 8 lifts per minute and box sizes of 12, 18, and 24 inches (30.5, 45.7, and 61.0 cm, respectively) in the sagittal plane. A series of job stress indices (variations of the ratio of weight lifted to individual lifting capacities aggregated across tasks) were developed in an effort to predict lost time resulting from injury. None of these indices was strongly correlated with the injury experience, due in part to a small sample size. A more recent study by Liles et al. based on psychophysical strength norms is more supportive of such an evaluation procedure.[42]

Dynamic Strength Analysis

Recently a large number of machines have become available for strength testing under dynamic conditions. The most popular kinds of machines are isokinetic (constant speed) or isodynamic (constant load). In an early study of isokinetic testing, Hasue, Fujiwara, and Kikuchi found that under isokinetic conditions abdominal muscles were weaker than dorsal muscles, and there was a decrease of strength with age.[25] Lee and Langrana gave further reports of isokinetic strength in both sitting and standing.[41] Parnianpour et al. used a triaxial isometric dynamometer and found that with fatigue the dorsal and abdominal muscles are compensated with secondary muscles.[49] This means that there is increased coupled motion with fatigue in a flexion extension motion. Although they are convincing, these new techniques do not completely simulate reality due to the complexity of "real" manual tasks. These dynamic tests are, however, able to give a better understanding of which characteristics of the motion (velocity, range of motion, torque, power, or work output) are deficient.

Load Pushing and Pulling

In general, pushing and pulling capabilities have been studied within a more limited scope. Furthermore, estimates of the number of injuries that occur during pushing or pulling of loads are not complete, although approximately 20% of overexertion injuries have been associated with such acts.[46]

The previous work of Fox[20] and Kroemer and Robinson[39] shows that the effect of friction on static strength capability when pushing and pulling is of primary importance. They collectively showed that healthy young males could exert an average force of approximately 42.9 lb (200 N) when the coefficient of friction was about 0.3. With a friction coefficient greater than 0.6, the mean push or pull strength capability increased to 64.3 lb (300 N) for the same group, according to Kroemer and Robinson.[39] Bracing one foot and using the back to apply force (rather than using the hands) further increased the static push force capabilities.[20,38]

Martin and Chaffin,[44] Ayoub and McDaniel,[1] Lee,[40] and Davis and Stubbs[15] reported that the vertical height of the handle against which one pushes and pulls is of critical importance. In an experimental study of strength by Ayoub and McDaniel[1] the elbows and rearward knee were kept straight for the exertions. They recommended that the optimal height for pushing or pulling a handle should be approximately 35.8 to 44 inches (91 to 114 cm) (i.e., about hip height) above the floor. Davis and Stubbs[15] developed recommendations for pushing and pulling limits based on abdominal pressure measurements. Martin and Chaffin[44] used a biomechanical model to predict the maximum push-and-pull forces for extreme postures. In this regard, Lee[40] performed a set of dynamic push-and-pull experiments and found that the predicted compression forces were less when the hands were approximately 42.9 (109 cm) above the floor than when they were either 59.8 in. (152 cm) or 26.0 in. (66 cm).

In short, there is a recognized need to understand pushing and pulling activities, since many overexertion injuries appear to be related to such activities. It is also clear that many biomechanical factors interact to alter push-and-pull capabilities. At present, however, there exists only a limited amount of data and modeling of these common activities, and so any limits must be interpreted carefully for job evaluation purposes.

Asymmetric Load Handling

Based on both biomechanical models and experimental strength studies, symmetric load handling (in which the load is moved in the midsagittal plane with both hands) is recommended. Unfortunately, the studies of asymmetric load handling are few because of the experimental and biomechanical modeling complexities associated with three-dimensional force analysis. Clearly, however, asymmetric load handling increases the stress on the spine and most muscle groups, and it can result in poor postural stability. Unfortunately, asymmetric motions are often most efficient in terms of performance time.

One recent study by Warwick et al.[62] compared symmetric and asymmetric pushing and pulling. In general, the activities in asymmetric postures resulted in decreased strengths (of about 20 to 25%). The effects were very dependent on the direction of motion and postures, as might be expected. Pope et al.[50] found that there was a great deal of antagonistic muscle activity in an isometric twisting activity. Thus many muscles contract around simply to maintain postural stability.

Job Posture Evaluation

An approach to recording potentially stressful postures, referred to as *posture targeting,* was developed by Corlett, Madeley, and Manenica.[13] This procedure requires the job analyst to observe a worker at random times during the workday and record the angular configuration of various body segments with the aid of the body diagram displayed in Figure 12.4. The angular data are recorded by simply placing a small "x" on each postural target when a body segment deviates from the erect anatomic position shown. The concentric circles on each target represent 45-, 90-, and 135-degree angular deviations of a joint from that shown, with the arrow at the center of the target indicating the front of the body. The radial lines indicate the amount of deviation from the sagittal plane as viewed from overhead. Counting the number of "x" marks in a certain zone of a diagram, or simply observing how the marks cluster together, provides insight into possible stressful postures.

Although the Corlett study did not combine these postural data with external load data for biomechanical analysis,[13] such would be possible by noting the load magnitudes on the activity lists provided with the body diagram. In its simplest form, the procedure documents job postures in such a way that the analyst can easily identify the most frequent and potentially stressful ones for more detailed biomechanical analysis. Corlett and Manenica[14] have also demonstrated that this procedure is useful in evaluating workplace layouts when combined with worker reports of localized musculoskeletal pain obtained at several intervals during a workday.

It should be mentioned that Priel[51] proposed a system to allow postures to be numerically defined and recorded. From repeated observations of workers, the basic posture of the body

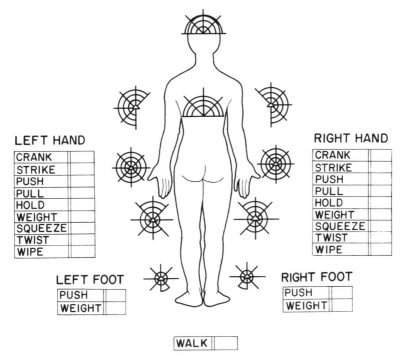

FIG 12.4.
Body diagram, showing each target adjacent to its associated body part. Deviations from the standard position shown are marked on the neighboring diagram, otherwise no mark is made with each observation of the worker. (Adapted from Corlett EN, Madeley SJ, Manenica I: Postural targetting: A technique for recording working postures. *Ergonomics* 1979; 22:357–366. Used by permission.)

within a three-dimensional coordinate system, the levels at which joints and limbs are located, and the direction and amount of movements are determined and graphed on a "posturegram."

In Finland the OWAS system was developed. The Ovaco working posture analysis system (OWAS) is a practical method of identifying and evaluating unsuitable working postures.[32,33] The method consists of two parts, the first being an observation technique for evaluating work postures. It can be used in time and motion studies of a daily routine and gives reliable results after a short training period for observers. The second part is a set of criteria for the redesigning of working methods and workplaces. The criteria are based on evaluations made by experienced workers and ergonomic experts. The criteria take into consideration factors such as health and safety, but the main emphasis is placed on the discomfort caused by sustained awkward working postures. This method has been extensively used by a steel company that participated in its development.

A method similar to OWAS is a technique developed by Berns and Milner for analyzing moving work postures (TRAM).[5] Both OWAS and TRAM record the postures at regular intervals on a recording sheet. By using various combinations of the basic posture a wide range of postures can be described. Included in the recording is an approximation of a weight or force acting externally on the body as well as longer static positions. A similar video-based postural recording method was developed, originally for recording shoulder torso postures, by Keyserling.[34,35] An analyst observing a videotape of a job uses an on-line personal computer to keep track of any deviations in postures. Keyserling's method has been compared with a more detailed biomechanical analysis and is currently being used in a large epidemiologic study of musculoskeletal injuries in industry (see Fig. 12.5).

A new Swedish system called ARBAN was developed by Holzmann.[30] ARBAN is a method for ergonomic analysis of work, including work situations involving greatly differing body postures and loads. The method consists of four steps: recording the workplace on videotape or film, coding the posture and load situation in a number of closely spaced "frozen" situations, computerization, and evaluation of results. A computer routine determines the total ergonomic stress for the whole body (as well as specified body parts) based on heuristic rules regarding the relative stress of specific acts. The results are presented as ergonomic stress/time curves, with the heavy load situation occurring as the peak of the curve. Kilbom, Persson, and Jonsson[36] developed a method called VIRA that clarifies body positions from a videotape. By means of a computer-aided procedure

Classifying Trunk Posture

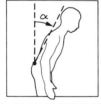

FLEXION/EXTENSION
α measured in the sagittal plane

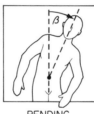

BENDING
β measured in the frontal plane

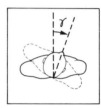

TWISTING
γ is rotation about the long axis of the trunk

Neutral occurs when the trunk is within 20 degrees of the vertical with less than 20 degrees of twisting

STANDARD TRUNK POSTURES	
1. Stand-Extension (α < -20°)	6. Lie-on Back or Side
2. Stand-Neutral	7. Sit-Neutral
3. Stand-Mild Flexion (20° < α ≤ 45°)	8. Sit-Mild Flexion
4. Stand-Severe Flexion (α > 45°)	9. Sit-Twisted/Bent
5. Stand-Twisted/Bent (β or γ > 20°)	

Classifying Shoulder Posture

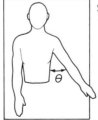

SHOULDER FLEXION/ABDUCTION is the included angle θ between the trunk and the humerus.

Neutral occurs when θ is less than 45 degrees

STANDARD SHOULDER POSTURES
1. Neutral (θ ≤ 45°)
2. Mild Flexion/Abduction (45° < θ ≤ 90°)
3. Severe Flexion/Abduction (θ > 90°)

FIG 12.5.
The Standard Posture Classification System used by Keyserling. (Adapted from Keyserling WM: Postural analysis of the trunk and shoulders in simulated real time. *Ergonomics* 1986b; 29:469–583.)

Keyserling compares actual postures recorded on videotape to a menu of standard postures.[34,35]

The observation techniques can be used together with discomfort/comfort scales[12] and various biomechanical analyses techniques. Grieve[24] has suggested a method to determine potential mechanical constraints during static exertions based on equilibrium (body balance) considerations reflected in a postural stability diagram.

Trunk Flexion Analysis

A measurement device for recording movements and postures in the sagittal plane has been developed by Nordin, Ortengren, and Andersson.[48] The instrument consists of a pendulum potentiometer as a transducer, a five-level analog-to-digital converter, control circuits, and nine digital registers. Together the unit forms a portable battery-powered system that weighs 2.1 lb (1 kg) and can be worn on the back in a small harness. Although the analyzer has the potential for measuring movements of any body segment, it has so far been adapted only for measuring trunk movements in the sagittal plane (forward flexion).

The range of flexion is divided into five intervals. Flexion greater than 90 degrees is recorded in the interval 73 to 90 degrees. The analyzer also records the total amount of time the worker spends in each interval of flexion as well as the number of times that the amount of flexion changes between one interval and another in one direction of flexion. The flexion analysis has been tested and found to be accurate and simple to use.[31,48]

More recently The Rehabilitation Engineering Center at the University of Vermont has developed a multiaxis goniometer system capable of measuring flexion-extension, lateral bend, and axial rotation. The device is shown in use in the construction industry in Figure 12.6. These data are recorded and preprocessed so that they are "binned" by time in a specific posture in Figure 12.7.

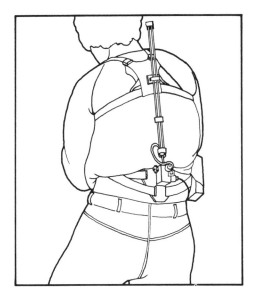

FIG 12.6.
Multiaxis goniometer system capable of measuring flexion-extension, lateral bend, and axial rotation. The device is shown in use in the construction industry.

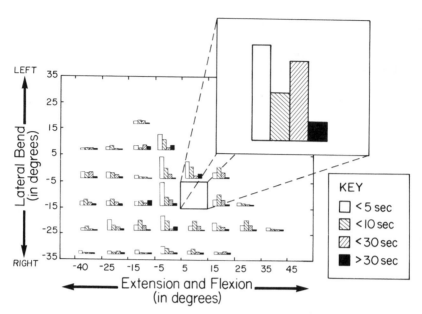

FIG 12.7.
Data measured by the goniometer are recorded and preprocessed so that they are "binned" by time in a specific posture.

Changes in work techniques and work design can easily be measured and quantified. Continuous recording can be made without an observer, but this is not recommended, since valuable information about the work cycle is lost. The advantage of the flexion analyzer is that it is noninvasive, reliable, and easily transported, and results are obtained immediately. The limitations of these instruments are obvious: they measure only posture and do not measure external body loading. A system like this, however, can be combined with a force grip strain gauge and thereby give an estimate of the external body loading.

EVALUATION OF WORKPLACE VIBRATION

The U.S. standard for vibration measurement is given by SAE J1013 (SAE). Accelerations are measured by a molded rubber disc 8 inches (250 mm) in diameter. The disc has a maximum height of 12 mm and contains a cavity for the accelerometers. The accelerometers should be capable of 0.1 m/sec² to 10 m/sec² (acceleration) measurements. The disc is designed to sit comfortably between the ischial tuberosities. The acceleration is usually analyzed in one-third octave band levels or by means of a ride meter. Most ride meters compute and assign a weighting factor to the overall RMS acceleration based on the published SAE tolerance curves. This gives one number that is representative of the vibration exposure. The advantage of one-third octave band analysis is that it shows intensity as a function of frequency and is thus more useful for analytic and design purposes.

Typical vibration levels as a function of frequency are given in Chapter 6. It should be noted that extremely high levels are found in earth-moving equipment and off-highway (military, agricultural, and recreational) vehicles.

Experience has shown that attention to some special protocols helps to ensure good data.

A low-pass filter with a cutoff frequency of less than 100 Hz should be used. Turning the accelerometer by 90 degrees from the vertical to the horizontal plane provides a 1-g calibration line if the accelerometer is not a piezoelectric type. This should be done before and after the test to allow scaling of the data. Prior to taking the data, the operator (test subject) should sit with the disc in place for 30 minutes. This time period allows for mechanical and temperature stabilization. In special cases in which the performance of the tasks may be affected by vibration, it may be necessary to establish vibration transmission to the head. In these cases, a bite bar or helmet-mounted accelerometer may be employed.

The test site should be carefully specified and the grade, speed, and distance to be traveled specified. The road surface (or other surface) and other test conditions should be chosen to be representative of those used during the normal work week.

Determining the complex exposure of the human to standing or seated vibration is made simpler using the three-tiered approach described by the ISO 2631-85 standard. The final presentation is a single number that combines critical parameters, such as the body's sensitivity to the frequency range and direction of vibration, at each of the three vibration axes. If the single combined number seems large, it can be broken up into its three components to show which axis provides the greater vibration. If there is further interest in the three axes, they can be further broken down into their respective spectra of RMS acceleration (m/s^2) versus frequency. This description is the reverse of what actually must be done with triaxial accelerometer data to obtain the single, final value.

SUMMARY

Traditional work measurement systems are limited in their ability to provide the data necessary to evaluate and improve the biomechanical aspects of various jobs.[10] Even the most detailed predetermined motion-time systems such as MTM-1 do not include data on posture and load-handling factors. Despite these limitations, however, it must be realized that these traditional motion-time analysis systems provide the fundamental data structure and procedures necessary to evaluate potential job-related biomechanical problems. The traditional systems emphasize a rigorous analysis. By including postural and load data, excellent biomechanical evaluations can be performed. Vibration measurements should be done using a disc-mounted accelerometer placed between the ischial tuberosities. The terrain and driving conditions should be carefully selected.

Unfortunately, it is not possible at this time to specify an optimal analysis method for future studies. From the limited attempts to develop such a system it would appear that several different job analysis schemes will be desirable in the future. Chaffin and Andersson have proposed the following considerations to assist in the choice of future analysis procedures.[10]

1. The degree of standardization of the tasks comprising a job.
2. The length of repetitive work cycles in a job.
3. The proportion of a workday involved in manual effort that is potentially overstressful to the musculoskeletal system.
4. The available time to observe and record manual activities (i.e., an MTM-1 analysis may require an analyst to spend 350 times the length of a job's cycle time to perform, according to Magnusson[44]).
5. The degree of sophistication to be utilized in evaluating the biomechanical job data.

6. The expected end use of the analysis, for example, redesigning a machine, tool, or layout; selecting and placing workers; modifying work methods; or setting productivity standards.

BIBLIOGRAPHY

1. Ayoub MM, McDaniel JW: Effect of operator stance on pushing and pulling tasks. *AIIE Transactions* 1974; 6:185–195.
2. Ayoub MM, Bethea NJ, Deivanayagem S, et al: Determination and modeling of lifting capacity, DHEW(NIOSH) Final Report R01 OH 00545-02, 1978.
3. Barnes RM: *Motion and Time Study: Design and Measurement of Work,* ed 6. New York, Wiley and Sons, 1968.
4. Battié MC: *The Reliability of Physical Factors as Predictors of the Occurrence of Back Pain Reports: A Prospective Study within Industry* (thesis). Gothenburg, Sweden, University of Goteborg, 1989.
5. Berns TAR, Milner NP: TRAM—A technique for the recording and analysis of moving work posture, in NP Milner (ed): *Methods to Study Work Posture.* Stockholm, Sweden, ERGO-LAB, Report 80:23, pp 22–26.
6. Borg GAV: *Physical Performance and Perceived Exertion.* Copenhagen, Ejnar M Munksgoard, 1962.
7. Borg GAV: Perceived exertion: A note on "history" and methods. *Med Sci Sports* 1973; 5:90–93.
8. Caldwell LS, Smith RP: *Subjective Estimation of Effort, Reserve, and Ischemic Pain.* Ft Knox, Ky, US Army Medical Research Lab Report No 730, 1967.
9. Caldwell LS, Grossman EE: Effort scaling of isometric muscle contractions. *J Motor Behavior* 1973; 5:9–16.
10. Chaffin DB, Andersson GBJ: *Occupational Biomechanics.* New York, Wiley and Sons, 1984.
11. Copley FB: *Frederick W. Taylor,* vol 1. New York, Harper and Bros, 1923.
12. Corlett EN, Bishop RP: A technique for assessing postural discomfort. *Ergonomics* 1976; 19:175–182.
13. Corlett EN, Madeley SJ, Manenica I: Postural targeting: A technique for recording working postures. *Ergonomics* 1979; 22:357–366.
14. Corlett EN, Manenica I: The effects and measurement of working postures. *Applied Ergonomics* 1980; 11:7–16.
15. Davis PR, Stubbs DA: Safe levels of manual forces for young males: 3. Performance capacity limits. *Applied Ergonomics* 1978; 9:33–37.
16. EEC: Proposal for a council directive on the minimum health and safety requirements for handling heavy loads where there is a risk of back injury for workers. *Official J Europ Communities C* 1988; 117:8–10.
17. Emanuel I, Chafee J, Wing J: *A Study of Human Weight Lifting Capabilities for Loading Ammunition into the F-86H Aircraft.* Wright Patterson Air Force Base, Ohio, US Air Force WADC-TR 056-367, 1959.
18. Evans WO: *A Titration Schedule on a Treadmill.* Fort Knox, Ky, US Army Medical Research Laboratory, Report No 525, 1961.
19. Evans WO: *The Effect of Treadmill Grade on Performance Decrement Using a Titration Schedule.* Ft Knox, Ky, US Army Medical Research Laboratory, Report No 535, 1962.
20. Fox WF: Body Weight and Coefficient of Friction Determinants of Pushing Capability, in *Human Engineering Special Studies Series,* No 17. Marietta, Ga, Lockheed Co, 1967.
21. Garg A, Chaffin DB: A biomechanical computerized simulation of human strength. *AIIE Transactions* 1975; 7:1–15.
22. Gilbreth FB: *Motion Study: A Method for Increasing the Efficiency of the Workman.* New York, D Van Nostrand, 1911.

23. Gilbreth FB: The present state of the art of industrial management. *Trans ASME* 1912; 34:1224–1226.
24. Grieve DW: The postural stability diagram (PSD): Personal constraints on the static exertion of force. *Ergonomics* 1979; 22:1155–1164.
25. Hasue M, Fujiwara M, Kikuchi S: A new method of quantitative measurement of abdominal and back muscle strength. *Spine* 1980; 5:143–148.
26. Herrin GD: A taxonomy of manual materials handling hazards, in C Drury (ed): *Safety in Manual Materials Handling*. National Institute for Occupational Safety and Health, Publ No 78-185, 1978, pp 6–15.
27. Herrin GD: Standardized strength testing methods for population descriptions, in Easterby R, Kroemer KHE, Chaffin DB (eds): *Anthropometry and Biomechanics—Theory and Application*. NATO Conference Series Vol 16. New York, Plenum Press, 1982.
28. Herrin GD, Jaraiedi M, Anderson C: Prediction of overexertion injuries using biomechanical and psychophysical models. *Am Ind Hyg Assoc J* 1986; 47:322–330.
29. Holzmann P: ARBAN—A new method for analysis of ergonomic effort. *Applied Ergonomics* 1982; 13:82–86.
30. Houghton FC, Yagloglou CP: Determination of the comfort zone. *J Am Soc Heating Ventil Eng* 1923; 29:515–536.
31. Hultman G, Nordin M, Ortengren R: The influence of a preventative educational program on trunk flexion in janitors. *Applied Ergonomics* 1984; 15:127–133.
32. Karhu O, Kansi P, Kuorinka I: Correcting working postures in industry: Practical method for analysis. *Appl Ergonomics* 1977; 18:199–201.
33. Karhu O, Harkonen R, Sorvali P, et al: Observing working postures in industry: Examples of OWAS application. *Appl Ergonomics* 1981; 12:13–17.
34. Keyserling WM: A computer aided system to evaluate postural stress in the workplace. *Am Ind Hyg Assoc J* 1986a; 47:641–649.
35. Keyserling WM: Postural analysis of the trunk and shoulders in simulated real time. *Ergonomics* 1986b; 29:469–583.
36. Kilbom A, Persson J, Jonsson B: Risk factors for work related disorders of the neck and shoulder with special emphasis on working postures and movement. Presented at the International Symposium in Ergonomics of Working Posture, Zadas, Yugoslavia, 1985.
37. Koyl FF, Marsters-Hanson P: *Age, Physical Ability and Work Potential*. Washington, DC, Manpower Administration, US Dept Labor, 1973.
38. Kroemer KHE: *Push Forces Exerted in 65 Common Work Positions*. Wright Patterson Air Force Base, Ohio, AMRL-T-68-143, 1969.
39. Kroemer KHE, Robinson DE: *Horizontal Static Forces Exerted by Men Standing in Common Working Postures on Surfaces of Various Tractions*. Wright Patterson Air Force Base, Ohio, AMRL-TR-70-114, 1971.
40. Lee K: *Biomechanical Modelling of Cart Pushing and Pulling* (thesis). Ann Arbor, Univ of Michigan, 1982.
41. Lee NA, Langrana NA: Lumbosacral spinal fusion. *Spine* 1984; 9:574–581.
42. Liles DH, Deivanayagam S, Ayoub MM, et al: A job severity index for the evaluation and control of lifting injury. *Human Factors* 1984; 26:683–693.
43. Magnusson K: The development of MTM-2, MTM-V, and MTM-3. *J Methods Time Measurement* 1972; 17:11–23.
44. Martin JB, Chaffin DB: Biomechanical computerized simulation of human strength in sagittal-plane activities. *AIIE Trans* 1972; 4:19–28.
45. Mundel ME: *Motion and Time Study*, ed 5. New Jersey, Prentice-Hall, 1978.
46. NIOSH (National Institute for Occupational Safety and Health): *Work Practices Guide for Manual Lifting*. Cincinnati, Ohio, Division of Biomedical and Behavioral Science, Tech Report 81-122, 1981.
47. Niebel BW: *Motion and Time Study*, ed 5. Homewood, Ill, RD Irwin, 1972.
48. Nordin M, Ortengren R, Andersson GBJ: Measurement of trunk movement during work. *Spine* 1984; 9:465–469.

49. Parnianpour M, Nordin M, Kahanovitz N, et al: The triaxial coupling of torque generation of trunk muscles during isometric exertions and the effect of fatiguing isoinertial movements on the motor output and movement patterns. *Spine* 1988; 13:982–992.
50. Pope MH, Svensson M, Andersson GBJ, et al: The role of prerotation of the trunk in axial twisting efforts. *Spine* 1987; 12:1041–1045.
51. Priel VZ: A numerical definition of posture. *Human Factors* 1974; 16:576–584.
52. Smith P, Armstrong TJ, Lizza GD: IE's can play crucial role in enabling handicapped employees to work safely, productively. *Indus Eng* 1982; 14:98–105.
53. Snook SH: The design of manual handling tasks. *Ergonomics* 1978; 21:963–985.
54. Snook SH, Campanelli RA, Hart JW: A study of three preventative approaches to low back injury. *J Occup Med* 1978; 20:478–481.
55. Stevens JC, Cain WS: Effort in muscular contractions related to force level and duration: Perception psychophysics 1970; 8:240–244.
56. Stevens SS: The direct estimation of sensory magnitudes loudness. *Am J Psychology* 1956; 69:1–25.
57. Stevens SS: The psychophysics of sensory function. *American Scientist* 1960; 48:226–253.
58. Stobbe TJ: *The Development of a Practical Strength Testing Program for Industry* (thesis). Ann Arbor, Univ of Michigan, 1982.
59. Switzer SA: *Weight Lifting Capabilities of a Selected Sample of Human Males.* Wright Patterson Air Force Base, Ohio, AMRL-AD-284054, 1962.
60. Taylor FW: *The Principles of Scientific Management.* New York, Harper and Bros, 1929.
61. US Dept of Labor: *Handbook for Analyzing Jobs.* Washington, DC, US Govt Printing Office, No 2900-0131, 1972.
62. Warwick D, Novack G, Schultz A: Maximum voluntary strengths of male adults in some lifting, pushing, and pulling activities. *Ergonomics* 1980; 23:49–54.

13

Worker Selection

Gunnar B.J. Andersson, M.D.
J. Duncan G. Troup, M.D.

INTRODUCTION

The purpose of worker selection is to match the worker with the appropriate job. Ideally, the requirements of all jobs should be such that worker selection and restricted placements are not required. This is not the case today, however, and will not be so for some time to come because of the large variability in the performance capability of the population and the fact that many jobs cannot be redesigned. Thus, selection is one method of reducing possible harmful physical effects of work created by a mismatch of worker capabilities and job requirements.

This chapter reviews several options and general criteria for worker selection. Job classification schemes to match subject capabilities are discussed in Chapter 14.

In this chapter screening is defined as the use of examinations or tests to detect previously unrecognized or unreported risk factors for low back pain. Screening can be used in preemployment examinations to determine work capacity and future risk in a proposed job. An applicant is hired or not based on screening results and on the jobs to be filled. Preplacement screening is used after a worker has been hired, sometimes on deployment to a new job. Based on the result, restrictions in placement or workplace modifications can be instituted.

Before a preemployment screening procedure is recommended, the general principles discussed in Chapter 11 should always be considered. The most pertinent questions follow.

- Is the screening procedure safe?
- Does the screening procedure have a good probability of predicting the risk of future low back pain or injury?
- Is the screening procedure practical?
- Is the screening procedure legal?

Safety

Clearly, a screening program aimed at reducing work hazards must be safe. The risks vary from none (in obtaining a medical history) to substantial, when radiographs or strength-testing programs are used.

Predictive Value

Three factors must be considered about a procedure's ability to predict a good match of worker and job.

- Is the test sensitive?
- Is the test specific?
- What is the frequency of positive results in the population?

These aspects are discussed in Chapter 11. For reference, the most important definitions are repeated in abbreviated form in Table 13.1.

Practicality

The practicality of a given screening test varies considerably and has a different meaning to different people involved in the screening procedure. A medical history can always be obtained with little effort and time, but a strength-testing program can be quite cumbersome, expensive, and difficult to implement correctly. From the management point of view, practicality includes cost effectiveness, that is, decreasing compensation claims and number of lost workdays and providing protection to the worker.

Ideally, a screening test should be simple, inexpensive, and highly predictive of future risk.

SPECIFIC SCREENING TESTS

Medical History

The most important part of the screening medical history is the identification of previous back problems. In fact, some physicians maintain that it is the only useful predictor of risk in the medical history.[35,81] Recurrent episodes of low back pain (LBP) appear to be almost part of the natural history of LBP. Rowe found that 83% of those with LBP had recurrent attacks.[70] Patients with sciatica had a recurrence rate of 75%.[71] Similar recurrence rates have been reported by Dillane, Fry, and Kalton;[28] Horal;[43] Hirsch, Johnsson, and Lewin;[42] Leavitt, Johnston, and Beyer;[53] Gyntelberg;[36] Pedersen;[64] Troup, Martin, and Lloyd;[85] Biering-Sorensen;[10] and Biering-Sørensen, Thomsen, and Hilden.[11]

A few studies specifically consider previous back problems in terms of risk of having a recurrence. Chaffin and Park found a threefold increase in risk in subjects with a previous history of back pain,[23] and Bergquist-Ullman and Larsson reported that 62% of their group of 217 workers with acute LBP had recurrences within a year, and another 18% had recurrences within two years.[9] Pedersen;[64] Troup, Martin, and Lloyd;[85] and Biering-Sørensen[10] all found a history of sciatica to be a risk indicator, in contrast to an earlier report by Dillane, Fry, and Kalton.[29] Magora and Taustein found that persons who had had

TABLE 13.1
Concepts in Screening Tests

Accuracy	The ability of a test to provide a true measure of a quantity or quality
Sensitivity	The ability of a test to identify workers who will develop a disease
Specificity	The ability of a test to identify workers who will not develop a disease
Predictive value	The ability of a test to predict the presence or absence of future disease. This value is determined by the sensitivity and specificity of a disease and by the prevalence of the disease in question.

sciatica in the past had more and longer sickness absence periods than those with a previous history of pain in the lower back only,[60] a finding confirmed by Andersson, Svensson, and Oden.[2]

Biering-Sørensen performed a cross-sectional survey of 558 men and 583 women 30 to 60 years of age.[10] He found a significantly increased risk of LBP in the year following examination in subjects who, in the year immediately before the study, had had either (1) many episodes of back pain, (2) many sickness absence days because of LBP, (3) short intervals between episodes, or (4) an aggravated course of LBP. Thus, information not only about the occurrence of previous LBP but also about its severity has predictive value. In a recent recalculation, Biering-Sørensen, Thomsen, and Hilden used a stepwise logistic regression model to identify the most important combinations of predictors.[11] Low back pain in the past, worsening of the pain from its onset, and sciatica were all risk indicators in men, while aggravation of low back pain when standing was a risk indicator in women.

Pedersen found that a history of more than three previous episodes of LBP was ominous because new episodes were both longer and more severe.[64] Acute onset of LBP, irrespective of cause, results in a longer duration of the pain episode.[9,11,64] Troup, Martin, and Lloyd, on the other hand, found that truly accident-related previous LBP did not predict recurrences.[85]

In a prospective study Lloyd and Troup found four factors to be of predictive value concerning risk of recurrent low back pain in patients returning to work after LBP: residual leg pain on return to work, falls as a cause for back pain, sickness absence of five weeks or more, and a history of two or more previous attacks.[55] The greater the number of these factors, the higher the risk of a recurrent attack.

These studies confirm the value of obtaining a medical history as part of the preemployment program. Snook, Campanelli, and Hart found that simply obtaining a medical history for prior back pain was not enough to reduce back injury rates.[77] They advocated a more comprehensive approach (including workplace changes and personnel training). Battié et al. performed a prospective study of 3,020 U.S. aircraft manufacturing workers over a four-year period.[4,5,6,7,8] Among many factors studied (some of which are discussed later in this chapter) previous back pain was one of the few associated with increased risk of future back pain reports.

Several problems arise from using a previous back pain history as a risk indicator. First, the applicant for a job may simply elect to give a dishonest answer. Second, the prevalence of back pain is so high that too many older workers would be refused employment, and in a young population the majority of future cases would still not be identified. Himmelstein and Andersson calculated the sensitivity of using previous low back pain as a screening tool for work applicants at age 30.[41] They assumed an age-related prevalence increase, a lifetime incidence of 75%, and that all those with previous back pain would have recurrences. Of 1,000 workers screened at age 30, 188 would be denied employment because of prior back pain, and 438 of 585 future back cases would not be identified. The sensitivity in this example is 0.25. A third problem is the difference in response that can result from the way the question about previous back pain is asked. A single question about previous back pain, in our opinion, is useless unless qualified by further questions about the nature of the pain, previous absence from work, the site of previous pain, and so on. It is important, then, to exclude from "previous back pain" aches arising on some occasion after unaccustomed work. It is also important to differentiate between the temporal patterns of pain experience, that is, isolated, periodic, or chronic, and then determine severity and location.[16]

Combining a history of previous back pain with other tests may be a way of increasing the predictive value. Indeed, Troup et al.[84] found this to be the case when the predictive value of a psychophysical test program was evaluated. The limitations discussed above would still apply.

Clinical Physical Examination

The purpose of the physical examination in screening is to detect signs of clinical dysfunction indicative of a risk of future problems. Where there is evidence of ongoing back pain, neoplastic lesions, spondylolisthesis, or severe postural deformities, more extensive medical investigations are indicated. General observation of posture, ranges of motion, and similar tests do not seem to be reliable prognosticators, as discussed in Chapter 8. Age and sex have some direct influence on susceptibility to LBP; the risk of LBP increases with increasing age and differs between women and men. The individual variability is so great within age and gender groups, however, that to deny a person employment based solely on age or sex would be insupportable and, at least in the United States, illegal.

Anthropometric data and measurements of the range of motion of the spine are easily obtained at the clinical examination but are often of limited value to the selection procedure without reliable data on the layout of the workplace. In retrospective surveys of possible risk factors for back pain, height, weight, and different indices based on those measures have sometimes been found to be associated with back pain and sometimes not. Gyntelberg found that tall men had a somewhat higher risk of future back pain and that the risk was also greater in the highest and lowest weight groups.[36] Biering-Sørensen, on the other hand, found weight and height to be of no predictive value.[10] In a prospective study of 3,020 aircraft manufacturing workers, Battié et al., found a small association between future back pain reports and greater standing height in men and greater weight and body mass index in women.[6] These associations were present, however, only among subjects who had a previous history of low back pain, which suggests interaction.

It should be obvious from the preceding chapters that the worker must be matched to the work task according to reach and space requirements. If a specific reach requirement is documented for a particular job, it is necessary to evaluate the applicant's capability in that respect. The job requirement also should be adjusted to the subject's range of motion. The worker should not have to stretch or bend even close to the normal limits of motion. A lack of mobility at one joint can cause comparatively greater stresses on another joint; for example, limited ranges of motion of the hips and knee can require more motion of the spine. Also, a rigid joint is less well adapted to absorb shock. It is well known that joint motion is impaired following injury. Biering-Sørensen found that reduced spine motion in subjects with previous LBP indicated an increased risk of a future pain episode.[10] In contrast, previously healthy subjects with less spine mobility had a decreased risk for future LBP. Though Troup et al. found loss of lumbar extension to be a comparatively poor predictor of future back pain, a significant decrease in sagittal flexibility was found in subjects with ongoing pain.[84] Battié et al. found no association between either great or limited flexibility and subsequent back pain.[8]

Other physical findings may be of predictive value. Lloyd and Troup found five physical signs to be of significant predictive value in patients returning to work after a back pain episode.[55] These were restriction of the pain-free range of straight leg raising (SLR); reproduction of pain caused by SLR; inability to sit up from the supine position (trunk flexor weakness); pain or weakness on resisted hip flexion tests with the patient sitting; and back pain on lumbar extension induced by passive flexion of the knees with the patient in the prone position. When more than one of these signs were present, the risk of recurrence increased further. Although Lloyd and Troup's data cannot be directly transferred to a general population, the data may have a role in secondary prevention and reassigning workers. Nonetheless, the tests were positive in 25% of those seen after spells of back pain.

Battié et al. found no predictive value in any of several clinical tests in subjects with no previous history of LBP.[6] In subjects who had had LBP in the past, positive straight leg raising (SLR) was found to be a significant predictor of future back pain. Very few of the subjects included in that study actually had previous LBP and positive SLR, and of those only one-fifth developed LBP, making the usefulness of this test questionable.

General Fitness

Individuals in a good state of general fitness have a low risk of chronic LBP and recover more rapidly after LBP. Cady et al. measured the flexibility, isometric lifting strength, and cardiopulmonary function in 1,652 fire fighters in Los Angeles from 1971 to 1974.[17,18] The fire fighters were divided into three groups. The most fit had the least back pain but the most severe injuries. Although these results are not sufficiently conclusive to permit exclusion of workers with poor physical fitness, these data should stimulate workers to upgrade their physical status for other than back-related reasons. This topic is important in the design of back schools, as discussed in Chapter 15. Svensson and Andersson[80] found LBP to be more common in men who were physically less active in their leisure time,[80] but Videman et al. found it untrue for nurses.[88] This relative inactivity could, of course, be the result of existent back problems as well as a factor in their persistence.

In their prospective study at the Boeing Company Battié et al. did not find cardiovascular fitness (as measured by maximum oxygen uptake [VO_2 max]) to be predictive of future back pain reports.[7] In another study flexibility measures were also found to be poor predictors of future back pain.[8] Although fitness has many positive effects, therefore, it may also have to be related to job requirements to be of any value as a screening procedure.

Radiographic Screening

The use of preemployment radiographic assessments of the lumbar spine is widespread. Of the many papers published on this controversial topic, a few are presented here for the purpose of further discussion. For reviews of the literature see Montgomery,[62] Troup and Edwards,[83] and Himmelstein and Andersson.[41] As with any preemployment screening procedure, predictive and safety factors must be considered.

Safety Aspects: A single lumbosacral x-ray probably does not carry a significant health risk. Repeated radiographs, however, can result in considerable irradiation of the gonads and the bone marrow. The addition of oblique x-rays to the standard anterioposterior (AP) more than doubles this exposure. Low back x-rays are the largest single contributor to gonadal irradiation in the United States.[69] Gonadal shielding is clearly possible in males but impractical in females. In women with unsuspected pregnancy these x-rays also carry significant risk for irradiation of the fetus, which can double the risk of subsequent childhood leukemia. Therefore, low back x-rays should always be considered a potential health risk, and any unnecessary use should be discouraged.

The Predictive Value of Low Back Radiographs: No prospective, well-controlled, longitudinal study exists now. Most investigations on the subject have used one of two approaches: searching for an increased prevalence of radiographic abnormalities in patients who have developed back pain (a case-control study) or searching for decreased incidence of LBP after an x-ray screening program has been implemented.

The first method requires a control group without LBP. In the past, either a control group has been selected for that purpose or a general population sample has been divided into groups with and without LBP and these two groups compared. Examples of studies in which control groups have been selected are those by Splithoff,[78] Horal,[43] Torgerson and Dotter,[82] Fischer, Friedman, and van Demark,[29] and LaRocca and Macnab.[50] Examples of population studies are those by Bistrom;[12] Hult;[45] Lawrence;[51,52] Connell;[26] Hirsch, Johnsson, and Lewin;[42] Rowe;[70,71,72] Magora and Schwartz;[57,58,59] Wiikeri et al;[88] and Frymoyer et al.[31] The difficulty of obtaining adequate control populations is obvious from most of these studies.

The second approach has been to measure incidence of LBP after preemployment x-rays. Unfortunately, all the published studies have used other screening techniques as well, and it is difficult to assess the value of x-rays per se. Examples of studies using this approach are those by Kelly;[46] McGill;[61] Leggo and Mathiasen;[54] Redfield;[67] Kosiak, Aurelius, and Hartfiel;[48] and Crookshank and Warshaw.[27]

Based on these studies, it is clear that so-called radiographic abnormalities are quite frequent and do not always indicate morbidity. Common x-ray findings and their relationship to LBP are discussed in Chapter 8. Tumors, fractures, and infectious and inflammatory diseases clearly were related to present or previous LBP. Spondylolisthesis and osteoporosis occur frequently in patients with no LBP.

Another study design was used by Gibson et al.,[4] who compared two retrospective cohorts (of steelworkers): one hired before and one after back x-rays were introduced into an otherwise identical preplacement medical program. The inclusion of low back x-ray screening did not significantly influence the subsequent incidence of LBP in this carefully conducted retrospective study.

Other studies have provided additional information useful to determine the value of preemployment radiographs. Unsuspected findings are rare,[15,73,75] and diagnosis and treatment are minimally affected by the findings.[69] The frequency of abnormal radiographic findings in the population is very high, making the use of radiographs for screening purposes of doubtful value.[30,37]

Low back x-rays therefore have low sensitivity and low specificity and, consequently, also low predictive value. Rockey, Fantel, and Omenn[68] have made some interesting calculations on a hypothetical cohort of workers that clearly show how misclassification can occur for this reason and the effects of those miscalculations.

Consensus on Preemployment Back X-rays: The enthusiastic endorsements of the preemployment screening radiograph in its early days have changed gradually over the years. In a review article Montgomery[62] questioned the evidence and advised against the use of preemployment back x-rays for determining future risk. LaRocca and Macnab,[50] Houston,[44] Hadler,[37] Gibson,[33] and Rockey, Fantel, and Omenn[68] came to a similar conclusion. In 1973, the American College of Radiology, the American Academy of Orthopaedic Surgeons, and the American Occupational Medical Association jointly concluded that the use of x-rays as the sole criterion for selection of workers was not justified and that more concern was needed to protect workers from unnecessary radiation in such examinations.[1]

The negative stand of those who consider routine preemployment radiography unjustified is epidemiologically defensible. The question is when radiography may be justifiable, and the criteria for this decision are clinical. If the nature of back pain or the medical history suggests some underlying disease other than a simple mechanical derangement in the lumbar spine, then x-rays must be done as a matter of course.

One factor has been suggested as having a theoretical predictive value: the space available for the cauda equina and nerve roots in the lumbar spinal canal and neural foramina. Narrowness has been associated with the severity of disc prolapse and of back symptoms both ultrasonographically[65,56] and radiographically,[40,87] but no prospective studies have been made. Ultrasonic scans can be made only in one plane. This is a disadvantage, considering that the various parameters of narrowness are independent, as this is only partly discounted by the absence of radiation risk.

Failure Strength

Brinckmann et al.[13,14] predicted the compressive strength of vertebrae from scanners of bone density and cross-sectional area. At present their method employs CT scans, but similar data have become obtainable from MRI imaging. Should this become reality it may be possible to adopt compressive vertebral strength as a screening test.

Laboratory Screening Procedures

There are no direct laboratory screening tests for LBP. Clinical interest, however, has been generated by the statistically significant association found between ankylosing spondylitis and a histocompatibility complex antigen HLA B-27. Although the sensitivity of the test is high (95%), the specificity is low,[19] making its use as a screening procedure of little value.[74]

Strength Testing

The use of preemployment strength testing to reduce the incidence and severity of musculoskeletal problems has been met with considerable enthusiasm over the past decade. The obvious goal is to ensure that only people with sufficient strength to perform a job safely are assigned to that job. It is clear from previous studies that strength varies enormously among people. Many jobs in industry do indeed require exertions that approach the maximal strength of individual workers. It is beyond the scope of this chapter to review the various muscle-strength evaluation methods and equipment. The reader is referred to Chaffin;[20,21] Kroemer;[49] Garg, Mital, and Asfour;[32] Stobbe;[79] and Chaffin and Andersson.[22] Static (isometric) strength-testing methods are available,[24,25,47,79] whereas dynamic strength tests have yet be further developed.[66] The problem with static strength tests is that most exertions are dynamic. Commercially, a number of alternative systems of dynamic strength testing are being marketed. They add isokinetic, isodynamic, or isotonic testing to the static mode. The newcomers may be of value and in some cases may allow closer simulation of the actual job requirements. So far, though, no prospective epidemiologic studies have been reported. The difficulty with all three testing modes for maximal strength—isometric, isokinetic, and isotonic—is that none are quite physiologic, and this may account for the associated morbidity. Submaximal levels of isometric activity are, of course, commonplace, but constant velocity and constant tension are not normal features of manual work. Tests of maximal dynamic strength have been reported only in a military setting for obvious reasons of safety.

The solution appears to lie with submaximal dynamic strength testing using the psychophysical approaches proposed by Snook,[76] Ayoub et al.,[3] and Troup et al.[84] The potential value of this approach lies partly in its safety but also in that it lends itself readily to job simulation.

Safety: Various types of physical strength and endurance tests must be carefully evaluated to ensure that they are safe. Previous history of musculoskeletal problems or cardiovascular problems may contraindicate testing of a specific person or at least require a modified test procedure. Some morbidity, though minor, can be expected from maximal isometric strength tests.[38]

Predictive Value: Some epidemiologic support exists for strength testing as a useful means of reducing back injury rates. Chaffin and Park[23] found a sharp increase in the low back injury rates in subjects performing jobs requiring strength that was greater or equal to their isometric strength-test values. In fact, the risk was three times higher for the weaker subjects. A second longitudinal study was performed by Chaffin et al. to make further determinations about the value of strength testing, and again the back injury incidence rate was found to be almost three times higher in the overstressed group.[24] In a later paper, Chaffin, Herrin, and Keyserling suggested that specific placement and selection programs should be undertaken by industry based on strength performance criteria.[25]

Another study by this group involved the application of strength tests and a simultaneous biomechanical job analysis in the rubber industry.[47] Subjects were strength tested, and jobs were biomechanically classified. The subjects were then assigned to jobs in such a way that some were overstressed and others were understressed. The medical records were followed for one year to determine musculoskeletal problems over that period. Although the follow-up interval was short, job matching based on strength criteria appeared to be beneficial.

Although none of these studies allows absolute predictive values to be computed for strength testing, there appears to be some beneficial value. In a prospective study Troup, Martin, and Lloyd found reduced dynamic strength of back flexor muscles to be a consistent predictor for recurrence or persistence of back pain, but it was not true for first attacks.[85]

Battié et al. tested 2,178 workers for static strength in standard lifting postures.[5] The workers were then followed over a three-year period. When considered alone, greater strength was associated with a higher risk of back claims, but when controlled for age, strength did not correlate to either increased or decreased risk of low back pain. While this study, on the surface, would seem to argue that strength is not a risk factor, a closer look reveals that the workers' lifting strengths were not related to their job demands. A mismatch between strength and job demands can be a risk factor, as suggested by the studies discussed above. Clearly the study suggests that a standardized preemployment strength-testing protocol is not successful in reducing back claims, emphasizing the need for prior workplace analysis and appropriate design of the test protocol.

Practicality: Because static strength testing requires equipment specific to a given work situation and familiarity with strength-test procedures, strength testing may not always be practical. Chaffin[20] has suggested the following three general guidelines for equipment and procedure: hardware capable of simulation of a variety of work situations, minimal administration time, and minimal time of instruction and learning. In addition, the workplace must be carefully analyzed so that the strength test can truly assess the strength capabilities that are important in a given job.

SUMMARY

The most important part of the screening medical history is the identification of previous back problems. General observations of posture and range of motion are not useful prognosticators of future LBP, but they may help to match the worker to the job. Workers should not be excluded from work on the basis of poor fitness, but physical fitness should be encouraged. Preemployment radiographs are not justified unless the clinical signs suggest possible disease.

Strength testing is in its infancy, and there is little consensus based on experience and predictive value. It appears that strength testing can be preventive, provided the testing procedure is specific to the job being sought by the worker. It remains unclear whether a well-matched worker will develop a problem from a heavy physical job should the exposure period be extended beyond one year. Muscle strength and tissue resistance to future stress may not be direcly related. In general, a worker should have at least the demonstrable strength required to perform a job prior to having to perform the job. It is at least as important to eliminate postural stress at work, including the postural stress in sedentary work.

BIBLIOGRAPHY

1. American College of Radiology: Proceedings of Conference on Low-Back X-Rays in Pre-Employment Physical Examinations, Tucson, January 11–14, 1973.
2. Andersson GBJ, Svensson HO, Oden O: The intensity of work recovery in low back pain. *Spine* 1983; 8:880–884.
3. Ayoub MM, Mital A, Bakken GM, et al: Development of strength and capacity norms for manual materials handling activities. The state of the art. *Human Factors* 1980; 22:271–283.
4. Battié MC, Bigos SJ, Sheehy A, et al: Spinal flexibility and individual factors that influence it. *Physical Therapy* 1987; 67:653–657.
5. Battié MC, Bigos SJ, Fisher LD, et al: Isometric lifting strength as a predictor of industrial back pain. *Spine* 1990; in press.
6. Battié MC, Bigos SJ, Fisher LD, et al: Anthropometric and clinical measurements as predictors of industrial back pain complaints: A prospective study. *J Spinal Disorders* 1990, in press.
7. Battié MC, Bigos SJ, Fisher LD, et al: A prospective study of the role of cardiovascular risk factors and fitness in industrial back pain complaints. *Spine* 1989b; 14:141–147.
8. Battié MC, Bigos SJ, Fisher LD, et al: The role of spinal flexibility in back pain complaints within industry. A prospective study. *Spine* 14:851–856.
9. Bergquist-Ullman M, Larsson U: Acute low back pain in industry. A controlled prospective study with special reference to therapy and confounding factors. *Acta Orthop Scand [Suppl]* 1977; 170:117.
10. Biering-Sørensen F: *The Prognostic Value of the Low Back History and Physical Measurements* (thesis). Copenhagen, University of Copenhagen, 1983.
11. Biering-Sørensen F, Thomsen CE, Hilden J: Risk indicators for low back trouble. *Scand J Rehab Med* 1989; 21:151–157.
12. Bistrom, O: Need degenerative changes in the spinal column entail back pain? *Ann Chir Gynaec Fenn* 1954; 43:29–44.
13. Brinckmann P, Johannleweling N, Hilweg D, et al: Fatigue fracture of human lumbar vertebrae. *Clin Biomech* 1987; 2:94–96.
14. Brinckman P, Biggeman M, Hilweg D: Fatigue fracture of human lumbar vertebrae. *Clin Biomech [Suppl]* 1988; 3:1–37.
15. Brolin I: Produktkontroll av röntgenundersökningar av landryggraden. *Läkartidningen* 1975; 72:1793–1795.
16. Burton AK, Tillotson KM, Troup JDG: Prediction of low-back trouble frequency in a working population. *Spine* 1989; 14:939–946.
17. Cady LD, Bischoff DP, O'Connell ER, et al: Strength and fitness and subsequent back injuries in fire-fighters. *J Occup Med* 1979; 21:269–272.

18. Cady L, Thomas P, Karwashy R: Program for increasing the health and physical fitness of firefighters. *J Occup Med* 1985; 27:111–114.

19. Calin A, Kay B, Sternberg M, et al: The prevalence and nature of back pain in an industrial complex: Questionnaire and radiographic and HLA analysis. *Spine* 1980; 5:201–205.

20. Chaffin DB: Functional assessment for heavy physical labor, in Alderman MH, Hanley MJ (eds): *Clinical Medicine for the Occupational Physician.* New York, Marcel Dekker, 1982.

21. Chaffin DB: Ergonomics guide for the assessment of human static strength. *Am Indus Hyg Assoc J* 1975; 36:505–511.

22. Chaffin DB, Andersson GBJ: *Occupational Biomechanics,* ed 2. New York, Wiley, 1990.

23. Chaffin DB, Park KYS: A longitudinal study of low-back pain as associated with occupational weight lifting factors. *Am Indus Hyg Assoc J* 1973; 34:513–525.

24. Chaffin DB, Herrin GD, Keyserling WM, et al: *Pre-employment Strength Testing in Selecting Workers for Materials Handling Jobs.* Technical Report No CDC-99-74-62, NIOSH Physiology and Ergonomics Branch, Cincinnati, Ohio, 1977.

25. Chaffin DB, Herrin GD, Keyserling WM: *Preemployment strength testing. An updated position. J Occup Med* 1978; 20:403–408.

26. Connell MA: Bony anomalies of the low back in relation to back injury. *Southern Med J* 1968; 61:482–486.

27. Crookshank JW, Warshaw LM: The lumbar spine in the workman. *Southern Med J* 1961; 54:636–638.

28. Dillane JB, Fry J, Kalton G: Acute back syndrome—A study from general practice. *Brit Med J* 1966; 2:82–84.

29. Fischer FJ, Friedman MM, van Demark RE: Roentgenographic abnormalities in soldiers with low back pain. A comparative study. *Amer J Roentgen* 1958; 79:673–676.

30. Foote GA: Pre-employment radiography of the lumbosacral spine. Radiology in health screening. *Australas Radiol* 1982; 26:25–29.

31. Frymoyer JW, Newberg A, Pope MH, et al: The relationship between spinal radiographs and LBP severity in males 18–55. *J Bone Joint Surg* 1984; 66a:1048–1055.

32. Garg A, Mital A, Asfour SS: A comparison of isometric strength and dynamic lifting capability. *Ergonomics* 1980; 23:13–27.

33. Gibson ES: The value of preplacement screening radiography of the low back. *Occup Med: State of the Art Reviews* 1988; 3:91–107.

34. Gibson ES, Martin RH, Terry CW: Incidence of low back pain and pre-employment X-ray screening. *J Occup Med* 1980; 22:515–519.

35. Glover JR: Prevention of back pain, in Jayson M (ed): *The Lumbar Spine and Back Pain,* ed 2. Tunbridge Wells, England, Pitman Medical, 1980.

36. Gyntelberg F: One year incidence of low back pain among male residents of Copenhagen aged 40–59. *Dan Med Bull* 1974; 21:30–36.

37. Hadler NM: Legal ramifications of the medical definition of back disease. *Ann Intern Med* 1978; 89:992–999.

38. Hansson TH, Bigos SJ, Worley MK, et al: The load on the lumbar spine during isometric strength testing. *Spine* 1985; 9:720–724.

39. Hansson T, Sandström J, Roos B, et al: The bone mineral content of the lumbar spine in patients with chronic low back pain. *Spine* 1985; 10:158–160.

40. Heliovaara M: Body height, obesity, and risk of herniated lumbar intervertebral disc. *Spine* 1987; 12:469–472.

41. Himmelstein JS, Andersson GBJ: Low back pain: Risk evaluation and preplacement screening. *Occup Med: State of the Art Review* 1988; 3:255–269.

42. Hirsch C, Jonsson B, Lewin T: Low back symptoms in a Swedish female population. *Clin Orthop* 1969; 63:171–176.

43. Horal J: The clinical appearance of low back disorders in the city of Gothenburg, Sweden. Comparisons of incapacitated probands with matched controls. *Acta Orthop Scand [Suppl]* 1969; 118:1–109.

44. Houston CS: Pre-employment radiographs of lumbar spine, editorial. *J Canad Assoc Radiol* 1977; 28:170.
45. Hult L: Cervical, dorsal, and lumbar spinal syndromes. *Acta Orthop Scand [Suppl]* 1954; 17:1–102.
46. Kelly FJ: Pre-employment medical examinations including back x-rays. *J Occup Med* 1965; 7:132–136.
47. Keyserling WM, Herrin GD, Chaffin DB: Isometric strength testing as a means of controlling medical incidents on strenuous jobs. *J Occup Med* 1980; 22:332–336.
48. Kosiak M, Aurelius JR, Hartfiel WF: Backache in industry. *J Occup Med* 1966; 8:51–58.
49. Kroemer KHE: Human strength. Terminology, measurement and interpretation of data. *Human Factors* 1970; 12:297–313.
50. LaRocca H, Macnab I: Value of pre-employment radiographic assessment of the lumbar spine. *Can Med Assoc J* 1969; 101:383–388.
51. Lawrence JS: Rheumatism in coal miners; occupational factors. *Brit J Indus Med* 1955; 12:249–261.
52. _____: Disk degeneration. Its frequency and relationship to symptoms. *Ann Rheum Dis* 1969; 28:121–138.
53. Leavitt SS, Johnston TL, Beyer RD: The process of recovery: Patterns in industrial back injury. Part 1. Costs and other quantitative measures of effort. *Ind Med Surg* 1971; 40:7–14.
54. Leggo C, Mathiasen H: Preliminary results of a preemployment back x-ray program for state traffic officers. *J Occup Med* 1973; 15:973–974.
55. Lloyd DCEF, Troup JDG: Recurrent back pain and its prediction. *J Soc Occup Med* 1983; 33:66–74.
56. MacDonald EB, Porter R, Hibbert C, et al: The relationship between spinal canal diameter and back pain in coal miners. Ultrasonic measurement as a screening test? *J Occup Med* 1984; 26:23–28.
57. Magora A, Schwartz A: Relation between the low back pain syndrome and x-ray findings. 1. Degenerative osteoarthritis. *Scand J Rehabil Med* 1976; 8:115–125.
58. Magora A, Schwartz A: Relation between the low back pain syndrome and x-ray findings. 2. Transitional vertebrae (mainly sacralization). *Scand J Rehabil Med* 1978; 10:135–145.
59. Magora A, Schwartz A: Relation between low back pain and X-ray changes. 4. Lysis and olisthesis. *Scand J Rehabil Med* 1980; 12:47–52.
60. Magora A, Taustein I: An investigation of the problem of sick-leave in the patient suffering from low back pain. *Indus Med Surg* 1969; 38:398–408.
61. McGill CM: Industrial back problems. A control program. *J Occup Med* 1968; 10:174–178.
62. Montgomery CH: Preemployment back x-rays. *J Occup Med* 1976; 18:495–498.
63. Nordgren B, Schele R, Linroth K: Evaluation and prediction of back pain during military field service. *Scand J Rehab Med* 1980; 12:1–8.
64. Pedersen PA: Prognostic indicators in low back pain. *J Royal Coll Gen Pract* 1981; 31:209–216.
65. Porter R, Hibbert C, Wellman P: Backache and the lumbar spinal canal. *Spine* 1980; 5:99–105.
66. Pytel JL, Kamon E: Dynamic strength test as a predictor for maximal and acceptable lifting. *Ergonomics* 1981; 24:663–672.
67. Redfield JT: The low back x-ray as a pre-employment screening tool in the forest products industry. *J Occup Med* 1971; 13:219–226.
68. Rockey PH, Fantel J, Omenn GS: Discriminatory aspects of pre-employment screening: Low back x-ray examinations in the railroad industry. *Am J Law and Med* 1979; 5:197–214.
69. Rockey PH, Tompkins RK, Wood RW, et al: The usefulness of x-ray examinations in the evaluation of patients with back pain. *J Fam Pract* 1978; 7:455–465.
70. Rowe ML: Preliminary statistical study of low back pain. *J Occup Med* 1963; 5:336–341.

71. _____: Disc surgery and chronic low back pain. *J Occup Med* 1965; 7:196–202.

72. _____: Low back pain in industry. A position paper. *J Occup Med* 1969; 11:161–169.

73. Runge CF: Pre-existing structural defects and severity of compensation back injuries. *Indus Med Surg* 1958; 27:249–252.

74. Sandström J, Andersson GBJ: HLA-B27 as a diagnostic screening tool in chronic low back pain. *Scand J Rehab Med* 1984; 16:27–28.

75. Scavone JG, Latshaw RF, Weidner WA: Anteroposterior and lateral radiographs: An adequate lumbar spine examination. *AJR* 1981; 136:715–717.

76. Snook SH: The design of manual handling tasks. *Ergonomics* 1978; 21:963–985.

77. Snook SH, Campanelli RA, Hart JW: A study of three preventive approaches to low back injury. *J Occup Med* 1978; 20:478–481.

78. Splithoff CA: Lumbosacral junction. Roentgenographic comparison of patients with and without backaches. *JAMA* 1953; 152:1610.

79. Stobbe T: Strength Testing. (Industr. Eng.) Ann Arbor, Univ Michigan, 1982.

80. Svensson H-O, Andersson GBJ: Low back pain in forty to forty-seven year old men: Work history and work environment factors. *Spine* 1983; 8:272–276.

81. Taylor PJ: Personal factors associated with sickness absence. A study of 194 men with contrasting sickness absence experience in a refinery population. *Brit J Indus Med* 1968; 25:106–118.

82. Torgerson WR, Dotter WE: Comparative roentgenographic study of the asymptomatic and symptomatic lumbar spine. *J Bone Joint Surg* 1976; 58:850–853.

83. Troup JDG, Edwards FC: *Manual Handling: A Review Paper.* London, Her Majesty's Stationery Office Health and Safety Executive, 1985.

84. Troup JDG, Foreman TK, Baxter CE, et al: The perception of back pain and the role of psychophysical tests of lifting capacity. *Spine* 1987; 12:645–657.

85. Troup JDG, Martin JW, Lloyd DCEF: Back pain in industry. A prospective survey. *Spine* 1981; 6:61–69.

86. Troup JDG, Videman T: Inactivity and the aetiopathogenesis of musculoskeletel disorders. *Clin Biomech* 1989; 4:173–178.

87. Vanharanta H, Korpi J, Heliovaara M, et al: Radiographic measurements of lumbar spinal canal size and their relation to back mobility. *Spine* 1985; 10:461–466.

88. Videman T, Nuriminen T, Tola S: Low back pain in nurses and some loading factors of work. *Spine* 1984; 9:400–404.

89. Wiikeri M, Nummi J, Riihimäki H, et al: Radiologically detectable lumbar disc degeneration in concrete reinforcement workers. *Scand J Work Environ Health* 1978; 4 [Suppl 1]:47–53.

14

Workplace Design

Don B. Chaffin, Ph.D.
Malcolm H. Pope, Dir. Med. Sc., Ph.D.
Gunnar B.J. Andersson, M.D., Ph.D.

INTRODUCTION

Approximately one-third of the workforce in the United States is required to exert nearly their maximum strength in the daily performance of their jobs.[14] This illustrates that gross manual activities, even if only infrequently performed in a job, are still required of a large number of people, placing them at high risk of incurring low back pain (LBP).[5,8] It has also been shown that LBP is often caused by slipping, tripping, and falling,[16] which emphasizes the need for greater care in the design and specification of floors and shoes. Growing evidence has accumulated to indicate that prolonged sitting without appropriate low back support or while subjected to vibration increases the risk of LBP.[9]

This chapter emphasizes the role of workplace design in the prevention of low back pain in industry. As discussed in Chapters 2 and 12, the magnitude of the loads handled, the postures assumed in material handling, and the frequency of strenuous exertions combine in a complex fashion to increase the risk of LBP. Designing seated work to reduce low back stresses and exposure to vibration is also presented.

One method of preventing LBP is to design the workplace in a manner that minimizes conditions believed to increase the mechanical stresses on low back tissues beyond their physiologic limits. Although the precise relationship between a specific set of work conditions and relevant tissue injury limits are not available at this time, the simple biomechanical models and epidemiologic data discussed earlier provide the basis for some general workplace design guidelines.

To design a workplace so that stresses on the low back are minimized, the following factors must be controlled: posture, external load (material and tools), movements, and vibration. Each of these is discussed in the chapter, but the reader is also referred to Chapter 2, which covers the occupational biomechanics of the spine.

POSTURE

Practical Considerations in Seat Design

Because there are many different opinions and user requirements, chairs vary widely. Compare, for example, the driver's seat in an automobile with an office chair or a work chair in a factory. Regardless of use, it is important to be able to adjust any chair to meet the basic anthropometric dimensions of its user. Different recommendations have been published for various populations. This is not surprising, since anthropometric dimensions vary greatly between populations of different countries. Rather than provide a list of all these data, we explain why different dimensions are critical, with the main emphasis on the specifications of office and industrial chairs.[4,11,12]

Some important office chair dimensions are shown in Figure 14.1a. Seat height should be adjustable for the individual user. The seat surface should be 1.2 to 2 inches (3–5 cm) below the knee fold when the lower limb is vertical. Foot supports can be used with higher than normal chairs. The width of the seat should be sufficient to accommodate the user population. The edges of the seat should not be detectable during ordinary sitting work.

The depth of the seat is also important. For the backrest to provide any benefit the seat must not be too deep. Pressure should be avoided on the back of the thigh near the knees. A free area between the back of the lower limb and the seat is also useful to facilitate arising and moving the legs. About 4 inches (10 cm) is suggested as the minimum clearance. The front part of the seat should be contoured. In some cases a forward slope is advantageous in reducing the load on the spine. This is particularly important for semisitting postures in raised chairs, which are not infrequent in industry. It can also be useful for performing desk work. More often, a backward slope of about 5° is suggested for normal sitting posture. This slope facilitates the use of the backrest and prevents sliding on the seat surface as the user moves around in the chair. Sliding can also be prevented by the choice of seat contour and seat cover materials with high surface friction. A proper choice of seat cover materials is important for climatic comfort (i.e., they should breathe in hot environments) and in the industrial setting where specific materials may be necessary (e.g., to avoid static electricity).

For the backrest the following dimensions are important: (1) top height, (2) bottom height, (3) center height, (4) total height, (5) width, (6) horizontal radius, and (7) vertical radius (Fig. 14.1b). Other factors are (8) pivoting and reclining possibility, (9) softness, (10) adjustability, and (11) climatic comfort. The choice of height of backrest depends on the use of the chair. A high backrest supporting the whole spine is always the choice in cars and trucks, where the backrest is typically reclined to 110 degrees or more. There is also evidence that this is the choice of operators of VDT terminals.[6,7] In other situations a high backrest may restrict movements. A lower (lumbar support) is always preferred. The backrest should be adjustable in both horizontal and vertical directions. It should support the lumbar spine without restricting movements of the spine and arms. The width should support the back completely without arm interference. The shape should be convex to the normal lumbar lordosis and concave from side to side to conform to human anatomy and support the occupant in the chair. A spring-loaded pivoting action can allow the backrest to follow natural body movements while maintaining body support, but it can be impractical in jobs that demand great precision. Most pivoting backrests offer support at different locations on the lumbar spine as a function of backrest angle; that is, the single pivot cannot follow the complexity of motion in flexion-extension. When reclining is permitted, a control system must be used so that there is firm support when the backrest is in the reclined position. Intervertebral disc loads are reduced if the backrest is inclined at 110 degrees, and lumbar support is provided. Other postures can lead to high disc loads.

Another chair feature is the armrest. Design considerations for the armrest include (1) length, (2) width, (3) height, (4) width between armrests, and (5) distance from armrest front to seat. In general, placement of the armrests is important to reduce pressure on the seat surface and load on the spine and shoulders and to facilitate rising from the chair. When armrests are too high the occupant must raise the shoulders and abduct the arms. This is also the case when the armrest-to-armrest width is too great. Too low an armrest, on the other

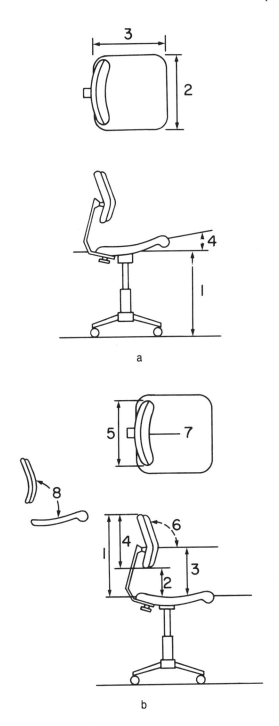

FIG 14.1.
(a) Seat dimensions: (1) seat height, (2) seat width (breadth), (3) seat length (depth), (4) seat slope. (b) Backrest dimensions: (1) backrest top height, (2) backrest bottom height, (3) backrest center height, (4) backrest height, (5) backrest width (breadth), (6) backrest horizontal radius, (7) backrest vertical radius, (8) backrest seat angle.

hand, does not permit use of the armrest unless the occupant slides forward or leans to one side to use it. The length and placement of an armrest should allow the chair to slide close enough to the table that the worker can sit erect using the backrest for support. Armrests may be impractical in such tasks as typing, where it is necessary to get very close to the desk.

Factors such as the number of feet on the chair, the base diameter, and the use of wheels or casters are necessary safety considerations. Five casters or feet are suggested, with a minimum radius of 12 inches (30 cm) to prevent tipping and a maximum horizontal radius of 15 inches (35 cm) to prevent tripping over the base of the chair.

The Table or Work Surface

To ensure that the worker does not have to bend unnecessarily or elevate the arms the work surface needs to be adjustable for two reasons. First, because factors such as the size of the workplace, motions demanded by work, and overall work layout vary, the height of the work surface cannot be the same for all types of activity. Second, the anthropometry of workers is variable, and therefore work surfaces must be adjustable to ensure proper individual fit. Some important work surface dimensions are (1) table bottom height, (2) table top height, and (3) table slope. The work surface also should be large enough to accommodate work objects without unnecessary clutter and have friction high enough to prevent objects from sliding. Too large a work surface, however, creates the problem of stretching and should be avoided. When controls are used they must be placed within an optimum work area in all planes.[9]

The work surface bottom height is critical to ensure sufficient leg room, particularly when sitting, while table-top height is important to ensure good posture and optimal reach conditions. Field of vision is of utmost importance, and table-top height should be chosen to prevent foward flexion of the neck and trunk. An eye focal distance ranging from 8 inches to 15 inches (20 to 40 cm) is common. The height of the table also should be related to the position of the elbow so as not to require abduction or elevation of arms and shoulder.[10] These requirements demand either an adjustable table or a high table and an adjustable footrest. Too low a table causes kyphosis of the lumbar spine, increasing the load. Too high a table, on the other hand, causes abduction of the arms and elevation of the shoulder as well as kyphosis of the neck and fatigue in the shoulder and neck muscles. Chaffin found a 15-degree angle at the neck acceptable.[2]

It is important to remember that the work-surface height is not always the table height. In using a typewriter, word processor, or computer, for example, it is the keyboard height that is important. Tilting the work surface toward the worker whenever possible is a good method of preventing unnecessary forward flexion of neck and back. In keyboarding, frequent rests prevent neck and back fatigue and reduce discomfort (Chapter 2).

MATERIAL HANDLING

Although several material-handling principles are reviewed in earlier chapters, other aspects of manual material handling related to the design of the workplace are discussed now.

General Manual Material Handling Considerations

If an object is large and heavy, a hoist or crane should usually be used to assist in its movement. If a hoist is used that is moved manually from one location to another, sufficient time or power assistance must be provided to the operator to avoid sudden jerking motions that can result in an uncontrolled swinging of the object being moved. It is not uncommon for hoist operators to suffer back injuries while attempting to stop an uncontrolled swing motion of an object supported by the hoist. It is also possible for an object to slip from the hoist or overload the hoist when swinging. For the latter reason, specific structural and safety specifications must be met if a hoist or crane is to be used. The reader is referred to American National Standard B30.2.0 and OSHA Regulation 1910.180.

Carts and manually powered trucks are also used to move heavy objects in the workplace. The risk of inducing low back pain by the use of such devices arises from two types of hazard. First, as in the use of a hoist, the overexertion hazard is associated with pushing or pulling on too heavy a load. The compressive forces on the L5–S1 disc become quite high, particularly when pulling a load.[13] To avoid this situation, it is important to ensure that the pushing or pulling hand force requirements are well below 50 pounds (225N) and that the hands are between hip and waist level when making a maximum exertion, thus minimizing the spinal load moments.

These requirements can be best satisfied in the design of a workplace by specifying a cart that (1) has vertical handles that can be grasped at varying heights, (2) has large rubber tires with good bearings that do not "hang up" on irregular surfaces, (3) has two wheels that easily pivot, and (4) is designed to handle the intended load. Furthermore, it is just as important to ensure that the floor surface be smooth, kept clean, and have a grade inclination of no greater than a few degrees. These concepts are illustrated in Figure 14.2.

The second hazard to the back when pushing or pulling carts comes from the increased risk of slipping during such activities. It is not uncommon for the required coefficient of friction (ratio of foot shear force divided by person's body weight) to exceed 1.0 during pushing and pulling activities. It is for this reason that the floor surface in areas on which pushing and pulling activities take place must be kept clean and dry and have high-traction surfaces, and that workers be instructed to use or be provided with high-traction shoes.

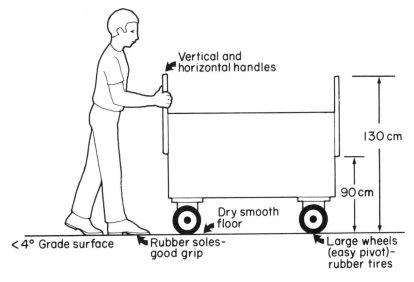

FIG 14.2.
Important specifications in a cart.

Container Design Considerations

The weight and dimensions of a load to be lifted are primary risk factors. In this context, *container dimensions* are important.

In general, if a container is designed to be compact, a worker can minimize the spinal load moment by keeping the object's center of mass close to the body. The effect of an object's center of gravity being lifted on spinal stress has been approximated in the NIOSH *Work Practices Guide to Manual Lifting*[14] (Fig. 14.3). The figure illustrates the necessity of having compact containers; the load moment arm H should be kept as small as possible.

The dimensions of a container are also important if a person must ascend or descend stairs while carrying the object. If the container is too large, it impairs vision, resulting in an increased risk of a trip or fall, as shown in Figure 14.4. In stair descent the hazard is even greater. In general, stair climbing in the workplace should never be done with large or heavy containers. As a general safety rule, one hand should always be able to grasp the stair handrail quickly to prevent a fall. This is especially important during descent. Carrying any containers on a stair seriously compromises this rule. Therefore, to move goods from one level to another, hoists, platforms, lifts, and elevators should be used.

If a container must be lifted from the floor and it is too large to pass between the knees, the person must lift the object in front of the knees. Such an action causes a larger spinal load moment than would result if the object could be lifted between the knees. (This concept is discussed in Chapter 2). Any object wider than about 12 inches (30 cm) cannot easily be lifted between the knees, and so the H distance is increased, as Figure 14.3 shows.

Container design must also include the means of firmly grasping it. This is important not only for lifting the container properly but also for avoiding sudden spinal inertial loads that

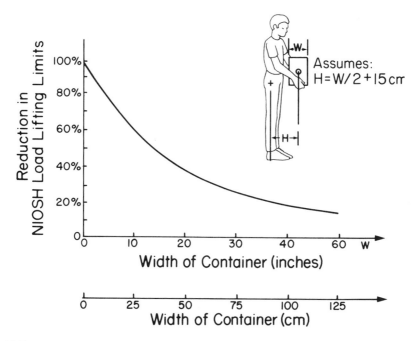

FIG 14.3.
Minimizing load moment H: The importance of compact containers.

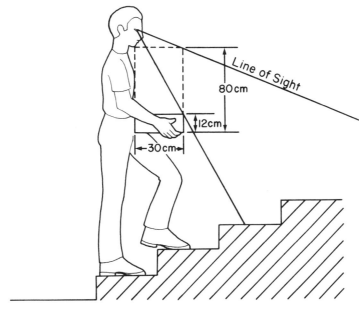

Maximum container size varies depending on task

FIG 14.4.
The importance of container size during negotiating of stairs.

occur when one attempts to regain control of an object slipping from the hands. In general, a forceful grasp of an object is provided by either a hook grip, whereby the fingers wrap around the object but without thumb opposition, or a power grip, in which the thumb assists in retention of the object by overlapping the fingers. The hook grip is used when grasping the bottom edge of a container and lifting. It is often adequate for moderate loads lifted for short periods, but it can entail excessive tension in finger flexor muscles as well as wrist flexor muscles and other upper extremity muscles to maintain the coupling between the hand and container.

If a proper handle is provided, a power grip can be used. This requires less upper extremity muscle action to maintain the coupling because the handle is fully secured between the fingers and the thumb. To provide such a handle requires consideration of hand anthropometry. Figure 14.5 illustrates the principal dimensions of concern. Finger depth clearance requires a minimum space of 1.2 inches (3.0 cm) for the bare hand of a large person. An additional 1.0 inch (2.5 cm) is suggested for cold-weather work gloves. Hand breadth minimum clearance of 5.0 inches (12.7 cm) is recommended for a larger person's bare hand. A heavy work glove could increase it by 1.0 inch (2.5 cm). The minimum radius of the handle to provide a low-pressure bearing surface for the fingers is about 0.75 inch (1.9 cm).

WORKSPACE DESIGN

One of the primary concerns when designing a workspace that will prevent low back disorders is to allow the worker to stand or sit erect while performing manual activities.

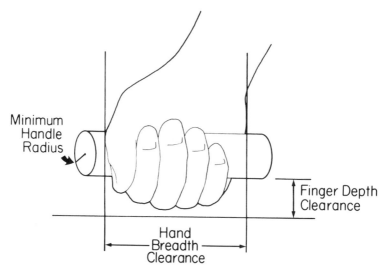

FIG 14.5.
Dimensions in handle design.

Workers should not have to reach beyond a comfortable arm reach in front and to the side of the body, especially if the manual activity required is lifting of heavy materials.

As discussed in the section on container design, the horizontal distance between the worker and the center of mass of an object being lifted (H) should be minimized. Obstructions over which a worker must lean to reach an object or place an object must be eliminated. If a heavy object is to be lifted, it should be located so that the worker can lift it without bending down or leaning forward. In practice, this may require the following:

1. Roller conveyors that allow objects to be pulled in toward the body before lifting (Fig. 14.6a) or powered conveyors to bring containers to the worker.
2. Gravity-fed slides (or shelves) that present items to the worker; such slides are used in airline baggage claim areas (Fig. 14.6b).
3. Machine designs that place the workpiece or part being manufactured close to the operator (Fig. 14.7).
4. Tilting of large stock bins to present parts closer to the operator (Figure 14.8).
5. Enough room for a worker to walk around large bins or pallets of parts to avoid having to reach and lean forward to remove parts from the opposite side.

It should also be remembered that when lifting loads above the shoulder, not only does fatigue in the shoulder and upper back muscles become important, but a person is more unstable because of the higher center of mass of the body and load combination. The NIOSH *Work Practices Guide for Manual Lifting* remedied this situation by including a vertical height factor in computing the load-lifting limits. The effect of this vertical correction is shown in Figure 14.9; it clearly indicates the disadvantages of lifting loads above shoulder height (the suggested limits are as much as 50% lower than if lifting loads at knuckle height).

It is also clear in Figure 14.9 that loads should not be lifted from below standing knuckle

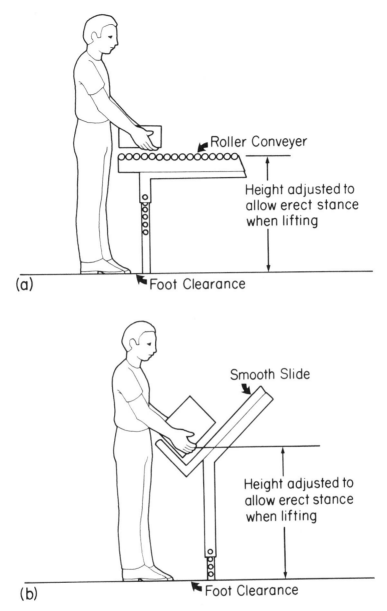

FIG 14.6.
Improvements of workplace design: (a) roller conveyors, (b) gravity-fed slide.

height: the lifting limits are 30% less for a lift from the floor than for a lift at knuckle height. To accommodate this requirement, use stock support tables that adjust vertically to allow the operator to maintain an erect trunk posture regardless of the remaining stock in a bin or on a pallet (Fig. 14.10). Another solution is the use of work benches and tables with adjustable height when a person is required to perform prolonged work on such surfaces. These are normally adjusted to about elbow height.

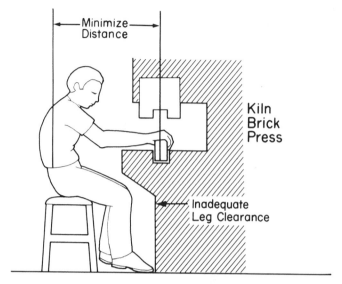

FIG 14.7.
Considerations in making task close to worker.

WHOLE-BODY VIBRATION

As discussed in Chapter 6, workers who drive vehicles are more likely to have LBP. Vibration is probably a major factor in the etiology, but postural stress, muscular effort, and shock and impact forces are also important. Many vehicles subject the driver to vibrations in the range of resonance of the spine and, due to cyclic muscle firing, muscle fatigue also

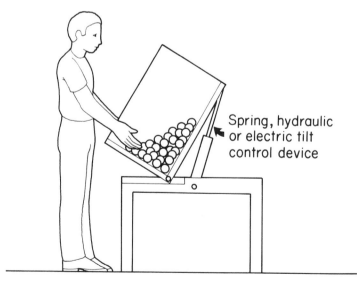

FIG 14.8.
Tilting of bins gets work close to worker.

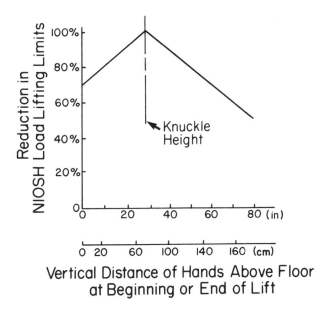

FIG 14.9.
The effect of vertical height in NIOSH load-lifting limits.

occurs in a vibrational environment. Recently, means have been sought to reduce these risks, including the use of postural supports, cushions, and vibration dampening devices.

One method of reducing whole-body vibration is to reduce the vibration input. This can be done by the appropriate choice of vehicle, by training operators to choose the terrain over which they drive, and by modifying operators' speed and style with the objective of reducing the magnitude of vibrations. Much of this is within the control of the operator.

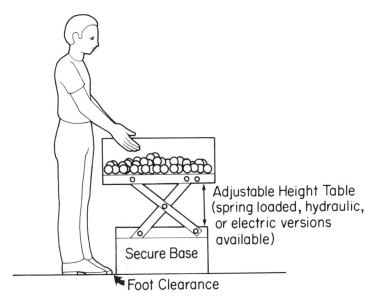

FIG 14.10.
The use of an adjustable height table.

Many of the principles presented in the context of static sitting are of equal importance in dynamic sitting. Andersson and Ortengren showed that disk load can be minimized in the seated subject if the backrest inclination is 110 degrees and there is additional level support at the third lumbar vertebra level.[1] There are other advantages in inclining the backrest at 110 degrees. If the trunk is upright or leaning forward when accelerated vertically, the head and shoulders bend further forward. This flexor torque adds to the net spinal stress. The psoas muscle activity is reduced, and on vertical acceleration the load is distributed over the backrest as well as the seat. Thus, an extension position is as favorable in vibration as it is in static situations. However, care must be taken to avoid the imposition of bending vibrations ("backslap") directly to the spine. Backslap can be reduced if the seat has a scissors mechanism rather than a forward-placed pivot.

Wilder et al. have shown that various postural supports can markedly affect the spine's vibrational response.[17] Lumbar, arm, and foot supports are helpful, and a contoured seat pan to minimize pelvic rocking was particularly promising.[15] Much of the vibrational response is due to the rocking of the pelvis, which can be minimized by a contoured seat.

To reduce vibrations to less harmful frequencies and to reduce vibration amplitude, soft cushions should be replaced with firm ones. The seat should be suspended and damped to give it a natural frequency of less than 1.5 Hz (Fig. 14.11). Suspension seats made to this specification are readily available commercially and do, in fact, reduce deleterious vertical vibrations. The marked isolation of a suspension seat as compared to a conventional seat is shown in Figure 14.12. The intensity of vibration from unsafe to safe levels is defined in the guide published by the International Standards Organization (ISO 2631). Figure 14.13 shows the ISO standard for horizontal vibration. Horizontal vibrations are extremely important in certain environments, such as trains, ships, and trams. (See also Chapter 6.) It is logical to attempt to reduce vibration levels to below the levels in ISO 2631.

The following guidelines are based on ISO-2631-1978 and ISO 2631/DAM 1-1980. The level of vibration in the ISO guidelines is expressed as acceleration (m/sec^2) root mean squared. The limits are given in terms of (1) reduced comfort boundary, (2) fatigue-

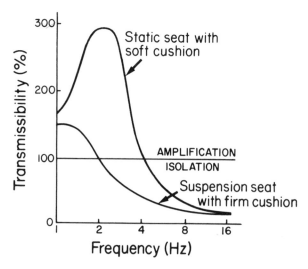

FIG 14.11.
Natural frequency of typical suspension seat.

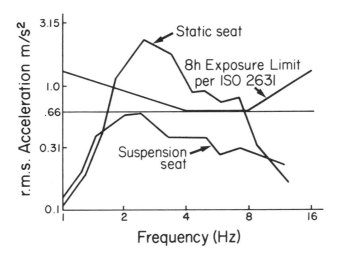

FIG 14.12.
Suspension seat behavior as compared to ISO standard.

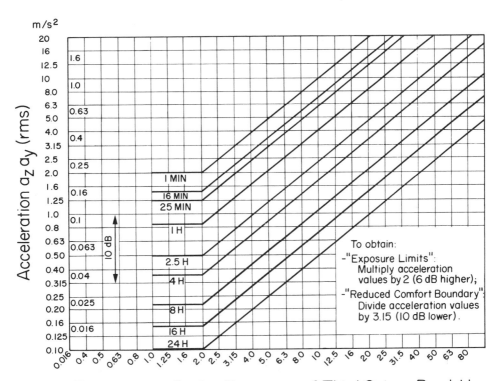

FIG 14.13.
The ISO standard for horizontal vibration.

decreased proficiency boundary, and (3) exposure limit. Different values exist for vertical and horizontal vibrations.

The reduced comfort boundaries are obtained by dividing the fatigue-decreased proficiency limits by 3.15 (a decrease of 10 dB). Exposure limits are obtained by multiplying the fatigue-decreased proficiency limits by 2 (an increase of 6 dB). The 1985 supplement of the standard suggests that to estimate reduced comfort and proficiency a filtered vibration signal over the entire frequency range should be used. Since prolonged exposure to a vibration environment leads to muscle fatigue, lifting directly following a long period of driving should be avoided. Drivers should be encouraged to stretch and exercise during a trip to reduce postural fatigue.

These data suggest that the following features should be provided in the ideal vehicle seat:

1. Three-axis damping of seat pan to levels below the ISO 8-hour exposure
2. Firm, contoured rather than soft seat cushions
3. Lateral support to reduce lateral flexor activity
4. Damped but firmly rigid lumbar support
5. Adjustability of forward posture and height
6. Tilted seat pan
7. Seat back in a position of extension
8. Adjustability of damping for different driver weights
9. Adequate travel, so that the seat does not "bottom out."

SUMMARY

Sitting in the workplace is currently the most common posture in the industrial world. Although sitting offers many excellent advantages, the seat design needs to be thought out carefully to avoid causing musculoskeletal problems to workers. This chapter offers some guidance in this area, but to be fully effective it must be supplemented by the information on workplace design and function available in many ergonomics texts. With attention to detail in design, layout, and work method, seated work can be made less stressful to the low back than it is currently in many offices and factories.

Manual exertions in a standing posture can stress the low back if care is not taken in the design and layout of the workplace and the objects that are handled (containers, materials, handling devices, and carts). Once again, allowing the worker to remain in a stable, upright posture with the load held close to the body is essential. A significant proportion of the U.S. workforce has to exert forces close to their maximum strength daily. Container dimensions should be small to minimize spinal load moments and to improve visibility. Hoists, articulated arms and carts should be used when possible. Loads to be lifted should never be placed near the floor. Pushing and pulling forces of various materials handling devices (e.g. carts) should be well below 50 pounds and the carts should be designed to move easily. In general, workplace design should allow the worker to stand or sit erect and not force the worker to reach beyond a comfortable distance or twist the torso while lifting.

Cyclic loadings due to vibration should not exceed the ISO requirements. Vibration isolation seats should be used when possible, and padded seat pans and backs that effectively support the lumbar region and arms should be employed. Lateral motions should be minimized. With the present technology, there is no reason that the workplace should not be adjustable to fit any individual.

BIBLIOGRAPHY

1. Andersson GBJ, Ortengren R: Lumbar disc pressure and myoelectric back muscle activity during sitting. III. Studies on a wheelchair. *Scand J Rehab Med* 1974; 3:122.
2. Chaffin DB: Localized muscle fatigue—definition and measurement. *J Occup Med* 1973; 15:346.
3. Chaffin DB, Andersson GBJ: Occupational biomechanics. New York, Wiley Interscience, 1984.
4. Chaffin DB, Andersson GBJ: Occupational biomechanics. New York, Wiley Interscience, 1990.
5. Frymoyer JW, Pope MH, Costanza MC, et al: Epidemiologic studies of low back pain. *Spine* 1980; 5:419.
6. Grandjean E, Hünting W, Wotzka W, et al: An ergonomic investigation of multipurpose chairs. *Human Factors* 1973; 15:247.
7. Grandjean E, Hünting W, Pidermann M: VDT workstation design: Preferred settings and their effects. *Human Factors* 1983; 25:161.
8. Herrin GD, Chaffin DB, Mach RS: Criteria for research on the hazards of manual materials handling. Workshop proceedings on contract CDC-99-74-118, Cincinnati, Ohio, US Dept of Health and Human Services (NIOSH), 1974.
9. Kelsey JL, Hardy EJ: Driving of motor vehicles as a risk factor for acute herniated lumbar intervertebral disc. *Am J Epid* 1975; 102:63.
10. Kroemer KHE: Über die Höhe von Schreibtischen. *Arbeitswissenschaft* 1963; 2:132.
11. Kroemer KHE: Seating in plant and office. *Am Ind Hyg Ass J* 1971; 32:633.
12. Kroemer KHE, Robinette JC: Ergonomics in the design of office furniture. *Ind Med Surg* 1969; 38:115.
13. Lee K: *Biomechanical Modeling of Cart Pushing and Pulling* (thesis). Ann Arbor, Univ of Michigan, 1982.
14. National Institute for Occupational Safety and Health: *A Work Practices Guide for Manual Lifting.* Tech Report No 81–122. Cincinnati, Ohio, US Dept of Health and Human Services (NIOSH), 1981.
15. Pope MH, Wilder DG, Seroussi RE: Trunk muscle response to foot support and corset wearing during seated, whole-body vibration. *34th Ortho Res Soc* Atlanta, Ga, 1–4, Feb 1988, p 374.
16. Troup JDG: Driver's back pain and its prevention. A review of the postural, vibratory, and muscular factors, together with the problem of transmitted road shock. *Appl Ergonomics* 1978; 9:207.
17. Wilder DG, Frymoyer JW, Pope MH: The effect of vibration on the spine of the seated individual. *Automedica* 1985; 6:5.

15

Education and Training

Margareta Nordin, M.D.
Michelle Crites-Battié, M.D.
Malcolm H. Pope, Dir. Med. Sc., Ph.D.
Stover Snook, M.D.

INTRODUCTION

Education and training are commonly used in industry to prevent low back pain (LBP). Typically, safety and personnel departments have responsibility for instructing employees in proper methods and work procedures. Training in safe lifting procedures has been a part of safety programs in industry for over 50 years. In recent years, increased emphasis has been placed on strength and fitness training and the use of back schools. The training of supervisors and other management personnel to respond appropriately to the low back-injured worker is a relatively new use of education and training to minimize the impact of low back disorders. In this chapter, two main strategies for education and training are reviewed: primary and secondary prevention. Primary prevention aims at reducing the occurrence of low back pain. Secondary prevention aims at minimizing disability through education and training.

PRIMARY PREVENTION THROUGH EDUCATION AND TRAINING

The basic challenges in a primary prevention program are many. Since most back problems occur during prime productive years, they are a health concern to the individual. Back problems are also a significant economic problem, particularly for heavy industries and occupations exposing the individual to prolonged constrained postures, repetitive motion, and vibration. Yet the cause-effect relationship is not clearly established between the precipitating factors and the anatomic structure of the spine giving rise to the pain. Current scientific knowledge on how to decrease occurrence is therefore limited. Nevertheless, several attempts to reduce and prevent low back pain have been made. The most common attempts include safe lifting instruction, strength and fitness training, and back schools, each of which are reviewed here.

Training in Safe Lifting

Lifting is the most common event associated with the onset of compensable LBP complaints.[2,12,15,67] Consequently, there has been a major effort within industry to train workers to lift safely; but the rationale, particularly the effects of the education programs, and the compliance with them are controversial.

The most common type of manual lift in industry is from the floor or close to the floor.[65] The original concept of safe lifting required the worker to maintain a straight back, bend the knees to lower the body, and then lift with the leg muscles. It was recognized that the intervertebral disc could better withstand the compressive forces of straight-back lifting than the shear forces of bent-back lifting.[35] If the load is bulky, however, the bent-knee lift results in greater load moments on the lower back.

Other principles of safe lifting have been added to the original concept. Holding the object close to the body is as important, if not more important, than keeping a straight back.[3] Slow, smooth lifting without jerking tends to minimize the effects of acceleration on the lower back. Turning with the feet instead of twisting the trunk reduces the torsional loads on intervertebral discs and back muscles.[35]

The correct positioning of feet, chin, arms, and hands is emphasized in the "kinetic lifting"[1] currently recommended by the International Labour Office[35] and the National Safety Council in the United States.[52] Kinetic lifting is defined as a lift whereby the worker adds kinetic energy either to a horizontally moving load or to the vertically moving body before actually lifting the load vertically. This is done by imparting some velocity to the object. There is not always consensus about the elements of a safe lifting program, however. For example, some authorities emphasize bending the knees,[63] but others place greater importance upon maintaining a straight back.[33]

Lifting with straight back and bent knees places the quadriceps muscles at a severe mechanical disadvantage and requires greater energy expenditure than lifting with bent back and straight knees. Perhaps this is why workers seldom use straight-back and bent-knee lifting in industry, even after programs in safe lifting are conducted.[14,28] Most workers use a combination of bent back and bent knees, depending on the characteristics of the lifting task and the workplace design. Keeping the back straight to prevent shear forces appears to have merits, but it is difficult to enforce. Workers who have or have had LBP have been found to be more likely to keep their backs straight when lifting.[65] Consequently, it may be more appropriate to teach the straight-back lift to such workers, since they may accept the trade-off of shifting the load to the knees rather than the back.

The National Institute of Occupational Safety and Health (NIOSH) observes that many safe lifting programs have tended to rely on a dogmatic style of instruction, and sets of rules for safe lifting are common. The drawback is that literal application of some of these rules has led to some unsafe lifting practices. For example, the rule to always lift with the knees is often impractical and may, in fact, be dangerous in some circumstances. In some people, the extensor muscle of the knee may be insufficient for the task at hand. Moreover, this lifting posture applied unselectively can lead to lifting bulky objects at arm's length in front of the knees, thus creating more stress on the spine than the straight-legged stoop posture. Any rules used as memory aids should at least teach a basic aim or principle. What matters is that the trainee is led to a proper understanding of the problem and not merely expected to remember a set of catchphrases.[71] To achieve these goals, NIOSH recommends that training in safe lifting should include the following information:[24]

1. the risks to health of unskilled lifting
2. the basic physics of lifting
3. the effects of lifting on the body
4. individual awareness of the body's strengths and weaknesses
5. how to avoid unexpected physical factors that might contribute to LBP
6. the development of handling skills
7. the use of handling aids

Despite these practical and commonsense guidelines, the effect of training in safe lifting on the reduction of LBP and disability has not yet been adequately studied. Several studies have found a 65 to 70% reduction in reported low back disability,[29,46] but other studies have discovered little or no effect.[14,21,66] Unfortunately, these studies have been neither controlled nor of sufficiently long duration. Many authorities recommend a minimum experimental observation period of three years because of the cyclic nature of low back disability in industry and the Hawthorne* effect of many training programs. Two studies have investigated the biomechanical aspects of lifting with straight back and bent knees versus lifting with bent back and straight knees. One study concluded that straight back/bent knees should be recommended only for small, compact objects that can be lifted between the knees and close to the body.[56] The other study could find no clear biomechanical rationale for deciding between the two lifting postures.[28]

Several studies have looked at the efficacy of training in patient handling, which requires specific skills since the "materials" are human. In a geriatric hospital, Wood combined a personnel program aimed at prompt improvement in communications following back injuries with an instructional program in patient-handling techniques.[75] The program proved to be cost effective. Wood found that compliance with existing safety rules was essential to the success of the program.[75] Training alone is insufficient to increase compliance. Supervisor involvement in the form of feedback has been shown to elicit the highest compliance rates. When feedback is removed, compliance returns to baseline levels.

Videman, Rauhala, and Asp introduced an educational component of lifting for nursing students and compared their subsequent back injury rates to those in a previous class of nurses who had not been exposed to special training.[73] While the two groups did not differ in back injury rates overall, nurses with poor patient-handling skills had an increased risk of back injury.[73] This suggests that improved patient-handling skills may prevent some injuries. Efforts to alter lifting techniques solely through education, however, have met with little success. In the main, such techniques have lacked long-term reinforcement.[21,54,69,73]

NIOSH agrees that the value of any training in safe lifting is open to question because there have been no controlled studies showing a consequent long-term drop in LBP.[71] "Yet so long as it is a legal duty for employers to provide such training or for as long as the employer is liable to a claim of negligence for failing to train workers in safe methods of . . . [lifting], the practice is likely to continue despite the lack of evidence to support it."[71] Until manual materials handling is looked upon as a skill; i.e, practiced on-site, taught by model workers, and reinforced periodically, the concept of training of safe lifting will continue in an unstructured way yielding disappointing results.

Strength and Fitness Training

Strength and fitness training variably emphasizes factors such as musculoskeletal strength, aerobic capacity, endurance, and flexibility. Exercises to increase these physical capacities have been a part of LBP treatment programs for many years, but in recent years various exercise programs have been advocated in industry to reduce or prevent the onset of LBP. Yet, the efficacy of strength and fitness training as a technique for prevention is debatable. It must also be recognized that in industry the enforcement of training is difficult. In most cases, industry must rely on voluntary compliance.

The Hawthorne effect is improvement merely because there has been an intervention of some kind.

The work most frequently cited to support the view that individuals with higher fitness levels are at lower risk of sustaining injury, specifically back injury, is that of Cady et al.[15,17] They reported the effects of strength and fitness on compensable LBP in Los Angeles fire fighters. A five-point fitness index was used, consisting of endurance, strength, flexibility, exercise blood pressure, and recovery heart rate. Fire fighters were evaluated and grouped into three categories of most fit, middle fit, and least fit. Over a period of four years, 7.1% of the least fit group, 3.2% of the middle fit group, and 0.8% of the most fit group suffered compensable LBP. These findings led them to the conclusion that "physical conditioning and fitness of fire fighters are preventive of back injuries." Unfortunately, the effects of other factors, such as age, were not controlled during the analyses, making interpretation of the study results less clear. Two other prospective, longitudinal studies failed to reveal a similar association.[6,31] A recently reported prospective study of back pain complaints in aircraft manufacturing workers did not find an association between fitness level (measured in oxygen consumption level) and back pain reporting.[6]

Several other studies have indicated a positive role for strength and fitness training in reducing the likelihood of an LBP episode. A study at the Eastman Kodak Company investigated the relationship between LBP and abdominal muscle weakness and that between LBP and trunk stiffness.[64] Although a definite relationship was found, it could not be determined which came first—the muscle weakness/trunk stiffness or the LBP. Such retrospective studies clarify the need for prospective, longitudinal studies in the identification of risk indicators. Otherwise, the chicken-and-egg dilemma cannot be resolved.

The relationship between preemployment strength testing and musculoskeletal injuries has also been investigated. Chaffin and Park reported a longitudinal study of low back pain in association with isometric lifting strength and occupational lifting requirements.[18] Isometric lifting strength in relation to job demands was evaluated among 400 individuals employed in 103 different jobs. During the one-year follow-up, 25 low back incidents were reported to the company medical department. The incidence rate was approximately three times greater in individuals who were unable to demonstrate strength equal to or greater than that required by the job. This difference was not reported as statistically significant, however, perhaps because of the small number of subjects and back pain incidents involved. Subsequently, another prospective study of isometric lifting strength with respect to job requirements and injury reports has been published.[38] In this study too few back problems were reported to allow for analysis of this subset of musculoskeletal complaints.

Two other prospective studies have examined general isometric lifting strength in relation to reported back pain complaints.[5,70] Both studies concluded that isometric lifting strength was a very poor predictor of such complaints. The study of aircraft manufacturing workers actually found a trend for greater strength to be associated with more back pain reporting, although the finding did not hold when age was controlled.[5,6] Except for situations of extreme physical demands, where it is likely that an individual will not be able to meet the demands of the job without specific strength training, there is little scientific evidence to support isometric strength testing as a means to reduce back problems. Furthermore, generic isometric strength measurements of back muscles were not related to the incidence of LBP in Danish factory workers.[59] Measurements of muscle strength in adults with and without LBP also yielded little or no difference between the two groups, leading the authors to conclude that the strength of spinal and abdominal muscles are of doubtful importance for the prevention of LBP.[9,50]

Isometric trunk strength testing has been criticized for failure to simulate the actual job task, especially if the task is dynamic. Dynamic and static trunk muscle strength and endurance are poorly correlated.[53,57] Also, in dynamic fatigue testing of the trunk muscles, healthy subjects displayed significantly less motor control, which may lead to an inability to compensate for perturbation in the load or position of the trunk. This in turn may lead to a loss of ability to protect the passive elements (discs and ligaments) susceptible to industrial and recreational injuries.[58] Dynamic devices allowing measurement of subject-generated torque throughout three-dimensional ranges of motion are available for the trunk; but no prospective controlled long-term study has yet been completed to predict low back pain occurrence in industry. Dynamic trunk strength and endurance measurements are potentially more informative, but correlation with job requirements is complicated.[36]

A common public perception is that greater spinal flexibility is associated with improved back health and lower risk of "injury." In recent years, this belief has been evidenced by the promotion of stretching programs within the workplace.[42] The premise of such programs lacks a solid scientific foundation. Although the few prospective studies examining spinal flexibility and future back pain reports have yielded mixed results, all have agreed that flexibility measures are poor predictors of subsequent back problems.[4,10,11,70]

Although there are conflicting data on strength, fitness, and flexibility as they relate to back problems, other health benefits are associated with physical fitness. Several intervention studies introducing fitness programs into the workplace have reported sustained decreases in overall absenteeism and medical costs.[13,17] Several studies have demonstrated the psychologic benefits of exercise, such as reduced anxiety and depression.[27,30,48,49] Thus, while we are not yet in a position to claim that physical fitness prevents back problems, other benefits may make the introduction of fitness programs into the workplace worthwhile.

Back Schools in Industry

The concept of the back school can be traced to the teachings of Delpech in Toulouse.[60] The concepts of education on a one-to-one basis to control LBP in patients started in the late 1950s.[23,24] In 1969, the concept of back school was introduced more formally in Stockholm.[76] Early back schools were also developed in the United States.[32,43,45,47,55] The original concept of the back school was to educate patients who were already suffering (or had recently suffered) from LBP, that is, it was a form of treatment. A recent use of the back school is to educate workers in industry on how to prevent or reduce the severity of LBP.

Several attempts have been made in industry to determine the value of a primary-prevention back school. Two large-scale studies showed a decrease in the numbers of reported back injuries and days lost following such a program.[43,54] Confounding factors such as employee layoffs and randomization, however, made it difficult to credit the entire positive outcome to the back programs alone.

Other studies have been reported for preventive types of back schools, or education programs, in industry.[37,61] Unfortunately, they have not been controlled studies, and other types of preventive techniques were used concurrently. Therefore, it is not possible to assess the effects of the educational component on subsequent injury reporting.

In two more recent studies conflicting results were found. Ljungberg and Sanne introduced a primary-prevention back education program among 4,000 Swedish federal employees.[41] The results showed no impact on the reported injuries or lost work days. In contrast, a three-year prospective study by Versloot et al. of 400 bus drivers in Holland showed a significant decrease in absenteeism after a back injury prevention program was instituted.[72] The average decrease in lost work days was six days per employee per year. The difference in the impact of these two programs may be explained by variables such as company support, social security system, use of model teachers, and employee involvement, which characterized the latter study.

It is still not clear why some programs are successful and others are not, and further controlled prospective research is needed.

MINIMIZING DISABILITY THROUGH EDUCATION AND TRAINING

While the primary prevention of back pain remains a rather elusive goal, recent studies offer hope of secondary prevention programs focusing on preventing long-term back pain disability through more active early medical management, monitoring, and support at the workplace.[20,25,26,40]

Management Training

The use of education and training to prevent or reduce LBP in industry has been directed almost exclusively toward the worker. Equally important is the training of management. It must be recognized that within the current state of the art, LBP cannot be entirely prevented. Prolonged disability from back problems is often associated with adversary situations, litigation, and lack of follow-up and concern. Management can prevent many of these situations by appropriate training of foremen, supervisors, managers, engineers, and medical personnel.

An example of a program focusing on changing the attitudes of management toward back problems was reported by Fitzler and Berger.[25,26] They describe a program at American Biltrite in which management was trained in the positive acceptance of LBP. An atmosphere was created in which workers were encouraged to report all episodes of LBP (even minor episodes) to the company clinic. An immediate, conservative, in-house treatment was provided by the company nurse, including worker education. Attempts were made to keep the worker on the job, often with modified duties that were consistent with the worker's condition. If necessary, referrals were made to the company doctor, where treatment and progress were closely monitored. Over a three-year period, workers' compensation costs for low back claims were reduced from over $200,000 per year to less than $20,000 per year—a tenfold decrease. The results are impressive despite the fact that the study was uncontrolled.

Wood also reported on the effects of a personnel program directed at minimizing the impact of back problems among hospital workers.[75] He stresses early care management as well as management attitude and reinforcement of safety rules.

Company medical personnel should be trained in the benefits of early intervention, initial conservative treatment, patient follow-up, and job placement techniques. Medical personnel should be familiar with recent literature that objectively evaluates various types of treatment for LBP.[8,22,40,62,64,74] Medical personnel acquainted with the physical demands of jobs performed in the company are better prepared to place injured employees and new employees and to allow temporary modification. This may ensure a more timely return to the workplace following an episode of low back pain. Modifications to allow an early return to the workplace and training on site, in conjunction with an early activation program, have substantially reduced lost workdays.[40]

Data from the Weyerhaeuser Company indicate that workers with back injuries who are off work more than six months have only a 50% possibility of ever returning to productive employment. For more than one years' absence, the possibility is 25%; after more than two years' absence, the possibility of returning is almost nil.[44] Another study concludes that, with the passage of time following injury, patients increasingly elaborate and exaggerate their symptoms but are less truly depressed by their predicament.[7] Even if the physical disability remains constant, the patient's psychologic posture and the likelihood of returning to work changes. These studies emphasize the importance of providing modified work as a means of returning the worker to the job as quickly as possible. Unfortunately, modified work is not well accepted in industry, and management often refuses to return an employee to work unless the worker is 100% recovered, which is a statement physicians are often leary of making. The reluctance to accept modified work is costly to industry and unhealthy for the worker; it should be the focus of intensive management training.

Industrial and production engineers should be trained in the ergonomic principles of good job design. New techniques are available for identifying high-risk jobs and evaluating suggested job modifications.[65,71] Good job design may reduce the onset of low back episodes, allow the worker to stay on the job longer, and permit the injured worker to return to the job sooner. Although job redesign usually involves some cost, it is frequently less than the average cost of a single case of compensable LBP.

Management should be aware that no single approach can solve all problems surrounding LBP. All of the approaches described here are necessary for an effective program in controlling LBP. Well-directed, innovative education and training can produce beneficial results for both the employee and employer, but only through a commitment by management at the highest levels.

Education Following a Back Injury Report

The back school concept emphasizes the importance of involving the patient in his or her own care. Since the prognosis of most LBP episodes is favorable irrespective of the treatment prescribed, the most likely determinant of outcome may be how the back is used and cared for 24 hours a day rather than single physical therapy treatments.[68] Back schools attempt to convey two important messages. The first message is that the responsibility for recovery from LBP is shared by the patient and the practitioner. The patient has very definite responsibilities, and the most successful recovery results from meeting these responsibilities. The second message is that recovery may not mean complete absence of pain. Residual pain may remain, or pain may recur. The overall goal is to teach the student how to cope and function with LBP. The educated patient as his or her own therapist may be a more efficient mechanism to apply this principle. Although patients can be educated in the principles of back care by physicians, realistically, pressures of time may interfere. The formalized curriculum of a back school overcomes this problem. Learning is likely enhanced by the present notion of a school. That is, the patients attending a back school understand from the onset that their treatment and their outcome depend on learning. The back school ensures that pertinent aspects of a curriculum be covered. Ideally, the patient would be tested for comprehension before and after the educational program.

The content of patient education programs can vary widely, and these differences need to be well-defined when studying program efficacy. Instructors come from a variety of backgrounds and include physical and occupational therapists, psychologists, nurses, physicians, and chiropractors, among others. The back school is an attempt to educate the patient in many aspects of back care; it represents a comprehensive approach to self-care and commonly includes instruction in safe lifting, building strength, and physical fitness. Most back schools also include discussions on anatomy and physiology of the lower back, body mechanics, and posture. Some back schools offer advice on stress management, coping with pain, relaxation, drug use and abuse, first aid and acute care, epidemiology, activities of daily living, and vocational guidance. The style of teaching can range from informal demonstrations and discussions to structured classroom settings. Job simulation or actual visits to the workplace can also be a part of the back shool curriculum.

The type of learning that is emphasized may have one or more attributes of classic learning: cognitive, psychomotor, and affective experiences. Cognitive learning is purely informational, presented in a didactic, classroomlike atmosphere. The presented material may include printed brochures, audiovisual programs, or live professional instruction. Currently, there are many prepackaged low back schools available. Anatomy and function of the spine, posture, home exercises, epidemiology, and psychologic aspects of the pain experience are usually included in these instructional units.

The affective component of learning takes into consideration the importance of the patient's motivation. The back schools that have enjoyed the greatest success appear to have done so largely because their evangelistic teachers have the ability to sell concepts to patients and motivate them to use the methods taught.

There has been only one controlled study of the effectiveness of low back schools. Using the Swedish back school developed by Zachrisson-Forssell,[76] Bergquist-Ullman and Larsson investigated its effect on subacute LBP patients from the Volvo Company in Gothenburg, Sweden.[8] Patients were randomly assigned to one of three types of treatment: back school, physical therapy, or placebo. The back school consisted of four sessions, with six to eight patients in each class. Physical therapy was conducted on a one-to-one basis. The placebo group was given treatment with "short waves of the lowest possible intensity." Seventy patients completed the back school; 72 patients underwent physical therapy; and 75 patients were given placebos.

There was no statistically significant difference between the back school and physical therapy in terms of pain relief (days); both required significantly fewer days (significance level $[p] < 0.05$) than the placebo group. The number of days before return to work was significantly fewer for the back school ($p < 0.5$, 5 days less) than either the physical therapy or placebo groups.

The authors concluded that the back school is superior to the placebo treatment in time required for pain relief and return to work. Although there was no significant difference between the back school and physical therapy in terms of pain relief, the authors observed that the back school is economically superior because one therapist can treat more than one patient at a time.

The study did not investigate the effect of the back school on patients with chronic pain or the effect of the back school as a preventive technique for industrial workers. For example, Hall reviewed his experience with 6,418 participants in the Canadian Back Education Units.[32] Significant improvement occurred in 69%. The rate of success was influenced by duration of LBP, higher levels of education, and a recognition of the emotional levels of pain. Poorer results occurred in those patients with greater than six months' duration of LBP, sciatica, and workers' compensation.

To summarize the studies above, it is clear that education has a place following a back injury. Education in the form of a back school or back educational program emphasizes the benign nature of a low back pain occurrence and at the same time makes the patient an informed health care consumer. The back school is most successful if it encompasses a visit to the actual workplace, includes practical realistic training on the work site, or involves both of these measures. It must be remembered, however, that back schools have not been proved effective for chronic low back pain patients (> 6 months of back pain), as documented by Lankhorst et al.[39]

CONCLUSION

What can education and training be expected to accomplish? Fifty percent of compensable LBP is associated with lifting, but instructions for proper technique have frequently been faulty or incomplete. Most workers use a combination of bent back and bent knees. It is probable that those most likely to use safe lifting techniques are those who have had LBP. Strength and fitness training to prevent LBP has not yet proved beneficial, but industry should nonetheless encourage the general health benefits of improved physical fitness. Recently, back schools have been used to discuss such topics as how the back functions, lifting techniques, and general emotional and physical health. There are many models of the back school, but they all stress a shared responsibility for recovery, though recovery may not mean complete absence of pain. Controlled study shows that the back school is better than placebo and economically superior to physical therapy. There is some indication that preventive school can be helpful. Management training is also helpful. Company physicians should be trained in the benefits of early intervention and conservative treatment, follow-up, and careful job placement. Industrial engineers should be trained in ergonomic principles to provide for more optimal job design. All of these approaches require the enthusiastic and goal-oriented cooperation of an educated management for success.

BIBLIOGRAPHY

1. Anderson TN, McClurg R: Human kinetics in strain prevention. *Brit J Occup Safety* 1970; 8:248.
2. Andersson GBJ: Epidemiological aspects of low back pain in industry. *Spine* 1981; 6:53.
3. Andersson GBJ, Ortengren R, Nachemson A: Quantitative studies of back loads in lifting. *Spine* 1976; 1:178.
4. Battié MC, Bigos SJ, Sheehy A, et al: Spinal flexibility and individual factors that influence it. *Phys Ther* 1986; 6:653.
5. Battié MC, Bigos SJ, Fisher LD, et al: Isometric lifting strength as a predictor of industrial back pain. *Spine* 1989; 14:851.
6. Battié MC, Bigos SJ, Fisher LD, et al: A prospective study of the role of cardiovascular risk factors and fitness in industrial back pain complaints. *Spine* 1989; 14:141.
7. Beals RK, Hickman NW: Industrial injuries of the back and extremities. *J Bone Joint Surg* 1972; 51:1593.
8. Bergquist-Ullman M, Larsson U: Acute low back pain in industry. *Acta Orthop Scand [Suppl]* 1977; 170:1.
9. Berkson M. Schultz A, Nachemson A, et al: Voluntary strengths of male adults with acute low back syndromes. *Clin Orthop* 1977; 129:84.
10. Biering-Sorenson F: A one year prospective study of low back trouble in a general population: The prognostic value of low back history and physical measurements. *Dan Med Bull* 1984a; 31:362.
11. Biering-Sorenson F: Physical measurements as risk indicators for low-back trouble over a one-year period. 1983 Volvo Award in Clinical Science. *Spine* 1984b; 9:106.
12. Bigos SJ, Spengler DM, Martin N, et al: Back injuries in industry: A retrospective study: II. Injury Factors. *Spine* 1986; 11:246.
13. Bowne DW, Russell ML, Morgan JL, et al: Reduced disability and health care costs in an industrial fitness program. *J Occup Med* 1984; 26:809.
14. Brown JR: *Lifting as an Industrial Hazard*. Toronto, Labour Safety Council of Ontario, Ontario Department of Labour, 1971.
15. Cady LD, Bischoff DP, O'Connell ER, et al: Strength and fitness and subsequent back injuries in firefighters. *J Occup Med* 1979a; 21:269.
16. Cady LD, Bischoff DP, O'Connell ER, et al: Letters to the editor: Author's response. *J Occup Med* 1979b; 21:720.

17. Cady LD, Bischoff DP, O'Connell ER, et al: Strength and fitness and subsequent back injuries in firefighters. *J Occup Med* 1979; 21:269.
18. Chaffin D, Park K: A longitudinal study of low back pain as associated with occupational weight lifting factors. *Amer Indus Hyg Assoc J* 1973; 34:513.
19. Chaffin DB, Herrin GD, Keyserling WM: Preemployment strength testing: An updated position. *J Occup Med* 1978; 20:403.
20. Choler U, Larsson R, Nachemson A, et al: *Pain in the Back*. Stockholm, Spri Rapport, 1985.
21. Dehlin O, Hedenrud B, Horal J: Back symptoms in nursing aids in a geriatric hospital. *Scand J Rehab Med* 1976; 8:47.
22. Deyo RA: Conservative therapy for low back pain. *J Am Med Assoc* 1983; 250:1057.
23. Fahrni WH: Backache relieved through new concepts of posture. Springfield, Ill, Charles C Thomas, 1966.
24. Fahrni WH: Conservative treatment of lumbar disc degeneration: Our primary responsibility. *Orthop Clin Amer* 1975; 6:93.
25. Fitzler SL, Berger RA: The Chelsea back program: One year later. *Occup Health Safety* 1982; 7:52–54.
26. Fitzler SL, Berger RA: Attitudinal change: The Chelsea back program. *Occup Health Safety* 1983; 3:24–26.
27. Folkins C, Syme W: Physical fitness training and mental health. *Amer Psych* 1981; 36:373.
28. Garg A, Herrin GD: Stoop or squat: A biomechanical and metabolic evaluation. *AIIE Trans* 1979; 11:293.
29. Glover JR: Prevention of back pain, in Jayson M (ed): *The Lumbar Spine and Back Pain*. New York, Grune and Stratton, 1976.
30. Greist J, Klun M, Eischens R, et al: Running as treatment for depression. *Comprehensive Psychiatry* 1979; 20:1.
31. Gyntelberg F: One year incidence of low back pain among male residents of Copenhagen aged 40–59. *Dan Med Bull* 1974; 21:30.
32. Hall H: The Canadian back education units. *Physiotherapy* 1980; 66:115.
33. Hall HW Sr: "Clean" vs "dirty" learning, an academic subject for youth. *ASSE J* 1973; 20.
34. Hickey DS, Hukins DWL: Relation between the structure of the annulus fibrosus and the function and failure of the intervertebral disc. *Spine* 1980; 5:106.
35. Himbury S: *Kinetic Methods of Manual Handling in Industry*. Occupational Safety and Health Series No. 10. Geneva, International Labour Office, 1967.
36. Himmelstein JS, Andersson GBJ: Low back pain: Risk evaluation and preplacement screening. *Occup Med* 1988; 3:255.
37. Johnson CD: Safety forum. *Ind Safety Prod Nes* 1981.
38. Keyserling WM, Herrin GD, Chaffin DB, et al: Establishing an industrial strength testing program. *Am Ind Hyg Assoc J* 1980; 41:730.
39. Lankhorst GJ, Van de Stadt RJ, Vogelaar TW, et al: The effect of the Swedish back school in chronic idiopathic low backpain—A prospective controlled study. *Scand J Rehab Med* 1983; 15:141.
40. Lindstrom I, Ohlund C, Eek C, et al: Work return and LBP disability: Results of a prospective randomized study in an industrial population. Presented at ISSLS Annual Meeting, Kyoto, Japan, May 15–19, 1989.
41. Ljungberg P, Sanne H, Ryggbesvär: Goteborg, Sweden, Statshälsan, 1986.
42. Locke JC: Stretching away from back pain, injury. *Occup Health Saf* 1983; 52.8.
43. Mattmiller AW: The California back school. *Physiotherapy* 1980; 66:118.
44. McGill CM: Industrial back problems: A control program. *J Occup Med* 1968; 10:174.
45. Melton B: Back injury prevention means education. *Occup Health Safety* 1983; 20.
46. Miller RL: Bend your knees! *Nat Safety News* 1977; 57–58.
47. Mooney V: Alternative approaches for the patient beyond the help of surgery. *Orthop Clin N Amer* 1975; 6:331.
48. Morgan W: Anxiety reduction following acute physical activity. *Psychiatric Annals* 1979; 9:3.

49. Morgan W: Affective beneficence of vigorous physical activity. *Med Sci Sports Exercise* 1985; 17:94.

50. Nachemson A, Lindh M: Measurement of abdominal and back muscle strength with and without low back pain. *Scand J Rehab Med* 1969; 1:60.

51. National Institute for Occupational Safety and Health: *A Work Practices Guide for Manual Lifting*. Tech Report No 81-122, Cincinnati, Ohio, U.S. Dept. of Health and Human Servies (NIOSH), 1981.

52. National Safety Council. Human kinetics . . . and lifting. *Nat Safety News* 1971; 6:44–47.

53. Nicolaison T, Jorgensen K: Trunk strength, back muscle endurance and low-back trouble. *Scand J Rehab Med* 1985; 17:121.

54. Nordin M, Frankel V, Spengler DM: A preventive back care program for industry (abstract). Presented at International Lumbar Spine Meeting, Paris, May, 1981.

55. O'Donnel RJ: *Prevention of Back Injury*. Atlanta, GA, The Back School, 1981.

56. Park KS, Chaffin DB: A biomechanical evaluation of two methods of manual load lifting. *AIIE Trans* 1974; 6:105.

57. Parnianpour M, Nordin M, Moritz U, Kahanovitz N: Correlation between different tests of trunk strength. Proceedings. On Musculoskeletal Disorders at Work edited by P. Buckle, Taylor & Francis London, 1987.

58. Parnianpour M, Nordin M, Kahanovitz N, et al: The triaxial coupling of torque generation of trunk muscles during isometric exertions and the effect of fatiguing isoinertial movements on the motor output and movement patterns. *Spine* 1988; 13:982.

59. Pedersen OF, Petersen R, Staffeldt ES: Back pain and isometric back muscle strength of workers in a Danish factory. *Scand J Rehab Med* 1975; 7:125.

60. Peltier L: The back school of Delpech in Montpellier. *Clin Orthop* 1983; 179:4.

61. Pilcher OJ: Personal communication, 1979.

62. Quinet RJ, Hadler NM: Diagnosis and treatment of backache. *Semin Arthritis Rheum* 1979; 8:261.

63. Ring L: Facts on backs — A simplified approach to back injury prevention and control. Loganville, Ga, Georgia Technical Institute Press, 1981.

64. Rowe ML: Low back pain in industry: A position paper. *J Occup Med* 1969; 11:161.

65. Snook SH: The design of manual handling tasks. *Ergonomics* 1978; 21:963.

66. Snook SH, Campanelli RA, Hart JW: A study of three preventive approaches to low back injury. *J Occup Med* 1978; 20:478.

67. Snook SH, Campanelli RA, Ford RJ: A study of back injuries at Pratt and Whitney Aircraft. Hopkinton, Mass, Liberty Mutual Insurance Company Research Center, 1980.

68. Spitzer W, Leblanc F, Dupuis M et al: Report of the Quebec Task Force on Spinal Disorders. *Spine* [European Ed Suppl 1]; 1987, 12:(FS).S9–S59.

69. Stubbs D, Buckle P, Hudson M, et al: Back pain the nursing profession: I. Epidemiology and pilot methodology. *Ergonomics* 1983; 26:755.

70. Troup JDG, Foreman TK, Baxter CE, et al: The perception of back pain and the role of psychophysical tests of lifting capacity. *Spine* 1987; 12:645.

71. U.S. Department of Health and Human Services. *Work Practices Guide for Manual Lifting*. DHHS (NIOSH) Pub No. 81-122, 1981.

72. Versloot JM, Schilstra AJ, Tolen FJ, et al: Back school in industry, a prospective longitudinal controlled study (3 years). Presented at ISSLS Annual Meeting, April 13–17 Miami USA 1988.

73. Videman T, Rauhala H, Asp S: Patient-handling skill, back injuries and back pain. An intervention study in nursing. *Spine* 1989; 14:148.

74. Weber H: Lumbar disc herniation: A controlled, prospective study with ten years of observation. *Spine* 1984; 8:131.

75. Wood DJ: Design and evaluation of a back injury prevention program within a geriatric hospital. *Spine* 1987; 12.77.

76. Zachrisson-Forssell M: The back school. *Spine* 1981; 6:104–106.

PART V

Legal Aspects

16

Impairment Rating—The United States Perspective

John W. Frymoyer, M.D.
Scott Haldeman, M.D., Ph.D.
Gunnar B.J. Andersson, M.D., Ph.D.

OVERVIEW

The legal responsibility to compensate workers who are injured in the normal conduct of their occupation is a product of the industrial revolution. During the nineteenth century employers were not held responsible for injured workers on the premise that a worker accepts the inherent risk of a job upon voluntarily accepting employment. The employer was also held blameless if the employee in any way contributed to the condition through negligence or if a supervisor or "fellow servant" intervened in any way to prevent injury. Furthermore, an employee's action against an employer for alleged injury required a tort action. These stipulations effectively removed mechanisms for all but a few employees to be compensated for injury on the job. They prevailed in Great Britain and the United States until the late nineteenth and early twentieth century.

The first attempt at a social and legal mechanism for the injured worker to find redress from occupational injury was part of social reforms enacted in Germany in 1884. Great Britain passed similar legislation in 1897, but the first United States' workers' compensation statutes were not enacted until 1910 in New York. Each state subsequently passed such legislation, with Mississippi being the final state to enact such a law in 1949. Although there are considerable variations among individual state laws, the intent of all is to provide compensation for lost wages and medical care to workers who have suffered a personal injury on the job. In most states the injury must be accidental, which implies it is both untoward and unexpected.*

Initially, low back pain (LBP) was not viewed as an "injury," except when due to an obvious fracture. Prior to 1934, most low back conditions were viewed as arthritic and thus unrelated to the job. This situation was altered by Mixter and Barr's description of the clinical and anatomic features of lumbar disc herniation.[18] This initiated the "dynasty of the disc" and, from both lay and professional viewpoints, provided a plausible explanation for low back injury. The public perception of a traumatic causation is implicit in the terms "ruptured" and "slipped" applied to "disc." Subsequently, other injury mechanisms and unproved diagnoses have become acceptable, including lumbosacral sprain and strain, which explicitly indicate tissue disruption (injury) of ligaments or muscles. Further

---

*This discussion is based on a more detailed account in Hadler NH: Clinical Concepts in Regional Musculoskeletal Illness. Orlando, Fla, Grune & Stratton, 1987.

confusing the issue are the concepts of cumulative trauma and repetitive strain, as well as the use of the term *traumatogens*[19] to explain possible subclinical mechanisms of injury. Thus, vibrational exposures in drivers or the requirement for repetitive lifting could not only have acute effects but also may cause injury by repetitive exposure.

As part of other social legislation, entitlement programs such as Social Security Disability have provided yet another mechanism for the injured and diseased to obtain relief from medical costs as well as a replacement source of income.

Such legislation has important social, legal, and political ramifications. First, the existence of workers' compensation statutes shows that society believes the cost of injury to a worker should be included in the cost of production. Second, the existence of statutory programs such as Social Security Indemnity indicates that society must bear some of the cost of supporting disabled persons. Third, the evolution and current existence of impairment rating schemes, independent medical examiners, and compensation boards indicates that society needs an objective mechanism to determine causality and impairments resulting from injury rather than relying solely on individual self-assessment of the condition and its cause.

CURRENT CONCEPTS IN IMPAIRMENT AND DISABILITY ASSESSMENT

Most statutory programs clearly distinguish impairment from disability. The legal distinction is that impairment is a quantifiable anatomic or functional loss that may be temporary or permanent and that is solely the result of a medical condition. Disability, on the other hand, is the loss of capacity to engage in gainful employment caused by an impairment. The legal concept of disability takes into account the individual's education, training, experience, and such relatively unquantifiable factors as motivation and psychosocial situation. Stated another way, impairment is purely the result of a medical condition, and the rating of impairment is solely the responsibility of a medical expert. Identifying a disability is an administrative decision in which the objective assessment of impairment is but one dimension. Disability is a complex interaction between the disease condition and the social environment and psychologic condition of the patient, an interaction most apparent in the *chronic pain syndrome*. This point is also emphasized by analysis of the demographic, educational, and certain environmental factors associated with low back pain disability in the United States. An analysis of the National Center for Health Statistics data is graphically shown in Figures 16.1 to 16.5.

Impairment ratings are based on the "whole person" concept. A person's ability to engage in gainful employment depends on the sum of the person's anatomic parts and their functional capabilities. Thus, partial or even complete loss of a single function creates only partial impairment. A person assessed to have complete loss of spinal function (100% spinal impairment) has only partial impairment based on the "whole person."

Last, a central issue in the rating of impairment is the healing period. The healing period ends when the medical problem has resolved or when there is no longer reasonable progress toward resolution. In some low back conditions, such as fractures, these healing periods can be defined with relative accuracy. Similarly, there are fairly good data to establish when a person who has undergone a lumbar disc excision should have recovered. In other, less well-understood conditions such as lumbosacral strain and sprain and degenerative disc disease, definition of the healing period may be impossible to determine accurately. In these situations, the healing period is operationally defined as ended when there is no further

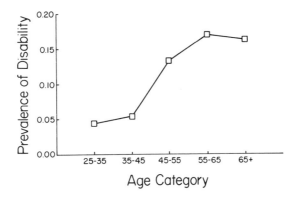

FIG 16.1–16.5.
Data are presented for the prevalence of disability (permanent or extended) by nationally based samples representative of the noninstitutionalized, adult United States population. All prevalence figures represent percentages of the population affected. For example, Figure 16.1 demonstrates a prevalence of 0.05 for the 35- to 45-year-old age group, which means 5% of the population in that age range has been disabled. (From Cats-Baril W, Frymoyer JW: Demographic factors associated with the prevalence of disability in the general population: Analysis of the NHANES I database. *Spine,* in press.)

FIG 16.1.
Disability is shown as a function of age. The slight decrease in disability from ages 55 to 65 may represent a response to entitlement programs, reduced work demands, or retirement programs that are heavily vested and thus keep the person at work until retirement age.

reasonable progress toward resolution rather than when there is no progress at all. The patient has reached "maximum medical improvement."

THE PHYSICIAN'S RESPONSIBILITY IN IMPAIRMENT AND DISABILITY DETERMINATION

The physician has four general responsibilities in the evaluation process. In some cases these responsibilities are established by law, and in other situations the responsibilities are established by tradition.

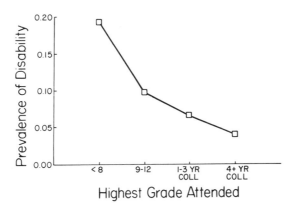

FIG 16.2.
An increasing level of education is associated with a significant reduction in disability.

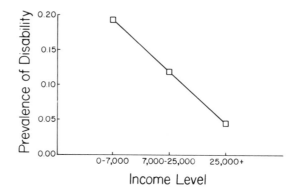

FIG 16.3.
Low income is a major determinant of disability, whereas high income is associated with a much lower rate of disability.

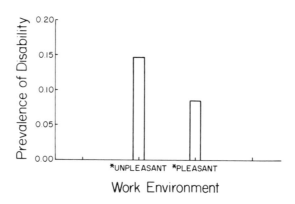

FIG 16.4.
This study describes an unpleasant work environment as one with excessive fumes, noise, or other factors associated with an increased risk of disability.

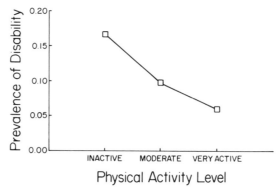

FIG 16.5.
Lack of physical fitness is associated with an increased rate of disability.

The physician's first responsibility under the workers' compensation law is to establish a causal relationship between the injury event and the resultant impairment. The process is also central to statutory or litigation cases outside of the work environment, such as personal injury claims. In other entitlement programs, such as Social Security, establishing causality is not central to the process. Currently, causality in the workplace can be categorized as direct or as an aggravation of some preexistent condition. A relationship ordinarily exists if the findings (impairment) could have been caused by the injury events with reasonable certainty. It is not the physician's role to question the patient's perception of the injury event but rather to record that perception and to assess the reasonableness of that perception with regard to the impairment. The employer or insurance carrier may challenge the patient's history and assessment of the injury event.

The second responsibility of the physician is to determine the end of the healing period. We believe that a treating physician should give an injured worker a reasonable estimate of the expected duration of the impairment as well as the potential for some permanence to the condition. The patient should also understand that the healing period will end when there is no longer reasonable progress toward the resolution of the problem. Ideally, the healing period should end when maximum anatomic or physiologic recovery occurs, but it is known that injured tissues continue to remodel to some degree over a period of one to two years. Also, in some low back conditions (e.g., herniated lumbar disks) patients may continue to improve over two to five years.[26-28] Thus, the treating physician has to chart a course for the patient, which on one hand promotes the earliest return to work and on the other hand permits sufficient healing to occur so that reinjury risks are minimized. Because many of the important parameters that guide this decision are unknown, most physicians tend to err on the side of extending the period of presumed disability. Such caution tends to promote a chronic pain syndrome and lessen the potential for eventual return to work. The uncertainties and biases of the treating physician can be overcome by a combination of the use of objective, outside physicians to monitor the patient's progress, appropriate and timely interventions, and more active and aggressive rehabilitation to minimize risks for future injury.

Significant social and legal barriers remain, however, even when an optimum approach is employed. For example, Haddad analyzed the return to work in injured workers who had an attorney and those who did not.[10] Of 2,517 cases, 2,169 were represented by counsel, and 348 were not. Only 9% of the patients with attorneys returned to work, whereas 77% of the patients not represented by attorneys returned to work. Thus, the presence of an attorney apparently delayed the "healing" time.

The third responsibility of the physician is to establish whether permanent impairment exists at the end of the healing period and, if present, to rate that impairment. A percentage rating based on the whole person concept, as recommended by the American Medical Association (AMA), is the most common way to accomplish this goal. Other systems, such as the California system, define disability as the percentage of the work force from which the injured worker is excluded. A particularly difficult and inexact part of this process is the assessment of the relative contribution of any preexistent condition to the impairment caused by the injury. This process, known as apportionment, is particularly critical to tort cases such as personal injury. In workers' compensation cases, however, either work-caused or work-aggravated conditions may ordinarily be compensable. In the approach taken by the AMA an aggravation of a preexistent condition must be substantive and not speculative. Five types of aggravation are identified.

1. An occupational disorder aggravated by supervening nonoccupational disorder

2. An occupational disorder aggravated by another supervening occupational condition arising out of and in the course of employment by the same employer
3. An occupational disorder aggravated by another supervening industrial condition arising out of and in the course of employment by a different employer
4. An occupational disorder aggravated by a preexisting nonoccupational condition
5. An occupational disorder aggravating a preexisting nonoccupational condition[2]

The judgment of the treating physician is rarely the sole determinant of impairment. The injured worker, employer, or carrier has the legal right to challenge an impairment rating and to insist on a second or third determination. The physician in the role of an independent medical examiner is an unbiased observer. The qualification of such individuals is highly variable, but in some states (e.g., California) an attempt has been made to define and certify independent medical examiners based upon strict criteria, including training and experience.

The fourth responsibility of the physician is to estimate work capacity or restrictions. Often this is done with only a general knowledge of the person's usual work, frequently based on information obtained from the patient. Nevertheless, the physician is asked to outline work restrictions and to determine if these restrictions are temporary or permanent. If the restrictions are temporary, the anticipated duration of such restrictions may be estimated. In the past, physicians usually gave their estimates of work restrictions in vague or subjective terms, for example, "The patient should do no heavy lifting." In the past decade numerous refinements have been developed with the goal of quantifying the patient's physical capacities. These "work-capacity evaluations" range from written questionnaires, which tap into incrementally rated lifting activities, sitting, standing, bending, and twisting restrictions (Table 16.1) to complex "objective" measurements of lifting capacity, muscle strength and endurance, and the use of obstacle courses and other simulations of the work environment. Although it is attractive to think of these work-capacity evaluations as more objective and thus defensible, few have been subjected to any form of rigorous validation. Indeed, the study by Clark et al. showed major variations between independent medical examiners when they were asked to rate the physical capacities of hypothetical patients.[5]

CURRENT LOW BACK IMPAIRMENT RATING SYSTEMS

The goal of all impairment rating systems is an objective system that quantifies the function of the injured body part. This idealized goal has been a major problem in the lumbar spine because of three broad issues. First, classifications of low back disorders into defined pathoanatomic etiologies does not account for the majority of workers with low back complaints (Chapter 3). Therefore, it is very difficult to establish the expected natural history of an uncertain physical condition or the resultant impaired function that could be anticipated from a particular pathologic process or diagnosis. Second, there is broad variation in the self-reported impairment experienced by individual workers. For example, patient A may have complete fusion of the lumbar spine from a spinal operation and yet function quite normally in a job that requires heavy lifting. Patient B, on the other hand, reports nonspecific low back pain and the inability to perform heavy work yet has minimal objective findings to substantiate the complaint. Third, the "objective" measurements utilized in impairment ratings of the spine are subject to a variety of inherent as well as observer errors.

TABLE 16.1

A Typical Form Used to Evaluate the Work Capacity of a Recovering Worker

<u>WORK CAPACITY RATING FORM</u>

Please complete the following items based on your evaluation of any item that you do not believe you can answer should be marked N/A.

In an 8 hour workday, the patient can: (Circle full capacity for each capacity).

										Continuously	With Rests
Sit	1	2	3	4	5	6	7	8	(hrs.)	———	———
Stand	1	2	3	4	5	6	7	8	(hrs.)	———	———
Walk	1	2	3	4	5	6	7	8	(hrs.)	———	———

	Never	Occasionally	Frequently	Continuously
		0% to 33%	34% to 66%	67% to 100%
Lift:				
10 lbs.	———	———	———	———
11–20 lbs.	———	———	———	———
21–50 lbs.	———	———	———	———
51–100 lbs.	———	———	———	———
Carry:				
10 lbs.	———	———	———	———
11–20 lbs.	———	———	———	———
21–50 lbs.	———	———	———	———
51–100 lbs.	———	———	———	———
Bend:	———	———	———	———
Squat:	———	———	———	———
Crawl:	———	———	———	———
Climb:	———	———	———	———
Reach above shoulder level:	———	———	———	———

Patient can use hands for repetitive actions such as:

	Simple Grasping	Pushing & Pulling	Fine Manipulating
Right	__Yes__No	__Yes__No	__Yes__No
Left	__Yes__No	__Yes__No	__Yes__No

Restriction of activities involving:

	None	Mild	Moderate	Total
Unprotected heights	———	———	———	———
Being around moving machinery	———	———	———	———
Exposure to marked changes in temperature and humidity	———	———	———	———
Driving automotive equipment	———	———	———	———
Exposure to dust, fumes & gases	———	———	———	———

Has patient reached a medical end result? _____ If not, when? _____

Date _____ Physician _____

As a result of these problems widely variable impairment ratings are given by different physicians for the same condition or even for the same patient. This general problem has been studied in four different environments. Brand and Lehmann surveyed 69 orthopedists from Iowa and identified wide variations in the usual ratings given for low back conditions.[3] Furthermore, in arriving at their rating the orthopedists were influenced by a variety of factors that theoretically are not part of the impairment process. These factors included personality of the patient, educational level, and social environment. The time lapse between date of injury or surgery and date of the rating was significant, averaging a minimum of 8.9 months following an injury and 9.7 months after an operation. Despite the wide variation in the operational criteria utilized by these examiners, the average impairment was 13% ± 8%. The authors found that the average impairment given in Iowa was remarkably similar to the disability awards given in the Province of Ontario by the

Workmen's Compensation Board (14 ± 11%).[29] Greenwood, in her survey of West Virginia doctors, found similar variations in physicians' practices and the type of rating schedule used.[9] The median low rating was 5%, and the median high was 35%. The mean for all ratings was 12%—again, remarkably similar to Brand and Lehmann's data and also in close correspondence with Burd's data.[4]

A far more comprehensive review of current impairment rating scales was performed by Clark and associates.[5] Their initial survey involved California independent medical examiners (IME), who represent physicians selected by training and experience and who can be considered more experienced in the impairment rating process than IMEs in states that have no qualifying standards. IMEs were asked to give an impairment rating based on hypothetical patient profiles. The variation was from 0 to 70% for the patient profile illustrated in Table 16.2.

In a second round of the survey, real legal reports were compiled so that the examiners had sufficient historic, physical, and radiologic data to assign an impairment rating. Again, unacceptably high variations were identified between examiners.

In the third portion of the study, a list of 82 factors was developed, and IMEs were asked to weight each factor in the order of its significance. Although there was some variation, the level of agreement was much higher, than in the other parts of the study as shown in Table 16.3.

After the factors were refined, the researchers developed a standardized scoring system with limiting criteria such that a yes or no response could be calculated. In the initial new survey intraobserver reliability using standardized case histories was still significant. With refinements and greater explanation of each criterion a resurvey identified reduction in the differences between examiners to 10 to 15 points.

IMPAIRMENT RATING SYSTEMS

The early rating schedules were simple and often based on accident insurance statistics.[16] Rapid evolution then took place in the distinction between impairment and

TABLE 16.2
Disability Rating of the Same Hypothetical Patient by 65 Independent Medical Examiners in a Specialty Dealing with Back Pain

"Assuming a 55-year-old person with uncomplicated laminotomy for disc at L4-5 and a successful L4-S1 fusion, x-rays show mild generalized osteoarthritis at L5-S1 disc space narrowing; operative result considered 'good': one year postoperatively, what do you think the disability rating should be according to our California Disability Evaluation Schedule?"

Number of IMEs selecting	Disability Rating
2	0%
1	10%
4	15%
5	20%
20	25%
13	30%
16	50%
3	60%
1	70%
Total 65	

Reproduced with permission from Clark WL, Haldeman S, Johnson P, et al: Back impairment and disability determination: Another attempt at objective, reliable rating. *Spine* 1988; 13:332.

TABLE 16.3

Weighting by Independent Medical Examiners (n = 73) of Initial List of Factors Considered in Disability Evaluation

Weight*	Factor	Weight*	Factor
History		Laboratory, Roentgenogram, etc. (cont.)	
1.2	History of previous back surgery, such as repeated surgery	2.5	Elevated sedimentation rate or abnormal white blood count and differential
1.5	History of previous back surgery, such as failed fusion	2.7	Disc narrowing increased over that usual for age
1.5	History of previous back surgery, such as disc space infections	2.9	Old compressed fractures
		3.0	Spondylolysis
1.6	History of previous back surgery, such as laminectomy	3.6	Vertebral margin osteophytes
		3.7	Asymmetrical sacralization/lumbarization
1.6	History of previous back surgery, such as fusion	3.7	Abnormal facet tropism
1.7	Pain with aciatic radiation with weight bearing	4.2	Four lumbar vertebrae
1.7	Work is heavy work involving lifting, bending, and twisting	4.3	Spina bifida occulta
		Specialized Tests	
1.7	History of previous back surgery, such as response to previous surgery	1.8	Myelogram "positive"
		1.9	Positive cystometrogram
1.8	History of previous back surgery, such as chymopapain	2.1	CAT scan "positive"
		2.4	EMG "positive"
2.1	History of previous back surgery, such as kind and location of residual pain	2.5	Anatomically reasonable response to differential spinal anesthesia
2.4	Current back pain not relieved by treatment	2.5	Positive response to epidural steroid injection
Laboratory, Roentgenogram, etc.		2.7	Discogram "positive"
1.2	Malignant tumor, primary or metastatic	2.8	Positive response to facet block
1.6	Fracture-dislocation through the intervertebral disc	3.0	Positive response to costovertebral joint block
		3.1	Venogram "positive"
2.1	Positive bone scan	3.1	Positive "bicycle" test
2.2	Positive brucellosis, typhoid, tuberculosis, or syphilis test	3.2	Muscle spasm—by EMG?
		4.7	Thermogram "positive"
2.4	Spondylolisthesis		
2.5	Osteoporosis—hormonal, corticoid		
2.5	Cerebrospinal fluid protein elevated		

*Weighting of "1" indicates factor considered very important, weighting of "5" indicates factor not considered important at all.

Reproduced with permission from Clark WL, Haldeman S, Johnson P, et al: Back impairment and disability determination: Another attempt at objective reliable rating. *Spine* 1988; 13:332.

disability, and the concept of the "whole person" developed. Over the past 50 years subsequent modifications have been evolutionary rather than revolutionary, without major change in fundamental concepts. A series of methods have been developed (Table 16.4) and used to varying degrees,[1,2,13,16,24] most recently the California impairment rating system. The method of the American Medical Association, updated in 1988, is considered the rating system most widely used.

The American Medical Association impairment rating system depends largely on the assessment of range of motion, to which are added modifiers based on pathoanatomic

TABLE 16.4

Comparison of Impairment (Disability) Rating Systems

System*	Symptoms	Range of Motion	Diagnosis	Other Physiologic†	Functional Evaluation
Social Security Disability	X	X		X	
California	X	X	X	X	X
Minnesota			X		
AMA		X	X		

*The "system" represents the individual elements that go into the four impairment ratings. For example, California's system uses all of the elements, whereas Minnesota's is based solely on diagnosis.

†Other physiologic refers to other health conditions which might influence the musculoskeletal complaint.

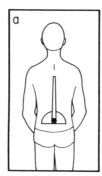 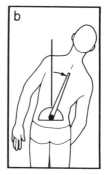

FIG 16.6.
The use of the goniometer in measurement of lateral bend.

diagnosis and surgical treatment. The third group of modifier is the presence of neurologic deficits. A fourth component, used in the rating of "chronic pain syndrome," is psychologic modifiers.

In the 1971 version of the AMA *Guides to the Evaluation of Permanent Impairment,* measurement of motion in the three planes (flexion-extension, rotation, and lateral bending) utilized the goniometer as the measuring instrument (Figure 16.6). The impairment rating derived from these measurements is given in Table 16.5.

TABLE 16.5
Impairment in Dorsolumbar Region as Measured by Trunk Rotation

Restricted Motion
Average range of ROTATION = 60 degrees
Value to total range of motion = 35%

	Degrees of Dorsolumbar Motion		Impairment of Whole Man
	Lost	Retained	
Right rotation from neutral position (0) to:			
0	30	0	5%
10	20	10	4
20	10	20	2
30	0	30	0
Left rotation from neutral position (0) to:			
0	30	0	5%
10	20	10	4
20	10	20	2
30	0	30	0
	Ankylosis		
Region ankylosed at:			
*0 (neutral position)			30%
10			40
20			50
30 (full right rotation)			60
Region akylosed at:			
*0 (neutral position)			30%
10			40
20			50
30 (full left rotation)			60

* position of function
Source, AMA guide to the Evaluation of Permanent Impairment

continued

Two issues are relevant to the measurement of spinal motion: the accuracy and reproducibility of the measurement and how nonmusculoskeletal conditions affect THE MOTION.

MEASUREMENTS OF RANGE OF MOTION

A variety of measurement devices have been utilized for spinal motion, such as fingertip-to-floor measures of spinal flexion, flexible rulers, and the change in length of tape measures placed down the bony spinous processes (Schober test),[6,22] but these methods have not been widely used in impairment rating systems. A more recent alternative is the inclinometer; it has been studied extensively and compared to other commonly used tests.[8,11,12,15,17,23] These comparisons are shown in Table 16.6.[8] The use of the double inclinometer technique is now being recommended or considered in impairment systems. This method separates the component of flexion-extension at the hips from the actual spinal motion. The device can also be used to measure the degree of elevation necessary to produce a positive straight leg raising test. Figures 16.7 and 16.8 show the use of this technique. Because axial rotation cannot be measured with accuracy by any easily standardized and cost-effective method, this measurement has been eliminated from the determination. To be considered reliable, the measurements must be repeated three times and be in agreement within a range of ±5 degrees. A validation criterion is also utilized whereby the sum of hip flexion and hip extension must fall within 10 degrees of the straight leg raising test on the

TABLE 16.5 (*continued*)
Impairment in Dorsolumbar Region as Measured by Lateral Flexion

Restricted Motion
Average range of LATERAL FLEXION (lateral bending) = 40 degrees
Value to total range of dorsolumbar motion = 25%

	Degrees of Dorsolumbar Motion		Impairment of Whole Man
	Lost	Retained	
Right lateral flexion from neutral position (0°) to:			
0°	20	0	4%
10°	10	10	2
20°	0	20	0
Left lateral flexion from neutral position (0°) to:			
0°	20	0	4%
10°	10	10	2
20°	0	20	0
	Ankylosis		
Region anyklosed at:			
*0° (neutral position)			30%
10°			45
20° (full right lat. flex.)			60
Region ankylosed at:			
*0° (neutral position)			30%
10°			45
20° (full left lat. flex.)			60

*position of function
Source: AMA guide to the Evaluation of Permanent Impairment.

TABLE 16.6
Repeatability of Measurements Used in the Determination
of Lumbar Spinal Motion*

Test	Coefficient of Variation	
	Standing	Sitting
Fingertip-to-floor flexion	14.1	—
Modified Schober flexion	0.9	1.5
Modified Schober extension	2.8	2.9
Modified Schober erect	3.2	4.2
Upper inclinometer flexion	33.9	27.3
Upper inclinometer extension	3.6	2.8
Upper inclinometer erect	2.3	4.3
Lower inclinometer flexion	9.3	6.9
Lower inclinometer extension	4.7	4.4
Lower inclinometer erect	1.7	6.2
Hip angle flexion	2.9	6.7
Hip angle extension	0.7	1.8
Hip angle erect	1.7	1.5
Lumbar spine angle flexion	6.0	22.3
Lumbar spine angle extension	12.4	11.3
Lumbar spine angle erect	7.0	10.8

* Repeatability is expressed as the coefficient of variation
Reproduced with permission from Gill K, Krag MH, Johnson GB, et al: Repeatability of four
clinical methods for assessment of lumbar spinal motion. *Spine* 1988; 13:50.

tightest side. An example of impairment, from loss of spinal flexion is determined by the
1988 AMA guidelines, is shown in Table 16.5.

One problem with joint motion evaluation is that it can be influenced by pain and the
"pain experience," by subject motivation, and by psychologic factors.[7,21,30] Patients who
have elevation of certain MMPI scores have less motion than patients who do not have these
elevations. The Waddell signs,[25] abnormal pain drawings,[20] and other measures of illness
behavior and psychosocial distress may help to clarify some of these contributors to reduced
spinal motion. The influence of nonorganic factors on functional testing is acknowledged in
Appendix B of the 1988 *Guides to the Evaluation of Permanent Impairment*. How to use

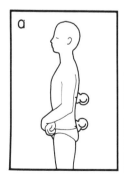 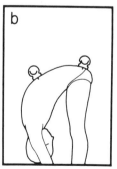 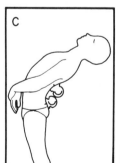 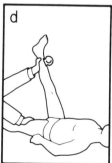

FIG 16.7.
The use of the inclinometer in **(a)** the neutral position, **(b)** flexion, **(c)** extension, and **(d)** straight leg
raising. *Guides to the Evaluation of Permanent Impairment,* ed 3. Chicago, American Medical Association, 1988. Used by permission.)

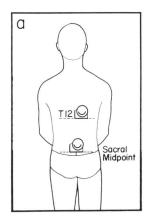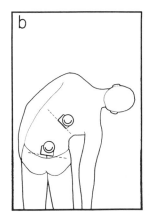

FIG 16.8
The use of the inclinometer in the measurement of lateral bend. Notice that the position of the two inclinometers at T12 and the sacral midpoint are the same in flexion and extension. (From *Guides to the Evaluation of Permanent Impairment,* ed 3. Chicago, American Medical Association, 1988.)

these mental and behavioral conditions in assigning impairment is less clear, although the AMA guide visualizes them as occurring along a continuum, as shown in Table 16.7.

DIAGNOSED PATHOANATOMIC CRITERIA

The other component of the AMA guide is the diagnostic-related criteria, which are restricted to a limited number of pathoanatomic conditions. The type of treatment and the result of that treatment are also considered. This information is displayed in Table 16.8.

The California system evolved from analyzing how independent medical examiners rate individual patients and the generation of weighted factors that most correspond to how

TABLE 16.7
Impairment Due to Mental and Behavioral Disorders

Areas of Function	Class 1 No Impairment	Class 2 Mild Impairment
Activities of Daily Living	No impairments noted	Impairment levels compatible with most useful function
Social Functioning		
Concentration		
Adaptation		

Class 3 Moderate Impairment	Class 4 Marked Impairment	Class 5 Extreme Impairment
Impairment levels compatible with some but not all useful function	Impairment levels significantly impede useful function	Impairment levels preclude useful function

Reproduced with permission from American Medical Association: *Guides to the Evaluation of Permanent Impairment,* ed 3. Chicago, 1988.

TABLE 16.8

Disorder	% Impairment of Whole Person		
	Cerv	Thor	Lumb
I. Fractures			
A. Compression of one vertebral body			
0%–25%	4	2	5
26%–50%	6	3	7
>50%	10	5	12
B. Fracture of posterior elements (pedicles, laminae, articular processes, or transverse processes)	4	2	5
Note: Impairments due to compression of the vertebral body and to fractures of the posterior elements are combined using the Combined Values Chart.			
Note: When two or more vertebrae are compressed or fractured, combine all impairment values.			
C. Reduced dislocation of one vertebra	5	3	6
Note: If two or more vertebrae are dislocated and reduced, combine the impairment values using the Combined Values Chart.			
Note: An unreduced dislocation causes temporary impairment until it is reduced; then the physician should evaluate permanent impairment on the basis of the subject's condition with the reduced dislocation. If no reduction is possible, then the physician should evaluate impairment on the basis of restricted motion and concomitant neurological findings in the spinal region involved, according to the criteria in this Chapter and in Chapter 4.			
II. Intervertebral disc or other soft tissue lesions			
A. Unoperated, with no residuals	0	0	0
B. Unoperated with medically documented injury and a minimum of six months of medically documented pain, recurrent muscle spasm or rigidity associated with none-to-minimal degenerative changes on structural tests	4	2	5
C. Unoperated, with medically documented injury and a minimum of six months of medically documented pain, recurrent muscle spasm, or rigidity associated with moderate to severe degenerative changes on structural tests, including unoperated herniated nucleus pulposus, with or without radiculopathy	6	3	7
D. Surgically treated disc lesion, with no residuals	7	4	8
E. Surgically treated disc lesion, with residual symptoms	9	5	10
F. Multiple operative levels, with or without residual symptomatology	Add 1%/level		
G. Multiple operations ("failed back surgery") with or without residual symptoms:			
1. Second operation	Add 2%		
2. Third or subsequent surgery	Add 1%/operation		
III. Spondylolysis and spondylolisthesis, unoperated			
A. Spondylolysis or Grade I (1%–25% slippage) or Grade II (26%–50% slippage) spondylolisthesis, accompanied by medically documented injury and a minimum of six months of medically documented pain, recurrent muscle spasm, or rigidity	7	4	8
B. Grade III (51%–75% slippage) or Grade IV (76%–100% slippage) spondylolisthesis, accompanied by medically documented injury and a minimum of six months of medically documented pain, recurrent muscle spasm, or rigidity	9	5	10
IV. Spinal stenosis, segmental instability, or spondylolisthesis, operated			
A. Single level operation, with no residuals	8	4	9
B. Single level operation, with residual symptoms	10	5	12
C. Multiple levels operated, with residual symptoms	Add 1%/level		
D. Multiple operations ("failed back surgery") with residual symptoms:			
1. Second operation	Add 2%		
2. Third or subsequent surgery	Add 1%/operation		

Note: List impairments separately for cervical, thoracic, and lumbar regions (Figures 83a–c).
Note: All impairment ratings above should be combined with the appropriate values of residuals, such as:
1. Ankylosis (fusion) in the spinal area or extremities
2. Abnormal motion in the spinal area (i.e., objectively measured rigidity) or extremities
3. Spinal cord and spinal nerve root injuries, with neurologic impairment (see Upper Extremity and Lower Extremity sections of Chapter 3 and Peripheral Nervous System section of Chapter 4)
4. Any combination of the above using the Combined Values Chart.
Reproduced with permission from American Medical Association: *Guides to the Evaluation of Permanent Impairment*, ed 3. Chicago, 1988.

IMEs actually analyze impairment. The final list of factors is shown in Table 16.9. This method depends minimally on calculations of range of motion, being more heavily weighted to clinical, radiographic, and diagnostic-related criteria. The validation of this method and its widespread utility has yet to be established, but it represents a new and potentially important departure from historic methods.

IMPORTANT FACTORS IN THE RATING OF LOW BACK IMPAIRMENT

Lehmann and Brand[14] recommended an overall approach to rating low back impairment that is based on the following facts.

1. The likelihood of return to work decreases with increasing time after injury.
2. Patients *and* doctors misunderstand current rating systems, which leads to wide variability.

TABLE 16.9
Proposed Listing of Factors with Point Scores for Low-back Impairment Rating

Factor No.	Points	Factor*	Factor No.	Points	Factor*
History			**Roentgenograms**		
1.	5	Moderate/severe pain more than 90 days	16.	1	L4–L5 disc space narrower than L3–L4
2.	3	2 disabling attacks in previous 5 years	17.	3	Spondylolisthesis, Grade 1 or more
3a.	5	Surgery, "good result"	18.	1	Segmental instability/7% translation
3b.	10	Surgery, significant residuals	19.	5	Severe spinal stenosis
4.	5	History of strenuous work 5 years	**EMG**		
Present Complaints			20a.	10	Moderate/markedly positive EMG
5.	5	Radicular pattern leg pain now	20b.	5	Slightly positive EMG
6.	3	Moderate/severe pain with long standing/sitting/driving	20c.	0	Questionably positive EMG
Physical Examination			**Work Capacity Evaluation**		
7.	2	Anatomically logical tenderness/pain	21a.	5	Lifting capacity decreased 25%
			21b.	10	Lifting capacity decreased 50%
8.	5	Restricted standing lumbar flexion	22.	5	Cardiovascular fitness below 25th percentile
9a.	5	Extension or lateral bending prevented by pain	**Neurogenic Disease Disorder**		
9b.	2	Extension or lateral bending causing pain	23.	3	Arachnoiditis with symptoms
10.	3	Legs dysfunction producing abnormal back motion	24a.	10	Neurogenic claudication
11.	10	Straight-leg raising positive	24b.	15	Neurogenic claudication and confirming electrodiagnostic studies
12.	3	Deep tendon reflex reduction			
13.	2	Hypoesthesia, anatomical pattern	25a.	10	Partial bowel/bladder incontinence
14a.	2	Minimal muscle weakness	25b.	5	Bladder retention requiring catheterization
14b.	3	Slight/moderate muscle weakness			
14c.	5	Moderate muscle weakness	26a.	3	Minor reflex sympathetic dystrophy
14d.	10	Severe muscle weakness	26b.	10	Major reflex sympathetic dystrophy
15a.	5	Trunk extensor muscles weaker than trunk flexors	**Modifying Factors**		
			M1(a).	5	Correlating MRI/myelogram/CAT scan
15b.	−5	Trunk extensor muscles stronger than trunk flexors	M1(b).	−5	Negative myelogram/CAT scan/MRI
			M2.	−10	If one or more of (a) positive Waddell test, (b) pain drawing score 3, (c) multiple previous injury litigation, (d) chronic intractable benign pain syndrome. NOTE: Psychological evaluation may be appropriate.

* Factors are listed in brief. Full definitions of each factor will be sent on request.
Reproduced with permission from Clark WL, Haldeman S, Johnson P, et al: Back impairment and disability determination: Another attempt at objective reliable rating. *Spine* 1988; 13:332.

3. Because many instances of low back pain do not have a ready pathoanatomic diagnosis, decisions are often deferred in the hope that the problem will resolve with time.
4. The treating doctor often has difficulty telling a patient he has a 10% impairment when the individual has been out of work for two years and feels he is 100% disabled.

When approaching the patient for an impairment rating, four critical elements should be kept in mind: (1) Early medical decisions are necessary, (2) delay in administrative decisions should be avoided, (3) frank, open discussion should be initiated with the patient about his or her medical condition and the disability process, and (4) the patient must understand both the patient's role and the doctor's role in the disability process. To this approach should be added a commitment of all parties (doctors, patient's insurers) to early rehabilitation when the patient is failing to recover as expected. The patient should be made aware that a "healing period" exists and that progress will be measured against that expectation. Doctors should carefully explain alternatives for surgical intervention, when appropriate indications exist, and educate the patient about how healing will progress postoperatively. The pitfall of seeking multiple opinions and performing numerous tests can significantly delay this process, so we advocate a single carefully modulated definitive workup whenever possible. Although this process does not make the actual impairment rating more reliable, it does create an environment and "tempo" in which the patient's expectations can be tempered with reality and the doctor-patient relationship can be preserved.

SUMMARY

In this chapter we have traced the history of workers' compensation laws, evaluated some of the practical and philosophic issues in the impairment rating process, and attempted to establish the treating physician's role in managing the patient and the process. It is clear that impairment rating is far from an exact science, although newer measuring systems and scales appear to be reducing the wide discrepancies that exist between examiners. In this process the treating physician can reduce some of the delay and confusion by the careful management of the "tempo" of treatment and by open, honest discussion of the nature of impairment rating with the patient.

BIBLIOGRAPHY

1. American Academy of Orthopaedic Surgeons: *Manual for Orthopaedic Surgeons in Evaluating Permanent Impairment*. Chicago, American Academy of Orthop. Surgeons, 1966.
2. American Medical Association: *Guides to the Evaluation of Permanent Impairment,* ed 3. Chicago, American Medical Association, 1988.
3. Brand RA, Lehmann TR: Low back impairment rating practices of orthopaedic surgeons. *Spine* 1983; 8:75.
4. Burd JG: The educated guess: Doctors and permanent partial disability percentage. *J Tenn Med Assoc* 1980; 73:441.
5. Clark WL, Haldeman S, Johnson P, et al: Back impairment and disability determination: Another attempt at objective, reliable rating. *Spine* 1988; 13:332.

6. Frost M, Stuckey S, Smalley LA, et al: Reliability of measuring trunk motion in centimeters. *Phys Ther* 1982; 62:1431.

7. Frymoyer JW, Rosen JC, Clements J, et al: Psychologic factors in low-back pain disability. *Clin Orthop* 1985; 195:178.

8. Gill K, Krag MH, Johnson GB, et al: Repeatability of four clinical methods for assessment of lumbar spinal motion. *Spine* 1988; 13:50.

9. Greenwood JG: Low-back impairment-rating practices of orthopaedic surgeons and neurosurgeons in West Virginia. *Spine* 1985; 10:773.

10. Haddad GH: Analysis of 2,932 workers' compensation back injury cases: The impact on the cost to the system. *Spine* 1987; 12:765.

11. Hart FD, Strickland D, Cliffe P: Measurement of spinal mobility. *Ann Rheum Dis* 1974; 33:136.

12. Keeley J, Mayer TG, Cox R, et al: Quantification of lumbar function. Part 5. Reliability of range of motion measures in the sagittal plane and an in vivo torso rotation measurement technique. *Spine* 1986; 11:31.

13. Kessler HH: *Disability Determination and Evaluation.* Philadelphia, Lea and Febiger, 1970.

14. Lehmann TR, Brand RA: Disability in the patient with low back pain. *Orthop Clin N Amer* 1982; 13:559.

15. Loebl WK: Measurements of spinal posture and range in spinal movements. *Ann Phys Med* 1967; 9:103.

16. McBride E: *Disability Evaluation.* Philadelphia, Lippincott, 1963.

17. Mayer TG, Tencer AF, Kristoferson S, et al: Use of noninvasive techniques for quantification of spinal range of motion in normal subjects and chronic low back dysfunction patients. *Spine* 1984; 9:588.

18. Mixter WJ, Barr JS: Rupture of the intervertebral disc with involvement of the spinal canal. *N Engl J Med* 1934; 211:210.

19. National Institute for Occupational Safety and Health: *Proposed National Strategies for the Prevention of Leading Work-Related Diseases and Injuries: Musculoskeletal injuries.* Assoc of Schools of Public Health, National Institute for Occupational Safety and Health, Cincinnati, OH, Report #DHHS/PUB/NIOSH-89-129 1986.

20. Ransford AO, Cairns D, Mooney V: The pain drawing as an aid to the psychologic evaluation of patients with low-back pain. *Spine* 1976; 1:127.

21. Ritter MA, McAdoo WG: A method for determining success following total hip replacement surgery. *Clin Orthop* 1979; 141:44.

22. Schober P: Lendenwirbelsaule und Kreuzschmerzen. *Munch Med Wochenschr* 1937; 84:336.

23. Troup JDG, Hood CA, Chapman AE: Measurements of sagittal mobility of the lumbar spine and hips. *Ann Phys Med* 1968; 9:308.

24. US Bureau of Disability Insurance: *Disability Evaluation Under Social Security. A Handbook for Physicians.* US Government Printing Office, Washington, DC, 1970.

25. Waddell G, McCulloch JA, Kummel E, et al: Nonorganic physical signs in low-back pain. *Spine* 1980; 5:117.

26. Weber H: Lumbar disc herniation. A prospective study of prognostic factors including a controlled trial. Part I. *J Oslo City Hosp* 1978; 28:33.

27. Weber H: Lumbar disc herniation. A prospective study of prognostic factors including a controlled trial. Part II. *J Oslo City Hosp* 1978; 28:89.

28. Weber H: Lumbar disc herniation: A controlled prospective study with ten years of observation. *Spine* 1983; 8:131.

29. White AVM: Low back pain in men receiving workmen's compensation. *Can Med Assoc J* 1969; 101:61.

30. Wise A, Jackson D, Rocchio P: Preoperative psychologic testing as a predictor of success in knee surgery. A preliminary report. *Am J Sports Med* 1979; 7:287.

17

Workers' Compensation

John D. Kemp
Malcolm H. Pope, Dir. Med. Sc., Ph.D.

HISTORY

Worker's compensation laws represent social legislation that creates a compromise between the right of the injured worker to sue an employer and the right of the employer to use common-law defenses against the employee. Each state and federal law is written with the intent that it shall be construed liberally in favor of the injured worker.

Before the present system was introduced, workers who suffered injuries on the job had to sue their employers to recover lost wages and medical expenses. Employers used the common-law defenses of contributory negligence, assumption of risk, and the fellow-servant rule (the negligence of an employee is not passed to the employer).[7]

The consequences of the old system were unsatisfactory in the burgeoning economy of the United States in the late nineteenth century. Employees were required to prove the negligence of their employers, often an expensive and time-consuming legal battle. Often the worker could not afford these expenses, and if the employee won the case, the amount recovered was usually small. From that award, attorney's fees were deducted and medical bills paid. It was also common for an injured worker who won the legal battle to lose his or her job. Those who lost their legal battles often became burdens on their families and society. Employers were also unhappy and considered the system disruptive and expensive. Although the system provided them with strong defenses against many of the claims, it left them guessing about their true exposure in any situation involving an injury to a worker.

The movement toward industrialization brought ever-greater pressure on society to change the system. In 1884, Germany passed the Sickness and Accident Law, the modern foundation for workers' compensation laws. A number of other European countries followed suit before the United States passed its first attempt at a workers' compensation law. Unlike other nations, the United States adopted laws state by state rather than on a national basis.

A number of workers' compensation laws were tested in the U.S. courts for constitutionality. The issues litigated concerned the loss of the rights of the parties to a liability suit. Both the plaintiffs and the defendants compromised their legal rights in exchange for a quick, reliable, and, for the most part, fair solution to an injured worker's medical and financial problems.

In the early part of the century many occupations were excluded from coverage in the United States.[12] The types of injury and disease covered were narrowly defined. Injuries had to arise out of and occur in the course of employment.[6] Injuries not caused by a specific accident were not covered. A worker whose back injury was the result of continuous trauma would not be compensated. Many diseases were arbitrarily excluded. In 1973, however, the report of the National Commission on State Workmen's Compensation Laws[13] recommended that states should have both medical and claim benefits unlimited as to duration and sum.

WORKERS' COMPENSATION BENEFITS

Claim

A common problem for injured workers is their relative lack of knowledge about workers' compensation benefits. Since 1960, unions have been making a concerted effort to inform members of their rights. Attorneys began representing large numbers of injured workers, and many court decisions have liberalized the application of the law. Although many states require employers to help injured workers understand their benefits, most workers look to physicians, friends, or attorneys to help them determine "what they should get."[16] The increase in the number of lawyers, state-assisted legal aid programs, and worker sophistication has made legal help more available.

Temporary Total (TT) Benefits

A worker who sustains a compensable injury or disease is entitled to compensation for wages lost as a result of the injury or disease. A waiting period of three to six days is usually required, but the benefit is then payable from the first day of injury in most states. The TT benefit is equal to two-thirds of the injured worker's salary up to a maximum set by law. Some states tie the maximum to the state's average weekly wage; others set the amount by statute. In 1982, maximum temporary benefits ranged from $112 per week in Mississippi to $940 per week in Alaska.[18] Since 1975, many states have been changing their maximum benefit annually to keep pace with inflation.

Temporary total benefits are payable for as long as a person is totally disabled and for as long as the condition has not been declared permanent. The nature of back injuries makes it difficult to determine when a condition has become permanent. As a consequence, employers and insurance companies are anxious to have doctors report any change in status as soon as that information is available.

Permanent Partial (PP) Benefits

When an injured worker, in the opinion of the attending physician, will not improve further, but a partial disability remains, the worker may be entitled to a permanent partial benefit. These benefits have been a source of controversy since their inception.

Permanent partial benefits are usually classified as scheduled or nonscheduled. Scheduled benefits require a physician to rate the permanence of an injury in terms of percentage loss of function of that body part. The doctor's estimate is applied to the state schedules, and an award is calculated. Despite many attempts to simplify the administration of this benefit, tremendous variations exist in benefits paid for very similar injuries.[8] Rating the loss of function "to the body as a whole" is a difficult if not impossible task, yet it is one routinely demanded of doctors treating back-injured workers.[13] This problem is discussed in detail from a medical perspective in Chapter 16.

Nonscheduled permanent partial benefits attempt to compensate an injured worker for an earnings impairment as opposed to a physical impairment. These benefits may be based on actual lost wages, on an estimate of lost earning capacity, or on the degree of disability.[8]

Florida has made an attempt to defuse the PP problem by using the concept of wage loss. A number of states, including Louisiana and Pennsylvania, have a loss-of-earning-capacity provision, but it is more closely tied to loss of function than actual loss of earning capacity. Florida also requires that rehabilitation services be provided for disabled workers who are unable to do their usual and customary work. Following rehabilitation services, benefits are paid as necessary to make up the difference between the average wages earned prior to the injury and the average earned after rehabilitation. Although this benefit is touted as being infinitely more fair to the injured worker and the employer, catastrophic injuries may pose special problems. For example, a paraplegic who is rehabilitated and goes to work as a computer programmer may earn the same amount of money she did prior to the injury. The insured worker would be entitled to no further wage loss benefits despite the fact that she may have to hire someone to paint the house or mow the lawn, both tasks having been well within the disabled person's capabilities prior to the injury.

Temporary Partial (TP) Benefits

The concept of wage loss is not new. Most states require that compensation be paid to injured employees who return to work at wages less than preinjury wages. This benefit provides an incentive for LBP patients to attempt part-time or slower-paced work. Unfortunately, the incentive is frequently overlooked. Doctors who are anxious to have their disabled but clinically improving patients return to some type of activity should consider this benefit. In most states, injured workers who return to a job with lower wages are entitled to two-thirds of the difference between preinjury and postinjury wages up to a maximum normally equal to their temporary total rate. The nontaxable benefit is usually paid when proof of earnings is submitted.

There are a number of ways to employ this benefit in helping low back-injured patients return to work. A worker may be released to return to work the normal number of hours but with frequent or prolonged rest breaks; another option is to have a shorter work week to allow the worker to recover. Yet another way is to return the injured worker to a lighter or modified job. The worker may earn less than before the injury, but modified work may strengthen the muscles and confidence while reducing the worker's financial burden. Doctors who consider helping their patients back to light or modified work are encouraged to seek information about such jobs directly from the employer or from the insurance company.

Although familiarity with the job site is preferable, a detailed job description should provide the physician with sufficient information to judge the appropriateness of the work. Recommendations for changes in the job should be made, when needed, to allow injured workers to return to the safest possible job. The job should be one that allows the patient to return to work as quickly as possible.

Permanent Total Disability (PTD) Benefits

Workers whose injuries permanently preclude their return to employment are entitled to PTD benefits. In some states, the injury must rule out a return to customary employment. In other states, it must preclude a return to any job for which the injured worker is qualified. Still other states mandate that a worker may be entitled to PTD benefits if rehabilitation services are unsuccessful in returning a disabled worker to work.

Many disability cases can have successful outcomes if the doctor, employee, employer, and insurance carrier work together. Too many back injury cases are ignored until the injured worker's chances of returning to work are nonexistent. A worker who believes he or she is permanently disabled usually does not return to work! (The point is stressed in Chapter 7.)

PTD cases are serious social and economic problems in the United States. Injured workers receive a periodic payment equal to a percentage of the preinjury wages. In some states this payment includes a cost-of-living increase. Many who have been declared permanently totally disabled are also eligible for Social Security disability income. The two benefits together have been assumed to make such a worker financially secure. Although that may be true, many of these "secure" people suffer from the emotional trauma that follows when a person is labeled permanently and totally "useless" in the working community. It is a challenge for both the workers' compensation system and the injured workers. Employers, doctors, lawyers, insurance companies, and legislators have failed to come to grips with the problem.

VOCATIONAL REHABILITATION

Vocation rehabilitation merits serious consideration by the injuried worker, employer, treating physician, and insurance carrier. The benefit is not limited to long-term training programs. It may involve counseling and assistance in developing job-seeking skills. It may involve a counselor working with an injured worker to identify a work-hardening program or to define interesting job opportunities within the worker's capabilities. On-the-job training may become the first step in a new career. These vocational rehabilitation services may be tailored to the injured worker's special set of circumstances.

Most people identify with the work ethic.[14] Injured workers who receive compensation benefits are stigmatized, at least in their own minds, because they are not part of the work force and are, therefore, outside the dominant segment of the community. Sometimes the failure to consider work as therapy results in the need for psychologic and psychiatric treatment.[15]

Even in states where vocational rehabilitation benefits are not widely publicized, most insurance companies are able to provide rehabilitation services for an injured worker who is unable to return to the usual employment but may be able to perform other types of duties.

MEDICAL BENEFITS

All workers' compensation laws provide for medical care for compensable injuries. Many states qualify which medical expenses must be paid with phrases such as "reasonable and necessary," "to cure and relieve," "tend to lessen the period of disability," and "usual and customary." Medical professionals dealing with workers' compensation cases for the first time may find the law arbitrary.

Generally, bills for standard medical and surgical treatments are paid at a rate that approximates the average within that community. New experimental techniques are challenged, as are fees substantially above the norm. In some states, for example, the employer or insurer may challenge repeated back surgery as excessive. In most states, a hearing may be held with the workers' compensation administrator to decide the appropriateness of the additional surgery. Although relatively few such cases occur, it is important to be aware of the potential in some jurisdictions for medical services to be challenged by the insurer.

Since the first workers' compensation laws were passed the list of approved medical services and providers has grown substantially. Medical doctors, podiatrists, chiropractors, physical therapists, psychotherapists, nurses, and many more specialists are reimbursed directly for services provided to injured workers. Arkansas, Connecticut, and Delaware are among a short list of states that recognize treatment by prayer or spiritual means!

A small number of states allow the employer or insurance carrier to choose the doctor who will provide services. In these states, an employee who chooses a doctor other than the one designated may be required to pay for the services (except in emergency situations). Georgia is one such state.

New York is an example of the opposite end of the spectrum. It is a misdemeanor for an employer or insurer to interfere with an injured worker's right to free choice of medical doctors. Most state laws fall somewhere in between these two extremes.

In every state the insurance carriers maintain the right to obtain an independent medical examination. These examinations have become a routine part of workers' compensation claims for low back pain. Attending physicians who are frustrated by chronic low back conditions often welcome an additional opinion.

Unfortunately, many independent medical examinations are said to be biased.[6] Reportedly, it has been common in Florida, for example, for a workers' compensation supervisor to find a "hired gun" to offset the opinion of a liberal physician concerning the extent of disability. Doctors were categorized and used for claims litigation by both sides. Ultimately, a judge would weigh both opinions and make a decision as to the percentage of disability to be used to calculate a permanent partial benefit award. Florida's law was substantially revised in 1979 to end the battle-zone mentality of workers' compensation claims administration, but a number of other states continue to operate in a litigious manner.

Generally, acute care for injured workers is covered by workers' compensation insurance without question if the claim is compensable under the law. That is, unless there is a question about whether the injury occurred within the jurisdiction of the workers' compensation law, acute care coverage is virtually guaranteed. Services such as ambulance transportation, emergency room care, first aid, doctors' office visits, and medication are paid without question for compensable injuries.

Coverage for chronic care is less straightforward. The patient who has undergone various conservative medical treatments and surgical intervention may find that the employer or insurer is beginning to scrutinize medical reports and bills. Doctors may be asked to be more specific about a prognosis or about the necessity of certain medications or tests. The chronicity of the patient's condition becomes the focal point of the frustrations of insurers and doctors.[4]

Medical rehabilitation is generally payable if it is provided or prescribed by a medical doctor. Rehabilitation hospitals may be regarded as an appropriate step after acute care. Outpatient physical and occupational therapy for a back-injured worker may also be strongly encouraged, at the appropriate time, following back surgery. Memberships at YMCAs have been paid to allow a back-injured person an opportunity to use swimming as physical therapy. Rarely, a low back injury is so severe that it involves a variety of overwhelming symptoms, in which case attendant care may be necessary.

Medical supplies and equipment such as braces and transcutaneous electric nerve stimulation (TENS) prescribed by a medical doctor to provide for a compensable injury are usually paid for under workers' compensation policies. Similarly, medications necessary for the treatment of injuries are covered under workers' compensation law. Although this provision may seem rather obvious, there is a considerable grey area. Consider, for example, a low back injury that requires long-term use of a certain medication. The medication may cause side effects that require additional treatment. It is relatively common for patients with long-term chronic back problems to experience reactive depression. Antidepressive drugs are covered by workers' compensation if the depression is linked to the back injury.

Psychiatric and psychologic care associated with LBP are covered under almost every workers' compensation law. The law requires that the employer or insurer must accept an injured worker as is. If preexisting emotional problems are exacerbated by a compensable workers' compensation injury, then treatment is covered.[19]

Another medical expense is reimbursement for travel care. Each state has its own set of rules about what travel to receive medical care is paid and at what rate. Generally, reasonable travel and other expenses for covered medical service are reimbursed to the injured worker. A low back-injured worker referred to an outpatient clinic some distance from home may receive an advance for mileage, meals, and room expenses, as appropriate.

INJURY TYPES

A wide variety of causes for LBP have been discussed in previous chapters of the book. A single trauma, cumulative trauma, disease, and psychologic strain may all relate to LBP. At one time, a compensable back injury was one related to a specific accident. Over the years, the scope of compensable injuries has grown considerably. Today, workers with LBP primarily caused by aging or disease are receiving workers' compensation benefits because their condition was "made worse" by their work.[1]

THE CLAIMS PROCESS

The injured worker must make a report to the employer to be compensated. At one time the injuries that were not reported within a specific time period following the accident were not compensable. If it can be shown that the employee's failure to notify the employer prejudiced the employer's case or that the employee intended to mislead the employer, the claim may be barred.[19] The courts are more lenient today, but it is always advisable to report all injuries as soon as possible.

The second step in this process is the employer's report to the insurance company. *Insurance company* is used here to refer both to companies that provide insurance coverages and companies that provide only claim services. The difference lies in the answer to the question, "Who actually pays the claim?" If insurance is provided, the insurance company pays the claim. If only service is provided, the employer is self-insured and pays all claims.

The 1973 report of the National Commission on State Workers' Compensation Laws provided the impetus for many states to impose penalties for errors in claim processing caused by late reporting.[13] Employers who fail to file reports quickly may be fined in some states if the insurance carrier had received no notice of the injury.

Rehabilitation services should be provided as needed to accomplish the highest-priority outcome.[11] First, workers should be helped to return to the same job with the same employer. Often, a misunderstanding of the requirements of the job results in a failure to consider this option. A poorly written or loosely interpreted job description may cause the attending physician to rule out heavy lifting, excessive bending or stooping, and the like.

The second priority is to return the employee to the same employer in a similar job or perhaps a modification of the same job, using reasonable accommodation principles promoting the employment of persons with disabilities. On-the-job training with the same employer should be considered at this stage of rehabilitation. An employee who knows the physical plant and the people generally experiences a less stressful return to work. An employer who takes back an injured worker avoids the costly training period that inevitably takes place with all new employees.

The third priority is to search for a similar job with a new employer. An injured worker who can use transferable skills to return to work experiences less turmoil than does the worker requiring formal training. This alternative may require a slight job modification, but such expenses can be paid as a vocational rehabilitation expense, particularly if the benefit-to-cost ratio is considered.

The fourth priority is to utilize on-the-job training with a new employer. If an injured worker has specialized skills and experiences, a new company may be anxious to employ him or her. It is ironic that a worker who may be considered marginal or worse by one employer may be very highly rated by a new employer.

The fifth priority involves extensive evaluation and consideration of available jobs requiring formal training. Such training may be accomplished at a technical school, a college, or special skill-training programs set up by a government agency. In addition to the other difficulties, an injured worker frequently completes a formal training program only to find that jobs are not readily available for that particular skill. Rehabilitation plans that involve formal training should be geared to provide the injured worker with skills that make the worker a good candidate in fields that have openings.

DOCUMENTING CONTINUING DISABILITY

A claim supervisor or adjuster must periodically document the file to substantiate continued payments. In several states, a worker who is no longer disabled but refuses to return to work may have a right to a hearing before compensation benefits are discontinued. A hearing may take several months to schedule.

At each review all involved parties should optimize return to work with the hierarchy of structures given above.

LITIGATION

Workers' compensation was designed to be a nonadversarial social program. An injured worker would report an injury to the employer, and the employer would report it to an insurance company for prompt payment. In fact, the system does work well for most injured workers and appears to be equitable for most injuries.

Litigation of workers' compensation claims has increased sharply over the past 15 years. A study by the California Workers' Compensation Institute was conducted in response to a 20% increase in litigation from 1973 to 1974.[16] The study showed that the most critical element in reducing litigation was information. Most injured workers went to an attorney because they felt they did not properly understand their state's workers' compensation system. The increase in complexity of workers' compensation laws has left many people, including doctors, confused about what benefits an injured worker should receive. In an effort to protect themselves, injured workers turn to lawyers. What some injured workers do not realize, however, is that the attorney's fees represent a significant percentage of the settlement.

Workers' compensation issues usually are litigated at first in an administrative forum with the possibility of appeal in the state's judicial system. A hearing officer or commissioner may decide cases in an informal manner. The appellate procedure may on occasion travel to the state's highest court. Considerable "new law" is made annually from these judicial decisions, which complicates the issue.

CLOSING FILES

There is considerable pressure to close workers' compensation cases as soon as possible. Large employers are liable for additional workers' compensation premiums based on estimates of claims and medical benefits to be paid on a case. Employers and insurance companies have come to realize that the longer an injured worker is paid compensation benefits, the more difficult it is for that person ever to return to work.

The usual closing of a file involves the injured worker recovering and returning to work. In some cases, the worker may be entitled to permanent partial benefits for loss of function. If the injured worker is found able to return to work but refuses to do so, the file may be closed because no further disability exists.[12] Cases may also be closed because an injured worker dies of injuries or disease unrelated to the workers' compensation case.

Other files are closed as a result of settlements. Cases may be settled as a compromise of a question of compensability or to provide the injured worker with capital to begin self-employment. Most files settled in this manner terminate the insurance company's liability for claims or medical benefits.

A number of states bar settlements of some or all types of benefits. California, for example, does not recognize settlement of vocational rehabilitation benefits. In some cases where settlements were arranged, injured workers subsequently were awarded rehabilitation benefits that included a weekly check equal to temporary total benefits. Thus, an inequity arose that allowed the injured worker to collect benefits twice.

SUMMARY

A growing problem with workers' compensation laws is that the injured worker tends to be unaware of the complexities of the system. A worker who sustains a compensable low back injury may receive temporary total benefits. This benefit is equal to two-thirds of the injured worker's salary up to a maximum defined by law. If a partial disability remains and there is no likelihood of further improvement, the patient may be entitled to a permanent partial benefit. Some jurisdictions use the concept of lost wages or lost earning capacity. Temporary partial benefits are designed to provide an incentive for chronic LBP patients to return to lighter work. Permanent total disability benefits are available for workers with low back injuries that permanently preclude a return to work. Medical rehabilitation and vocational rehabilitation benefits are usually paid at the average rate in the community. Acute care is usually covered without dispute. Continued disability must be documented. Insurance carriers exert considerable pressure to close workers' compensation cases as soon as possible.

BIBLIOGRAPHY

1. Burton CV: Conservative management of low back pain. *Low Back Pain* 1981; 168–183.
2. Crain L (ed): Aging, not job, causes many claims for cumulative trauma. *Business Insurance* 1978; ?:26.
3. Deneen LJ: Five studies/five sources. Presented at National American Personnel and Guidance Association Convention, Las Vegas, 1979.
4. Enelow AJ: The compensable injury. *Cal Med* 1967; 106:179–82.
5. Hirschfeld AH, Behan RC: The accident process. I. Etiological considerations of industrial injuries. *JAMA* 1963; 196:193–199.
6. Horowitz SB: *Injury and Death Under Workmen's Compensation Laws.* Boston, Wright & Potter Printing Co, 1944.
7. Larson A: *Workmen's Compensation for Occupational Injuries and Death.* New York, Matthew Bender, 1979.
8. Larson A: *The Law of Workmen's Compensation.* New York, Matthew Bender, 1982.
9. Linde S: *How to Beat a Bad Back.* New York, Rawson, Wade Publishers, 1980.
10. Lloyd D (ed): *Workers' Compensation Law Review,* vol 5. Buffalo, NY, William S Hein & Co, 1980.
11. Mattingly L: Role of the private rehabilitation supplier. Presented at the Institute of Continuing Legal Education Company. Atlanta, Ga, April, 1983.
12. Millus AJ, Gentile WJ: *Workers' Compensation Law and Insurance.* New York, Roberts Publishing Corp, 1976.
13. Mitchell FL: *Some Medical Issues in Workmen's Compensation. Supplemental Studies for the National Commission on State Workmen's Compensation Laws,* vol 2. Govt Printing Office, Washington, DC, 1973, 354–362.
14. Nemiah JC: Psychological complications in industrial injuries. *Arch Environ Health* 1963; 7:481–86.
15. Rubin SE, Roessler RT: Guidelines for successful vocational rehabilitation of the psychiatrically disabled. *Rehabilitation Literature* 1978; 39:70–74.
16. Tebb A: Litigation in Workers' Compensation. Presented at the State Workmen's Compensation Advisory Committee, San Diego, Calif, Oct 22, 1974.
17. Toufexis A: That aching back! *Time* 1980; 116:30–34.
18. U.S. Chamber of Commerce. *Analysis of Workers' Compensation Laws.* Washington, DC, 1982.
19. Wales JU, Ideson HA: *LLB Claims Law Worker's Compensation.* Basking Ridge, NJ, American Educational Institute, 1977.

18

Hiring Practices

John D. Kemp
Don B. Chaffin, Ph.D.

INTRODUCTION: LEGAL AUTHORITY

On July 26, 1990, President George Bush signed into law the Americans with Disabilities Act (ADA). This act extends civil rights protection to 43 million persons with disabilities. The scope of the law is impressive; it requires employers of 25 or more employees within two years, and employers of 15 or more employees within four years, to provide employment opportunities in a nondiscriminatory manner; it requires transit authorities to begin to make their transportation services accessible to persons with mobility limitations; it mandates that public accommodations, such as restaurants, movie theaters, and shopping malls, become accessible; and, finally, it requires telecommunications services to serve the needs of deaf and hearing-impaired persons through relay services. Several federal agencies are required to promulgate implementing regulations within two years for employment provisions, the Equal Employment Opportunity Commission; for transportation, the U.S. Department of Transportation; for public accommodations, the U.S. Architectural and Transportation Barriers Compliance Board; and for telecommunications services, the Federal Communications Commission.

The ADA builds on the progress made under the Rehabilitation Act of 1973, specifically case law and understanding arising out of Sections 503 and 504, discussed later in this chapter. The bill is certain to be at the center of many employers' agendas in the 1990s. No other country in the world has ever proposed to extend such civil rights protection to persons with disabilities.

Prior to congressional passage of Sections 501, 503, and 504 of the Rehabilitation Act of 1973 and Section 502 of the Vietnam Veterans Readjustment Act of 1974, persons with disabilities who experienced employment discrimination were left with no recourse. Statistical evidence indicates the disparity in employment opportunities for disabled and nondisabled workers, even during the 1980s: Labor force participation by people with disabilities is 33.1% of all disabled people; another third are capable of working competitively but cannot find work, and the remaining third are too severely disabled to be employed.[1] A dramatic trend in these years of disability enlightenment—1981 to the present—is the declining number of people with disabilities who are participating in the competitive work world.

Disabilities involving the low back, including pain, now cost society billions of dollars in medical and workers' compensation claims, lost days of work, and temporary or replacement personnel, not to mention the impact on the injured person of acquiring a disabling condition. Today, persons with low back injuries or pain enjoy limited protection from discrimination on the basis of handicap. These rights are founded in the Rehabilitation Act of 1973 and in recently amended state law.

The disability employment discrimination regulations promulgated according to Sections 503 and 504 of the 1973 act—the cornerstone of employment rights—are intended to remove the discriminatory aspects of hiring disabled persons and at the same time provide employers with workers who are qualified to perform essential job requirements.

COVERED EMPLOYERS AND APPLICABLE REGULATIONS

The 503 and 504 requirements for affirmative action and equal employment opportunities for "qualified handicapped individuals" apply to federal contractors and every recipient of federal financial assistance. A federal contractor is any entity that holds a contract or subcontract in excess of $2,500 to provide goods or services for the federal government or its contractor. A recipient that operates a health, welfare, or any social service program funded with federal assistance must comply with these provisions in developing and carrying out employment practices.

The regulations do not protect all applicants and employees with disabilities from discrimination on the basis of handicap. To be protected, a person must be a "qualified handicapped person," which is defined by the law as a "handicapped person who, with reasonable accommodation, can perform the essential functions of the job in question."[2]

Persons with communicable diseases, including AIDS are covered under the definition of "qualified handicapped person," as defined in regulations promulgated under Section 504 of the Rehabilitation Act of 1973. In light of this definition, the key issue concerning whether a "handicapped person" is qualified to perform a particular job is dependent on the *essential* functions of the job, that is, the basic qualifications necessary to perform the job.

For the purposes of Sections 503 and 504, the term *handicapped person* does not include an alcoholic or drug abuser whose current use of alcohol or drugs prevents the individual from performing the job and whose employment, by reason of the substance abuse, constitutes a direct threat to property or the safety of others.

Are there reasonable accommodations available that would enable the handicapped person to perform all the essential functions?

To date, neither the government nor the courts have clarified the meaning of the term *essential*. Because of the unlimited variety of circumstances under which an individual may be expected to perform a particular job, the determination of whether a particular job function is essential must be made on a case-by-case basis. When a question arises concerning the essential nature of a job function, it has been determined that the burden is on the employer to demonstrate that the job function is essential.

The ADA language used quite similar definitional language—for "handicapped individual" and "qualified handicapped individual," it uses "individual with a disability" and "qualified individual with a disability," reflecting society's heightened consciousness and regard for the person and clear distinction between externally imposed limits that "handicap" someone (physical barriers, preconceived stereotypes, etc.) and personal traits or conditions with which people learn to live in given environments.

The ADA defines "reasonable accommodation" to include making existing facilities used by employees accessible to and usable by individuals with disabilities, job-restructuring, part-time and modified work schedules, reassignment to a vacant position, acquisition or modification of equipment or devices, appropriate adjustment or modification of examinations, training materials or policies, the provision of qualified readers or interpreters, and similar accommodations.

How these obligations will be interpreted by various tribunals will further shape employers' duties, notwithstanding the impact of technology on improving disabled persons' control over their work environments.

Protected Employment-Related Activities

A contractor or recipient of federal financial assistance may not deny equal employment opportunities to qualified handicapped individuals. This requirement applies to *all* employment situations, including part-time employment. The most common employment-related activities covered include the following:[4]

- Recruitment, advertising, and processing applications for employment
- Hiring, upgrading, promotion, awareness of tenure, demotion, transfer, layoff, termination, right of return from layoff, and rehiring
- Rates of pay or any other form of compensation and changes in compensation
- Job assignments, job classifications, organizational structures, position descriptions, lines of progression, and seniority lists
- Leaves of absence, sick leave, or any other leave
- Selection and financial support of training, including apprenticeship, professional meetings, conferences, and other related activities, and selection for leaves of absence to pursue training
- Employer-sponsored activities, including social and recreational programs
- Any other term, condition, or privilege of employment
- Fringe benefits available by virtue of employment, whether or not administered by the recipient

With respect to decisions about providing fringe benefits, the final 504 regulations states:

> Section 84.11 simply bars discrimination in providing fringe benefits and does not address the issue of actuarial differences. The government believes that currently available data and experience do not demonstrate a basis for promulgating a regulation specifically allowing for differences in benefits or contributions.[5]

An employee may not be asked to waive rights to insurance or to bringing an action against the employer for any injury incurred regardless of a disability.

In addition to requiring that an employer make employment-related decisions free from discrimination, "an employer may not participate in contractual or other relationships that have the effect of subjecting qualified handicapped applicants or employees to discrimination on the basis of handicap."[6] This provision is based on the premise that a recipient or contractor may not do indirectly that which it cannot do directly. This requirement covers relationships with certain agencies or organizations, including the following:

- Employment and referral agencies
- Labor unions
- Organizations providing or administering fringe benefits to employees of the recipient
- Organizations providing training and apprenticeship programs

For example, a recipient has a contract arrangement with a private organization to provide a training program. The recipient requires that an employee complete a training program to be eligible for promotion. An employee with mobility limitations is prevented from taking the program because the organization's training site is inaccessible. The recipient cannot thereafter deny that employee a promotion based solely on the employee's failure to complete the training program.

A contractor or recipient cannot excuse noncompliance with the regulations because of the existence of a state law or policy that limits the eligibility of qualified handicapped persons to practice an occupation. Neither is an employer exempted because of the existence of a collective bargaining agreement containing provisions that conflict with the requirements of the regulations.

Reasonable Accommodation

A contractor or recipient, that is, a covered employer, must provide and pay for the accommodation to ensure equal employment opportunity to a qualified handicapped individual, that is, one who with reasonable accommodation can perform the essential functions of the job. This section also explains that a covered employer who is excused from providing the accommodation may not discriminate against a disabled applicant or employee who can provide the necessary accommodation to perform the essential functions of the job.

The regulations provide that a covered employer shall make reasonable accommodation to the known physical or mental limitations of an otherwise qualified disabled applicant or employee, unless it can demonstrate that the accommodation would impose an undue hardship on the operation of its program.[7] The covered employer is obligated only to make reasonable accommodation to the known physical or mental limitations of an "otherwise qualified handicapped applicant or employee."[8] If a disabled person is not "otherwise qualified," that is, he or she with reasonable accommodation cannot perform all essential functions of the job, the employer is under no obligation to hire or retain the disabled person and is therefore not required to provide the reasonable accommodation. For example, a person with a low back condition applies for a job that requires (a) several years' experience working with institutionalized persons, (b) significant amounts of travel, and (c) occasionally lifting persons or packages weighing more than 50 pounds. It is reasonable to arrange an accommodation that permits other persons to do the lifting, but the applicant does not have the requisite amount of experience. Even with an accommodation to meet an essential job requirement, the applicant is still not "otherwise qualified," that is, the applicant does not satisfy all the essential qualifications of the job. Thus, the employer is not obligated to hire the person or provide the accommodation.

Regarding all accommodation decisions, a covered employer must consider whether the provided accommodation renders the workplace safe in terms of the disabled employee and other employees and whether it creates a more functional, accessible work environment when other, nondisabled employees must use modified equipment or a changed environment. When a device that assists one person in one job is a barrier or is unsafe to others, then the accommodation may be unreasonable, especially in light of the business necessity defense available to the employer.

A covered employer must notify applicants and employees of its obligation under the regulations, including the obligation to make a reasonable accommodation (unless such accommodation would impose an undue hardship).[9] The burden then shifts to the disabled person to inform the employer that he or she is prevented by his or her limitations from performing nonessential job requirements and requires an accommodation. The regulations clearly state that employers are only obligated to make reasonable accommodation to the *known* physical or mental limitations of an otherwise qualified disabled person.[10] If the disabled person does not explain the nature of the handicap and does not request an accommodation, there is no violation of the regulations if the accommodation is not provided. For example, if an employee has a low back condition and has difficulty carrying weights of 25 pounds or more and does not inform the employer of the need for an accommodation when lifting such weights, the employer is under no obligation to provide one. Dismissal by the employer is not based on any discriminatory intent but solely on the basis of inability to perform essential job functions.

Once a qualified handicapped person informs an employer of his or her requirement of a reasonable accommodation, the employer may wish to solicit proposed accommodations from the disabled person. The employer is not required to provide the reasonable accommodation proposed by the disabled person if an alternative accommodation meets the requirements of the regulation, namely, that the accommodation be effective. Here are some examples.

- A low back-injured employee indicates that she needs a special type of ergonomic chair costing $400. The recipient locates another chair costing $100 that meets the needs of the disabled person.
- A blind man requests a reader as a reasonable accommodation. The employer determines that the necessary accommodation can be provided by restructuring job assignments so that a reader is unnecessary.
- A public health nurse who becomes blind requests as an accommodation that another nurse accompany him on home visits. The government concludes that an alternative job placement is comparable and, before making the placement, reviews the following factors in comparing the original and alternative job placements:
  - Salary scale (including fringe benefits)
  - Nature and scope of responsibilities
  - Potential of promotion
  - Seniority
  - Proximity to the existing work site
  It is unrealistic to expect an employer to pay two people to do one person's job.
- A sight-impaired woman who is otherwise qualified to perform the job of technician in a central supply department is not hired. The employer should have explored effective accommodations for the individual and, based on her needs, included the following suggestions:
  - Modification of gauges and equipment to give tactile readouts
  - The use of a stereoscope to read labels
  - The use of a light probe to enable the applicant to distinguish colors and shades of colors
  - Elimination of the inspection of linens from the job
  - The option to consult with and enlist the aid of an outside group such as the Agency for the Visually Impaired, which has expertise in accommodating jobs for blind persons.

The reasonable accommodation provision applies to all employment decisions made by a recipient, not simply to hiring and promotion decisions. For example, an employer may also be required to make a reasonable accommodation in its policies on job assignments, transfers, leave, and sick leave.

The government has received several inquiries concerning the applicability of the reasonable accommodation provision. One was from a teacher who was losing his eyesight. He was employed by the school district in a high school that was not close to his home. A job in his field, for which he was qualified, opened up at a high school that was within walking distance of his home. He was told that school must make reasonable accommodations with respect to job transfers and reassignments.[11]

A letter from the Office for Civil Rights, which enforces Section 504, explained that the regulation does not require that a recipient give preference during a reduction in force to a disabled employee unless it can be shown that the employer had previously engaged in systematic discrimination against disabled applicants or employees.[12]

Even when an employer knows of a handicapping condition, it is important to ascertain from the disabled employee whether an accommodation is required. The Education Department's Inflationary Impact Statement, which accompanied the department's notice of intent to publish a proposed Section 504 regulation, explained that "for the most combinations of types of handicapping conditions and job categories, reasonable accommodation will require either no or only minor outlays."[13] To provide an accommodation gratuitously may be unnecessary, costly, and in some cases, discriminatory.[14]

In a mid-1980s study of federal contractors' provisions of reasonable accommodations, over 80% of accommodations cost contractors less than $500, and many cost nothing at all.

Once it has been determined that, with reasonable accommodation an individual is a qualified handicapped person, the regulations require that the contractor or recipient make the accommodation unless "the accommodation would impose an undue hardship."[15] If an undue hardship can be shown, the recipient is excused from making the reasonable accommodation. In determining whether an accommodation would impose an undue hardship on the operation of a program, factors to be considered include the type of the recipient's operation, including the composition and structure of the recipient's work force and the nature and costs of the accommodation needed.[6]

The undue hardship provision attempts to place a reasonable cap on the costs that a contractor or recipient may incur in the process of ensuring equal opportunity for disabled applicants and employees.

As discussed, an employer may deny making a reasonable accommodation for two reasons: undue financial hardship and business necessity. Costs of the proposed accommodation must be considered, and more cost-effective alternatives to the proposed accommodation must be considered. Even when cost is considered, it is not, in and of itself, the sole determinant of undue hardship. The size and type of the recipient's program or activity must also be considered. The weight given to each factor in determining whether an accommodation constitutes undue hardship varies with the specific situation. And, when an employer cannot justifiably make an accommodation, nothing precludes the requesting applicant or employee from making independent arrangements to receive the accommodation from a third party or to provide it himself.

The business necessity defense of an employer to make a reasonable accommodation arises when the requested accommodation would unnecessarily disrupt the employers' flow of business operations, even though the cost of the actual accommodation is affordable.

Although cost is not a factor in determining reasonableness, it is clearly one of the factors to be considered in determining undue hardship. Even when cost is considered it is not, in and of itself, the sole determinant of undue hardship. The size and type of the recipient's program or activity must also be considered. The weight given to each factor in determining whether an accommodation constitutes undue hardship varies depending on the specific situation.

If a recipient employer can demonstrate that the provision of an accommodation would impose an undue hardship, it is excused from providing the necessary accommodation without violating Section 504. The recipient would be violating the regulations, however, if undue hardship were used as an excuse to deny the disabled individual the *opportunity* to be employed if the individual is able to provide his or her own accommodation. An individual is permitted to make independent arrangements to take advantage of an employment opportunity. These arrangements may include the provision of the accommodation by a public or private nonprofit agency or even, as a last resort, by the disabled individual alone.

DEFENSES AND LIMITATIONS

The BFOQ Defense

The general rule invoking the bona fide occupational qualification (BFOQ) defense is that an employer must look at the qualifications of *each* disabled person to determine whether, with reasonable accommodation, that *individual* is a qualified handicapped individual. There is one limited situation, however, where an employer that has determined that a certain job requires specific physical or mental characteristics could legitimately deny employment to a *class* of persons with disabilities who do not possess those characteristics; that is, the employer could determine that they are not qualified handicapped individuals.

Congress expressly recognized that, under Title VII of the Civil Rights Act, certain limited circumstances exist wherein an employer would be permitted to base a selection decision on characteristics common to the entire class rather than on the basis of individual qualifications. The concept is commonly referred to as the bona fide occupational qualifications provision.[17] The HHS's General Counsel's office concludes that there is BFOQ concept implicit in Section 504.

> The language "otherwise qualified" implies that differentiating on the basis of handicap is *not per se violative of Section 504 if the handicap goes to the essence of the job.* In such a case, a Section 504 BFOQ, which requires the absence of a particular handicap, would have to be narrowly construed in order to be consistent with the statute. *Thus, it would be applicable only to those situations in which the employer could demonstrate that the BFOQ would not preclude any handicapped individual from employment who could "otherwise qualify,"* i.e., who, with reasonable accommodation would perform the essential functions of the job if *individually tested.*
>
> Consistent with this conclusion, the section-by-section analysis, in the course of discussing the meaning of the phrase "otherwise qualified," explains that Section 503 or 504 would not prohibit, for example, a bus company from adopting a rule barring all blind persons from applying for a job as a bus driver.[18] By recognizing the legitimacy of such a practice, the Secretary has implicitly recognized the existence of BFOQ. The Section 504 BFOQ essentially presumes that there is no reasonable accommodation to overcome the limitations of this class of persons.[19]

The BFOQ defense is a limited one. Its narrow scope has been consistently upheld by the courts in dealing with employment discrimination on the basis of handicap. For example, in *Bevan v. New York State Teachers Retirement System,* the federal district court refused to accept the contention that blindness per se affects the ability to teach. The court further refused to accept the defendant's contention that the blind plaintiff would be incapable of carrying out incidental supervisory or administrative jobs:

> . . . none of these disciplinary, administrative or clerical duties related in the slightest degree to the basic qualifications of fitness to teach. These duties are incidental or peripheral; they are wholly unrelated to the essential ability to teach.[20]

In *Freitag v. Carter* the federal district court reached a similar conclusion concerning the denial of a chauffeur's license based on the existence of a fourteen-year-old psychiatric record. The court did not perceive even a tenuous connection between the antiquated medical diagnosis and the man's present ability to perform capably the duties of a chauffeur.[21]

It is unlikely that a BFOQ defense, normally a very narrowly drawn one, would be available to the class of persons with chronic low back pain who cannot lift weights in excess of 25 pounds. It is unlikely because many types of reasonable accommodation are available, such as task trading, task reassignment, or assistive lifting equipment. To apply a BFOQ defense to a class of people, all of them must be unable to perform an essential job task without any reasonable accommodations.

In sum, the BFOQ exception is applicable only to situations in which the employer can demonstrate that the exception would not preclude *any* handicapped individual from employment who could otherwise qualify, that is, a person who with reasonable accommodation could perform the essential functions of the job if individually tested. Thus, because the use of BFOQ results in the exclusion of a class of disabled persons from a particular job, it is extremely important to look at the reasonable accommodations available before determining that a BFOQ exists for that job. Even in situations where accommodations are not currently available, technological advances are occurring so quickly that BFOQs should become more and more rare.

Employment Tests and Criteria

Guidelines for Evaluating Jobs and Hiring Correctly

For the past ten years, employers have had to rely on dictum found in *E.E. Black, Ltd. v. Office of Federal Contract Compliance Programs* (OFCCP) of the U.S. Department of Labor to guide them on employee selection decisions. In *E.E. Black, Ltd.*, the court indicated that the employer bears the burden of proving there is substantial likelihood of imminent injury to occur in refusing to hire an applicant with given physical characteristics into a specific job; if the employer cannot sustain this burden of proof, discrimination on the basis of handicap might likely be found.[20a] For an employer to sustain this burden of proof requires extensive documentation and highly reliable job studies, detailing specific job functions and which physical characteristics applicants must have to perform the job safely. Most employers lack this data. To assist employers in evaluating jobs and making better hiring decisions, use this checklist:

1. A job evaluation or job analysis must exist for each specific job or job group, identifying:
   a. Frequency, intensity, and duration of each physical activity that is an essential job function (job related). (*Q:* What are a job's essential functions?)
   b. The level of previous job experience, training, or education needed to achieve competency in a reasonable amount of time.

   c. Tools, devices, aids, or computers needed for proficiency.
   d. Licensing, accreditations, certificates, and so forth.
   e. The environment in which the job is performed.
2. From this job analysis, develop a physical abilities checklist that identifies the baseline physical characteristics needed by applicants to perform the job.
3. Add to the list any health or physical restrictions based on safety concerns inherent in the job(s) or in materials handled.
4. Eliminate from the applicant pool those without the requisite training or experience requirements.
5. Using qualified health, medical, or safety personnel, select those who meet the checklist's requirements for the specific job. Decisions on those eliminated from the pool at this stage should be reviewed to determine whether reasonable accommodation principles could keep them in the pool. The employer or the screening firm acting as the employer's agent must believe that, for those eliminated from the pool, their employment in a specific job would likely cause injury to them or others, given their individual physical capabilities. This belief must be based on statistical profiles and qualified medical expertise.
6. The hiring official may make a conditional offer of employment to the most qualified candidate in the pool, subject to passage of a postoffer, preentrance medical examination. The use of such examinations are permitted so long as (a) the results are kept confidential and (b) *all* entering employees must take essentially the same examination.
7. If the results of the medical examination are satisfactory, that is, the applicant is capable of performing the essential job functions safely, hiring is complete. If the results are not satisfactory, determine if any reasonable accommodation principles would help the applicant (such as job restructuring); if not, job denial is not discriminatory.

The regulations contain a specific standard applicable to decisions concerning hiring and promotion. The provisions state: "A recipient may not make use of any employment test or other *selection criterion that screens out or tends to screen out handicapped* persons unless (1) the test score or other selection criterion, as used by the recipient, is shown to be job-related for the position in question, and (2) *alternative job-related tests or criteria* that do not screen out or tend to screen out as many handicapped persons are *not shown by the Director to be available*."[22] Based on this section, there is a clear method for determining whether a particular selection test or criterion is acceptable:

   1. It must be shown that the test or criterion "screens out or tends to screen out handicapped persons." In proposed regulations, a statistical showing or adverse impact on disabled persons is required to trigger a recipient's obligation to show that employment criteria and qualifications relating to a handicap are necessary. This requirement was changed in the final regulation because the small number of disabled persons taking tests would make statistical showings of "disproportionate, adverse affect" difficult and burdensome.[22]
   2. Once it is shown that an employment test has substantially and unnecessarily limited the opportunities of disabled persons, the recipient must show that the test (or test criterion) is job related to continue its use. For example, assume that school district A adopted a policy of not allowing blind teachers to teach sighted children. To sustain its policy, the school district is required to show that the selection criterion, sight, is related to the safe performance of the job of teaching. If the school district is unable to show the relationship between sight and teaching, the criterion is discriminatory. Assume that school district B uses a certain test to establish a priority list. Also assume that (1) the test substantially limits

the opportunities of disabled persons and (2) the school can demonstrate job relatedness. School district B has not violated Section 504 because the school district has met its burden of showing that the criterion is directly related to the performance and the ability to perform the job or is job related.

3. Once the recipient has shown the test of employment criteria to be job related, the burden shifts to the government to identify alternative job-related tests that do not screen out as many disabled persons.

The government relies heavily on the principle established under Title VII of the Civil Rights Act of 1964 in *Griggs v. Duke Power Company*.[24] The plaintiffs in *Griggs* challenged the defendant's employment criteria that an applicant have a high school diploma or attain a predetermined score on an intelligence test. The plaintiffs contended, among other things, that such criteria were not geared to measure the level of potential performance. The court concluded that since the company's testing and educational requirements had been shown to disqualify blacks at a substantially higher rate than whites, the burden shifted to the company to show that each requirement was demonstrably related to successful job performance.

> If an employment practice which operates to exclude Negroes cannot be shown to be related to job performance, the practice is prohibited.[25]

In addition to specifying the procedure for determining the legality of the selection criteria or tests used by the employer, the fact must be taken into account that some tests and criteria depend on sensory, manual, or speaking skills that may not themselves be necessary to the job in question but that may make it impossible for the person with a disability to pass the test.

The recipient must select and administer tests so as best to ensure that the test measures the disabled person's ability to perform on the job rather than the person's ability to see, hear, speak, or perform manual tasks, except, of course, where such skills are the factors that the test purports to measure. For example, a person with a speech impediment may be perfectly qualified for jobs that do not or need not, with reasonable accommodation, require the ability to speak clearly. Yet, if given an oral test, the person would be unable to perform in a satisfactory manner. The test results do not, therefore, predict job performance but instead reflect the impaired speech.

Preemployment Inquiries

In the past, employment application forms and employment interviews requested information concerning an applicant's physical or mental condition. This information was often used to exclude applicants with handicapping conditions, even before their ability to perform the job was determined. Reasons for this practice include myths about job capabilities and resistance to making reasonable accommodations, especially if accommodations were costly. Rejection of applicants with disabilities based on these discriminatory practices is often difficult to detect because the employers express nondiscriminatory reasons for rejection. Nor would the disabled applicant's failure to answer questions completely or honestly solve the problem of discrimination in hiring, since failure to answer all inquiries or to give truthful responses could just as quickly lead to rejection from further consideration for employment as would complete responses.[27]

The regulations limit the circumstances under which employers may make preemployment inquiries, including medical examinations. The purpose of the section is to minimize the likelihood that employers will practice discrimination on the basis of handicap. The preemployment inquiry prohibition is particularly useful in limiting discrimination against persons with handicaps that are not readily apparent, such as epilepsy, diabetes, emotional illness, heart disease, and cancer.

Also prohibited are preemployment inquiries concerning the existence of a handicap and the nature and severity of the handicap. The term *preemployment,* as used in this instance, means the period before which a conditional offer of employment has been made. For example, then HEW Secretory Califano, in a letter to the National Association of Chain Drug Stores concerning the applicability of Section 504 to the hiring of drug addicts, stated:

> In order to ensure that addicts are not hired for jobs which require access to controlled substances, an employer may routinely inquire, *after offer of the job is made,* whether the individual is addicted.[28]

In other words, a preemployment inquiry is prohibited only before an offer of employment not before the date of commencing employment. This offer of employment may be conditional on passing a medical examination or on determining that a reasonable accommodation would not cause an undue hardship to the operation of the recipient's program.

Thus, the following questions traditionally appearing on forms given to applicants at the initial stages of the interview process are unacceptable:

- Are you disabled? If so, to what extent?
- Were you disabled in a war?
- Have you ever had any of the following conditions: arthritis, diabetes, epilepsy?[29]

Since the purpose of the provision is to minimize discrimination on the basis of handicap rather than to require that covered employers hire unqualified persons, the regulations clearly state that an employer may make preemployment inquiry into an applicant's ability to perform job-related functions. The employer may also ask about a person's handicap if the person voluntarily refers to the handicap in a resume.

There are three exceptions to the general rule prohibiting preemployment inquiries. Preemployment inquiries can be made:

- In connection with remedial action obligations under Section 84.6(a) of the 504 regulations.
- When an employer is taking *affirmative action* under Section 503 of the Rehabilitation Act of 1973.
- When an employer is taking voluntary action, as outlined in Section 84.6(b) of the 504 regulations, to overcome the effects of conditions limiting opportunities for handicapped persons.[30]

If an employer makes inquiries for any of these three reasons, it must also satisfy the following conditions: The employer must include a paragraph preceding any questions about the existence of a handicapping condition stating that the information is intended for use solely in connection with one of the three purposes listed above. The paragraph must state that (a) the information is being requested on a voluntary basis, (b) it will be kept confidential, and (c) refusal to provide it will not subject the applicant to any adverse treatment.

Three types of inquiries are acceptable *after* a conditional offer of employment has been made: medical examinations, inquiries about the applicant's need for a reasonable accommodation, and questions relevant to a job requiring direct access to controlled substances. Descriptions follow.

Medical Examinations

Section 84.14(C) of the 504 regulations expressly permits a recipient to conduct a medical examination after a conditional offer of employment has been made. Nothing in this section prohibits a recipient from making an offer of employment conditional on the results of a medical examination conducted prior to the employee's starting the job, *provided that* (1) all entering employees are subjected to such an examination regardless of handicap and (2) the results of such an examination are used only to determine whether the applicant still satisfies the nondiscriminatory (job-related) employment criteria established by the employer.

The 503 regulations permit federal contractors to conduct preemployment medical examinations for applicants for a job or group of jobs, so long as they are job related and all other applicants for the job or job group are given the same examination.

Example: Assume that an employer subject to Section 504 asks Ms. Smith (age 30), an applicant for a job as a teacher, numerous questions to determine her qualifications. Based on a review of Ms. Smith's credentials, she is offered the job subject to the results of the medical examination. In the course of the medical examination, the applicant informs the doctor that she has diabetes, diagnosed when she was a teenager and always under control. The applicant transmits a letter from her doctor to this effect. The school district *cannot* deny Ms. Smith employment on the basis of the doctor's discovery that she has diabetes; to do so would be to discriminate against her on the basis of the handicap. Her condition does not affect her ability to perform the job, and the district has already concluded that she is qualified. If, instead of finding a preexisting condition that was under control, the doctor had discovered a new health problem that would affect her ability to perform essential job functions, for example, the existence of a contagious disease, the district could legally deny her employment at that time.[31]

Inquiries Related to the Need for a Reasonable Accommodation

A 504 employer may also ask whether the person has a disability, to determine (1) whether the person requires a reasonable accommodation and (2) the nature and extent of the accommodation, if one is required.

Although the government has never expressly stated that such inquiries are permissible after a conditional offer of employment, it is logical to ascertain before actual employment if a reasonable accommodation is required and whether that accommodation would result in an undue hardship.[32]

Inquiries Related to a Job Requiring Direct Access to Controlled Substances

The BFOQ defense allows all 504 employers to refuse to hire drug addicts for jobs requiring direct access to controlled substances.

> In order to ensure that addicts are not hired for such jobs, a 504 employer may routinely inquire, after a conditional offer of a job is made, whether the individual is addicted. The job offer may be withdrawn if the answer is affirmative. If addiction is denied and subsequently discovered, the offer may be withdrawn or the person discharged.[33]

Procedures Covering Use of Information About Handicapping Conditions

The regulations require that information provided or collected during preemployment inquiries about the disabled applicant's history or medical condition remain confidential. This information must be maintained on separate forms and "shall be accorded confidentiality as medical records," except that:

- Supervisors and managers may be informed about restrictions on the work or duties of disabled persons and about necessary accommodations.
- First-aid and safety personnel may be informed, where appropriate, if the condition might require emergency treatment.
- Government officials investigating compliance with the act shall be provided relevant information upon request.

CONCLUSION

Covered employers must be aware of their affirmative action and nondiscrimination responsibilities to disabled applicants and employees. Within two years of the passage of the Americans with Disabilities Act, employers of only 25 or more employees will be required to comply with nondiscrimination provisions in employment as well as in housing, public transportation, education, health care, and public accommodations, if such are applicable to their businesses. The ADA extends civil rights protection to 43 million Americans with disabilities. This chapter discusses employers' major duties and techniques for achieving compliance. For further information be sure to consult the "Resources" section of this book.

BIBLIOGRAPHY

1. Louise Harris & Associates, Inc.: *Self-Perception of 1200 Disabled Persons,* 1989.
2. Interview with John Wodatch.
3. The four points adopted from testimony by John D. Kemp of Kemp & Young, Inc., given before the S. 446 Report Hearings, June 1979.
4. 45 CFR 84.11(b) (1977).
5. 45 CFR 84.11(b) (1977).
6. 45 CFR 84.11(b) (1977).
7. 45 CFR 84.12(a) (1977).
8. 45 CFR 84.12(a) (1977).
9. 45 CFR 84.8(a) (1977).
10. 45 CFR 84.12(a) (1977).
11. Letter from David S. Tatel to Congressman Hawkins (June 22, 1977).
12. Letter from John Wodatch to Dolores D'Antonio (July 1, 1977).
13. "Discrimination Against Handicapped Persons: The Costs, Benefits, and Inflationary Impact of Implementing Section 504 of the Rehabiliation Act of 1973 Covering Recipients of Hew Financial Assistance," 41 FR 20312 (May 17, 1975).
14. The circumstances under which the gratuitous provision of accommodations are considered discriminatory are discussed in the next sections of this chapter.
15. 45 CFR 84.12(a) (1977).
16. 45 CFR 84.12(c) (1977).
17. U.S.C. Section 2000 e-2(e) (1970) (Section 703 of Title VI).

18. OCR Memorandum from Jeff Rosen to John Wodatch, "Employment Discrimination under Section 504—the Bona Fide Occupational Qualifications (BFOQ) Exception" (April 14, 1975).

19. Section-by-section analysis, 42 FR 22686, Col. 3, May 4, 1977.

20. 74 Misc. 2d 443, 345 N.W.S. 2d 921 (S.Ct. 1973), modified Empl. Prac. Dec. (CCH) 9590 (N.Y.S. App. Div. 1974).

20a. 497 F. Supp. 1088. 23 Fair Empl. Prac. Dec. (BNA) 1253. 24 Empl. Prac. Dec. (CCH) P31.260 (Sept. 5, 1980).

21. 489 F. 2d 1377 (7th Cir. 1973).

22. 45 CFR 84.13(a) (1977) (Emphasis added).

23. The discussion is based on the section-by-section analysis 42 FR 22688, col. 3 (May 4, 1977). (Emphasis added).

24. 401 U.S. 424 (1971).

25. 401 U.S. 424 (1971).

26. Section-by-section analysis, 42 FR22689, col. 1 (May 4, 1977).

27. In *Casias v. Industrial Commission of the State of Colorado*, No. 75-291 (Colo. Ct. App. Sept. 23, 1976), plaintiff appealed from denial of unemployment compensation benefits based on the determination of the Industrial Commission that claimant was properly discharged for falsification of his employment application. Plaintiff failed to disclose his condition of epilepsy. He had been, with the aid of medication, free from seizures for several years. The employer's physician stated that the employer had a policy to hire epileptics. The court held that the applicant would be entitled to employment benefits unless the falsification of an employment application is found to be material to the applicant's job performance.

28. HEW letter from Secretary Califano to Robert Bolger (Feb. 28, 1978).

29. OCR letter from Michael Middleton to Vincent De Shazo (June 19, 1978).

30. 45 CFR 84.14(b) (1977).

31. OCR Memorandum from Director, Division of Policy and Procedures to Cindy Brown, "L.O.F. in the *Bay State Medical Center, Springfield, MA* Case" (July 13, 1978).

32. Interview with John Wodatch.

33. 45 CFR 84.14(d) (1977).

19

Summary

Malcolm H. Pope, Dir. Med. Sc., Ph.D.
Gunnar B.J. Andersson, M.D., Ph.D.
Don B. Chaffin, Ph.D.
John W. Frymoyer, M.D.

Occupational low back pain is often described in pejorative terms such as "the albatross of industry" or "the nemesis of medicine." Such negative descriptions ignore the many positive ways of dealing with these patients. In most cases, injuries that cause low back pain are analogous to injuries that occur to any bodily tissue. With time the tissues heal, and their functional capacities remain. Physicians must recognize the causes of these injuries, develop methods for prevention, and reduce the cost of disability by taking a comprehensive team approach. Our book presents this hopeful, positive perspective—rather than a defeatist view—of the ubiquitous problem of low back pain in the occupational health environment.

In view of the variety of socioeconomic conditions among countries, the number of similarities in the epidemiology of low back pain is surprising. The incidence of low back pain ranges from 60 to 80% of the adult population worldwide, and back injuries average 20% of all compensable work injuries. The total direct and indirect costs of low back pain in the United States are over $100 billion per annum, and they have an important effect on the economy of other countries as well.

In this book we have defined low back pain and reviewed its functional anatomy, delineating the spine's complex roles of load bearing, mobility, and protection, on the premise that knowledge of the mechanical structure and function forms one basis for prevention. Overexertion causes 60% of low back pain cases. Most of those overexertion injuries are due to lifting, but a smaller number result from pulling and pushing activities. In general, an increased risk of low back pain follows the magnitude of the load moment and the frequency of lifting. Women in some physically heavy jobs have almost twice the incidence of low back pain as men. This statistic will become increasingly important as more women enter jobs traditionally held by men. The risk of back injury increases markedly as the requirements of the job exceed the worker's strength, although physical fitness alone has not yet been proved to prevent low back pain. Because of the strong association of lifting with low back pain there are many recommendations in the literature, often based on biomechanical models. These simple biomechanical models can assist in determining the variables that can produce injuries during lifting, and form one basis for modifying the workplace so that no worker is compelled to exert above actual strength limit.

Back pain also occurs in workers with sedentary occupations. Posture has a major effect on the load of the spine, and proper seat design can reduce disc loads and improve back comfort. Drivers of heavy vehicles are at an increased risk of serious low back pain, in part because vibration can affect the spine by causing fatigue of the tissue structures. This can be obviated by modification of the seat, the vehicle, or the driving style.

Once a person experiences low back pain, a major problem is the inability of the clinician to make a precise diagnosis. Two of the greatest problems of health care, in fact, are low back pain of unknown etiology and persistent symptoms of such a condition that do not respond to treatment. Patients with these problems demonstrate deconditioning and psychologic maladaption with time. New diagnostic approaches and early intervention are important advances to overcome these problems, but the evaluation of the worker with low back pain largely depends on an accurate history and physical examination. Sophisticated tests need only be performed when the clinical signs and symptoms indicate a serious disorder that requires specific therapy. Most workers improve in two to six weeks. The remaining ones pose the greatest problem in terms of management and cost. It is important that health professionals have a clear plan to manage the patient at the onset of symptoms, although the patient should be told that low back pain is a symptom with structural causes that often cannot be determined but that in most patients gradually disappears. The injured workers should be told that they themselves can influence their low back pain and should be charged with this responsibility. Back school can be very helpful in this regard.

Special attention to worker selection can help in matching the worker with the appropriate job. Management should consider, as a first priority, workplace modification to adapt the workplace to the worker. Placement programs are clearly secondary but still needed. Employment tests cannot legally be used unless the test is job related and there are no other job-related tests that are less discriminatory. Industry must also be aware that in the United States preemployment inquiries concerning the nature and severity of a handicap are prohibited by law.

Traditional work measurement systems appear to be limited in their ability to provide necessary data to prevent back injuries, but the new systems are promising. Evaluation to determine the severity of a disability is often required by statutory programs or by plaintiff's or defense attorneys in a worst case. Such evaluations are imprecise, however, and can be affected by examiner attitudes. The physician's role in this process should be to evaluate the relationship between injury and impairment, to determine the end of the healing period, and to identify any remaining physical restrictions. Evaluations should be rapid, and open discussions should be held with the patient.

It is important that the methods for dealing with low back pain be modified in the coming years. A partnership between worker, management, ergonomist, and medical professional is essential for solving the complex problem of occupational low back pain.

INDEX _____